BIOMEDICAL SCIENCE AND THE THIRD WORLD

UNDER THE VOLCANO

ANNALS OF THE NEW YORK ACADEMY OF SCIENCES

Volume 569

BIOMEDICAL SCIENCE AND THE THIRD WORLD

UNDER THE VOLCANO

Edited by Barry R. Bloom and Anthony Cerami

The New York Academy of Sciences
New York, New York
1989

Library of Congress Cataloging-in-Publication Data

Biomedical science and the Third World : under the volcano
/ edited by Barry R. Bloom and Anthony Cerami.

p. cm. — (Annals of the New York Academy of Sciences, ISSN 0077-8923 : v. 569)
Result of a conference held on Oct. 18-20, 1988 in New York, N.Y., sponsored by the New York Academy of Sciences and the L. W. Frohlich Charitable Trust.
Includes bibliographical references.
ISBN 0-89766-537-6 (alk. paper). — ISBN 0-89766-538-4 (pbk. : alk. paper)
1. Medical care—Developing countries—Congresses.
2. Medicine, Preventive—Developing countries—Congresses.
3. Medicine—Research—Developing countries—Congresses.
I. Bloom, Barry R., 1937- . II. Cerami, Anthony, 1940- . III. New York Academy of Sciences. IV. L. W. Frohlich Charitable Trust. V. Series.
[DNLM: 1. Developing Countries—congresses.
2. Health Services—congresses. 3. International Cooperation—congresses. 4. Research. W1 AN626YL v. 569 / WA 395 B615 1988]
Q11.N5 vol. 569
[RA441.5]
500 s—dc20
[362.1'09172'4]
DNLM/DLC
for Library of Congress 89-13585
CIP

PCP
Printed in the United States of America
ISBN 0-89766-537-6 (cloth)
ISBN 0-89766-538-4 (paper)
ISSN 0077-8923

ANNALS OF THE NEW YORK ACADEMY OF SCIENCES

Volume 569
December 8, 1989

BIOMEDICAL SCIENCE AND THE THIRD WORLD: UNDER THE VOLCANO [a]

Editors and Conference Chairmen
BARRY R. BLOOM AND ANTHONY CERAMI

CONTENTS

[a] This volume is the result of a conference entitled Under the Volcano: Biomedical Science and the Third World, sponsored by the New York Academy of Sciences and the L. W. Frohlich Charitable Trust, which was held on October 18-20, 1988 in New York, N.Y.

Part III. Strategies for Drug Design

Part IV. Implementation and Impact of Scientific Strategies

Major funding was provided by:

- CARNEGIE CORPORATION OF NEW YORK
- L. W. FROHLICH CHARITABLE TRUST
- JOHN D. AND CATHERINE T. MacARTHUR FOUNDATION
- MERCK & COMPANY

Preface

BARRY R. BLOOM

Department of Microbiology and Immunology
Albert Einstein School of Medicine
Bronx, New York 10468

The Third World is the place where 75% of the planet's population lives, where 86% of all children are born, and where 97% of all infant and childhood deaths occur. As the disparity between the quality of life in developed and developing nations widens, the forces of despair and disillusionment are building. At the same time, the revolution in biomedical sciences—and particularly in recombinant DNA technology, immunology, and structural biology—hints at unprecedented possibilities for development and application of scientific approaches to human problems. It is in this context that this conference was conceived, and we hope, in this volume, to provide a broad perspective on the dimensions of the burden of disease in different regions of the Third World and the opportunities provided by new scientific approaches to preventing and alleviating major diseases of the Third World. A major focus of this volume is the defining of scientific strategies for attacking major infectious disease problems of the Third World, including the development of vaccines and the design of new drugs. Major consideration is given as well to social and economic implications and to the impact of the new scientific technologies and their implementation.

This book derives from, and was enriched by, a conference in the series entitled Science and the Human Prospect, sponsored by the New York Academy of Sciences. A major biennial award, the L. W. Frohlich Award, administered by the New York Academy of Sciences, is associated with this conference series and is given to "the scientist whose singular achievements in research hold significant, direct promise for major improvements of human life, the promotion of human survival, and the creation of new economic or educational opportunities." The 1988 L. W. Frohlich Award was presented to Dr. Kenneth Warren. No one has made a greater contribution to the area of tropical disease research than Ken Warren: he has stimulated both ideas and people. As a physician-scientist he carried out important research in schistosomiasis, and established one of the leading centers in the world in Geographic Medicine at Case-Western Reserve University. As Director of Health Sciences for the Rockefeller Foundation, he had the vision and foresight to establish a major research effort, the Great Neglected Diseases Program, to apply the knowledge at the frontiers of biomedical science to the problems of the Third World. He has abundantly fulfilled the stipulations of the Frohlich Award, and is honored in this book by his colleagues for his contributions to science, his guiding spirit, and his indefatigable commitment to improving the quality of life of the poorest people on this planet.

A unique aspect of the L. W. Frohlich Award is that the awardee may select two L. W. Frohlich Fellows, who receive fellowships of $25,000 yearly for four consecutive years in order to continue the research activities begun by the awardee. In this way the valuable research tradition of the awardee is continued by a young investigator and the majority of the award goes into scientific research. Dr. Warren has given his award to support the research of two outstanding young scientists in tropical disease research in their countries in the developing world and in outstanding institutions in the United States for part of each year. He has designated Drs. Worachart Sirawaraporn of Thailand and James Ntambi of Uganda as L. W. Frohlich Fellows.

The conference and book could not have materialized without the support received from the L. W. Frohlich Charitable Trust as well as from the Carnegie Corporation of New York, the John D. and Catherine T. MacArthur Foundation, and Merck & Company. We are grateful to Dr. Joshua Lederberg, who generously offered the unique facilities of the Rockefeller University for the conference. On behalf of the participants, the editors wish to express our deep gratitude to Mr. William Golden, Chairman of the Board of Governors of the New York Academy of Sciences for his dedication to this project and his unstinting efforts in its behalf. We are grateful, too, for the tireless and professional work of organization done by Svetlana Kostic-Stone, Ann Collins Walsh, and Renée Wilkerson-Brown of the Academy. We also wish to thank the Editorial Department of the Academy for seeing this book through the press, and especially Sheila Kane for her assiduous labors on behalf of the book. Finally, we would like to thank the Rockefeller Foundation for providing funds for this book to be distributed by the World Health Organization to scientists in the developing world and to be translated into Spanish for further distribution in Latin America.

The vital force behind this project was Dr. Heinz Pagels. He was immediately engaged by it and was persuaded of its importance. Dr. Pagels, a brilliant physicist and Executive Director of the New York Academy of Sciences, was dedicated to making this conference happen. Because of his untimely death during its preparation, this book is respectfully dedicated to him in turn and honors his passionate commitment to the role of science in human survival.

Putting Biomedical Knowledge to Use in the Third World

JAMES P. GRANT

United Nations Children's Fund
Three United Nations Plaza
New York, New York 10017

I am delighted to address the L.W. Frohlich Award Conference, and especially pleased to do so during this ceremony in which the award will be presented to my highly respected friend, Kenneth Warren.

The power of the theme of this conference, "Under the Volcano: Biomedical Science and the Third World," derives from the potential to make a major difference in human well-being on a grand scale through accelerating the application of biomedical sciences to Third World health problems. This is, of course, the arena in which the considerable contributions of Dr. Warren's career have been made. By nature, the theme evokes one main and simple question: How do we get the fruits of the biomedical sciences into use for the poor majority in the Third World who need it the most?

NEGLECTED DISEASES

Two main paths toward this end, both well known, are ripe with possibility, yet both have been seriously neglected. First, there are the "diseases of the poor," about which relatively little research is being done even now, despite increased attention in recent years. Ken Warren has been a leader in focusing more attention by the scientific community on this issue through his persistent work, which is exemplified in his book[1] *The Great Neglected Diseases of Mankind;* through his work with the Rockefeller Foundation on the neglected diseases; in his work on schistosomiasis; and in his work with the Rockefeller Foundation on INCLEN, the international network dedicated to strengthening clinical epidemiology in the Third World through local training in these skills. These name but a few of his relevant contributions.

In this domain we see the great inequity between the quantity and quality of research done on diseases to which the rich are prone, such as cancer, and, "poor-prone" diseases such as, for example, the diarrheal diseases that still take the lives each year of 3.5 million primarily young children, the great majority of them among the world's poorer families, and schistosomiasis, which affects those such as paddy farmers and laborers working in infected waters. There are also, of course, the neutral-prone diseases such as AIDS, which strike without regard to economic boundary, but to which, so far, the medical "breakthroughs" have been decidedly rich-prone. As a pure science, biomedical research has a unique potential to unravel the secrets of diseases and reveal means to overcome their ravaging effects. Is this powerful tool meant to be used to explore only (or in gross disproportion) those diseases which affect rich people? The challenge in this sphere is to attract more and better research to the poor- and neutral-prone diseases, as well as to orient research to seek treatments that are applicable to the masses and not just largely to the rich.

MASS APPLICATION OF AVAILABLE KNOWLEDGE AND TECHNOLOGY

The second area of tremendous yet inadequately tapped potential—a second category of great neglect regarding diseases—involves massive health problems in which the biomedical sciences have already made breakthroughs, but that are greatly neglected in terms of application. It has long been acknowledged that one of the greatest health challenges of our times is to bridge the vital gap between existing knowledge and technologies and their actual use by those for whom they can make the life-or-death difference. I can remember my father, Dr. John B. Grant, a pioneer in Third World public health, writing more than forty years ago that the *use made of medical knowledge depends on social organization.* And it is a main principle of Primary Health Care, codified in the Declaration of Alma-Ata a decade ago. Yet in the early 1980s we were still slow in applying this principle in practice even though its rhetorical acceptance had soared since the meeting at Alma-Ata.

It was, in fact, following this second path of vastly expanding the availability to those most in need of existing health knowledge and technology that led in 1982 to the call for a "Child Survival and Development Revolution"(CSDR)—a call made possible by the combination of grossly underutilized low-cost/high-impact medical knowledge and technologies of mass applicability with the new capacity to communicate with and organize among the poor of the world. It was the synergistic convergence of these forces that led the global community concerned with children's health to dare to strive in earnest to achieve the unprecedented goal of *halving the 1980 infant and child mortality rates by the turn of the century.* Existing low-cost medical technologies with maximum capacity to affect children's health in poor countries were identified, and approaches for making these available and used on a massive scale were designed.

As Dr. Hiroshi Nakajima, the new Director-General of the World Health Organization, stated eloquently on August 28th to 1,500 health educators from around the world:

> We must recognize that most of the world's major health problems and premature deaths are preventable through changes in human behaviour and at low cost. We have the know-how and technology but they have to be transformed into effective action at the community level. Parents and families, properly supported, could save two-thirds of the 14 million children who die every year—if only they were properly informed and motivated. Immunization alone could save 3 million lives—and another 3 million deaths a year could be prevented by oral rehydration, a simple and cheap technology. . . .
>
> Society must make it possible for people to live healthy lives. A grand alliance of people, policy-makers and health professionals is necessary . . . to . . . empower people with knowledge and the relevant health skills to improve their own health.[2]

The actual medical and health techniques singled out in the CSDR are, of course, familiar to you all. They include *growth monitoring* to warn of impending malnutrition, *oral rehydration therapy* (ORT) to combat the lethal effects of diarrheal dehydration, *breastfeeding* combined with proper weaning practices, and universal *immunization* against the six main child-killing diseases—all of which are low-cost and adaptable to mass application. They also include *female education, family planning,* and *food supplementation* when necessary—measures which are either somewhat more costly or more difficult to implement, or both. As you are well aware, these are simple techniques which have been available for some time. Yet 10 years ago, only 5 percent of the world's children were immunized against the targeted diseases. And 10 years ago, despite the potential of ORT to save the lives of more than 10,000 children dying each day from diarrheal diseases, fewer than 1 percent of the developing world's children were being treated in this simple manner when they had diarrhea. As a result of CSDR activities (i.e., mass application efforts) by 1987 more than 20 percent of children with diarrhea were being treated with oral rehydration therapy, and as of August 1987, 50 percent of the world's children were immunized. Consequently, in the past 12 months *the lives of some 2.5 million children have been saved by these two interventions alone,* with a comparable number saved from lives of crippling disabilities due to the side-effects of childhood diseases. Unfortunately I must add that, lest we become complacent, nearly six million young children *still* die annually from causes preventable by these simple means.

These accomplishments are but the more visible aspect of a much larger picture of a shifting approach toward health. The picture offers, however, a glimpse of what is possible when low-cost/high-impact medical technologies are made available on a mass scale, and especially to those normally removed from channels of easy access.

You might well ask at this point: How has the CSDR fostered use of the benefits of medical sciences in the Third World? What is the prototype from which lessons can be applied on a broader scale?

A PIONEER IN HEALTH FOR ALL CHILDREN

Colombia was the pioneer, and it began with leadership from the top to persuade all sectors of society to participate in the child-survival revolution, beginning with universal immunization. Then-President Belisario Betancur mobilized the cooperation of the media, including the leading opposition press, and he recruited the Church and the Red Cross, the Rotarians and Lions, Scouts, schoolteachers, businesspeople, and all of his government ministries into what we might call a "Grand Alliance" for Colombia's children.

Together, they set out to do what had never been done before in history. In one 3-month period, through three national immunization days, a nation mobilized to immunize the great majority of its children against five major diseases then killing and crippling tens of thousands of Colombian children each year. There were more than 10,000 TV and radio spots; virtually every parish priest devoted several sermons to the importance of families' immunizing their children, and every school teacher was involved. President Betancur and other leaders personally immunized children.

The Campaign began in June 1984. By the end of that August, more than three-quarters of the under-fives had been fully immunized. For the children of the world, of whom more than 10,000 were dying each day from these six diseases, this unprecedented accomplishment in Colombia was far more significant than even man's landing on the moon 15 years before. Colombia illustrated the use of communications and social organization to close the gap between available knowledge and its widespread use in the community.

The results demonstrate how we can defend children against these brutal mass killers and cripplers, if only we fully mobilize to ensure that low-cost available health knowledge and technology is used by all of a population rather than by the relative few who traditionally enjoy easy access to such benefits. The great majority of Colombian children now have been immunized and a significant start has been made in teaching millions of mothers how to use oral rehydration therapy, thereby saving the lives of more than 10,000 children a year who would otherwise have died.

The effort in Colombia was sometimes referred to as Universal Child Immunization "to the third power"(UCI^3), because the goals were threefold: first, to immunize the children; second, to build "sustainability" into the program so that it would continue through the years; and third, to use it as an entry point for expanding support for other programs and the entire PHC effort at a time of economic constraints, when political forces are pressed for diversion of financial resources away from, rather than towards, PHC.

The "Trojan horse" of the "campaign" approach in Colombia in 1984 and 1985 provided the entry point and political will for strengthening the ongoing Primary Health Care infrastructures which have been vastly bolstered by intensive and complementary follow-up efforts. The primary school curriculum has been drastically revised to emphasize health education, and all high school students have to contribute 100 hours of "health scout" service as a pre-condition to receiving their graduation certificates. Television and radio spots and promotions now have a continuing supporting role. The Catholic Church has introduced a training program for priests: premarital counselling now includes health care of children (on the importance of immunization, ORT, and breastfeeding, among other items) as a major component. And, of course, all these measures have resulted *not* in higher costs for government services, but in the *saving* of many millions of dollars, as well as saving the lives of more than 10,000 children yearly and preventing the crippling and disabling of many thousands more.

Colombia's pioneering success at "going to scale"—UCI^3—has been joined by literally scores of countries. Medical scientists cannot do the task alone, but also it cannot be done without you.

In this second path of getting the benefits of biomedical sciences into use in the Third World—that of *expanding the application* of existing knowledge and technologies—Ken Warren's work has also made significant contributions. The "Good Health at Low Cost" conference that he organized through the Rockefeller Foundation in 1985 is considered by many a landmark in defining such approaches. He was the Rockefeller Foundation's active member of the Task Force for Child Survival beginning with its first meeting (which was hosted by the Foundation) in Bellagio, Italy in March 1984, and for the second meeting at Cartegena, Colombia, in October 1985. This spring the third "Bellagio" meeting, held in Talloires, France, gathered a dozen health ministers and health secretaries from most major developing countries of the world (Brazil, China, Colombia, India, Mexico, Nigeria, Pakistan); heads of major international organizations such as Barber Conable of the World Bank, Halfdan Mahler of WHO, and myself; plus major bilateral aid agency administrators such as Margaret Catley-Carlson of CIDA (Canada), Carl Tham of SIDA (Sweden), and Alan Woods of USAID; and private leadership from the Rockefeller Foundation and Rotary International. Out of this review of the world immunization/child survival effort came the exciting conclusion that, with a modest additional amount of political will, it *is do-able* by the end of this century—in twelve years—to reduce the 1980 child death rate by more than *half,* saving from death or disability in this process well over *one-*

hundred million children over the period, while slowing population growth as well, as families gain the confidence—through these means in which they participate—that the children they have will live.

The "Declaration of Talloires" proposes Year 2000 health goals that received consensus approval of participants. Achieving these ends will, of course, only be possible if biomedical scientists, and indeed much of the medical scientific community, takes an active leadership role in solving some of the problems which still remain. Of these goals, a useful "short-list" of do-able Year 2000 goals could be capsulized to include:

(1) halving the 1980 under-5 mortality rates, or reducing them to 70 per 1,000 live births, whichever is less;

(2) eliminating polio (endorsed by the World Health Assembly in May);

(3) achieving universal primary education (to which I would add 80 percent literacy among women of child-bearing age);

(4) achieving less than 1 percent severe malnutrition; and

(5) promoting expanded coverage of water supply and sanitation.

The accelerated health programs to which Ken Warren has contributed so much have brought a new political visibility, and consequently increased financial support, to PHC and other programs for children. It is the success of these politically attractive programs that has contributed so much to getting children placed, for the first time, on the political agenda of various summit meetings.

Within the last two years, the South Asian Association for Regional Cooperation (SAARC) Summit issued a Declaration on Child Survival; the heads of the seven Central American countries went on television together in behalf of the region-wide immunization campaign on World Health Day in 1987; and the Organization of African Unity (OAU) Summit in 1987 declared 1988 the Year of the African Child and issued a Declaration on Child Survival and Development. And this May in Moscow, at the USSR:USA Summit meeting of US President Reagan and USSR General-Secretary Gorbachev, their call for accelerated worldwide action to reduce childhood deaths from readily preventable causes was the only reference to development issues in the joint statement that the two leaders issued. The communiqué stated:

> Both leaders reaffirmed their support for the WHO/UNICEF goal of reducing the scale of preventable childhood deaths through the most effective methods of saving children. They urged other countries and the international community to intensify efforts to achieve this goal.

These health approaches for children have also contributed importantly to the growing support for the early adoption of the Convention on the Rights of the Child, which was first proposed in 1979, and which encompasses the protection and development as well as the survival of children.

UNDER THE VOLCANO: THE ROLE OF BIOMEDICAL SCIENCES

The historically unprecedented progress in Third World health which has just appeared on the horizon through the new perspective of the CSDR *can be attained.*

It is not a fanciful theory. But along with this revolutionary capacity comes a tremendous responsibility and challenge. For it will come about if—and only if—we are willing to travel two paths in ensuring that the biomedical sciences are put to use in poor countries and communities: using the resources at our disposal (including our scientific know-how) to tackle the health problems of the poor *and* ensuring that low-cost available knowledge is used *everywhere in the world.*

In Ken Warren's paper for the second Bellagio Conference he quoted an esteemed colleague who had written in 1963: "Never in the history of human progress has a better and cheaper method of preventing illness been developed than immunization at its best."[3] Ken went on to add that "In spite of the great potential power of vaccines, however, there has been little, if any, increase in support for vaccine research by most funding organizations," and he noted that research had to be conducted under contrived and "bootlegged" conditions. He continued:

> And herein lies the metaphor of the volcano. Given all of this subterranean activity, there are still relatively few new and better vaccines on the market. But the pressure is building up, and it is now inevitable that there will be a virtual eruption of vaccines within the next 15 years.[4]

Those who are committed to the improved health and well-being of the world's children, and especially its poor children, await eagerly the eruption of that volcano. We are ready to put to use the secrets hidden so closely beneath the surface. And we call for the shifting of priorities which will allow research to focus in this direction rather than so disproportionately toward the diseases and treatments of the rich. As you are well aware, we are close to having a rotavirus vaccine; a heat-stable measles vaccine would tremendously facilitate the prevention of that disease; and combining antigens against the six main child-killing diseases into one singly applied vaccine would be another major breakthrough. Can you, gathered at this conference—prominent leaders of the scientific community of the latter part of the twentieth century—take responsibility for producing before the year 2000, such a single-dose vaccine which could be taken orally? I add my voice to those who have issued such a challenge.

Another tremendous force lies close to the surface, a force that has just begun to be unleashed, and one that holds unprecedented possibility for the future. It is the volcanic potential of social organization, of mobilizing and empowering people to take greater charge of their own health.

Can we, as a gift from the twentieth to the twenty-first century, offer not only the eradication of smallpox, but the elimination of polio as well? Can we achieve in this time-frame the halving of child mortality rates worldwide? These are achievements that will require sophisticated research into both poor-prone diseases and into expanding our capacity in the new field of social mobilization. Scientists must demand that attention is focused on both of these arenas.

As it becomes increasingly undeniable that the capacity to save the lives of so many children, and to improve the health and well-being of so many more, is well within our reach, it becomes increasingly unconscionable *not* to act on these new possibilities. Never before has the scientific community been faced with the opportunity—and the challenge—to do so much, for so many, for so little.

As I said to the Convocation of Nobel Laureates in Paris in January, surely the time has come to put the mass deaths of children from immunizable diseases, from diarrhea and from other preventable causes, on the shelf—alongside slavery, colonialism, racism and apartheid—reserved for things that are no longer acceptable to humankind. Surely the time has come to say that it is obscene to let these preventable deaths continue day after day, year after year, as our civilization moves into the twenty-first century.

It is you, the world's leaders in the health sciences, who must take a leadership role in making these possibilities become realities throughout the world. And it is you, the readers of this volume, who must, each in your own field of expertise, support these efforts in your own country, whether of the first, second or third worlds. I urge all of you to take an even stronger, accelerated leadership in this peaceful revolution for the health of children, and of all the world's people.

NOTES AND REFERENCES

1. WARREN, K. 1988. The Great Neglected Diseases of Mankind: Biomedical Research Network, 1978-1988. The Rockefeller Foundation. New York.
2. NAKAJIMA, H. Health education: The grand alliance. Address to the XIII World Conference on Health Education, August 28-September 2, 1988, Houston, Texas.
3. DR. GEOFFREY EDSALL, Professor of Applied Microbiology at Harvard, 1963.
4. WARREN, K. 1986. Under the volcano: The inevitable new age of vaccines. Paper presented at the Bellagio II Conference: Protecting the World's Children. October 1985, Cartagena, Colombia. Task Force for Child Survival, Decatur; and The Rockefeller Foundation, New York.

Introduction

JOSHUA LEDERBERG

President, Rockefeller University
New York, New York 10021

It has been a manifest privilege for the Rockefeller University to have served as host for this scientific meeting on a subject of vital interest to the three-quarters of the population of this planet that reside in the Third World. In addition, it is a special privilege to honor Dr. Kenneth Warren, who has done so much for the cause of the science and its application to tropical diseases.

Fifteen years ago, biotechnology based on the genetics and molecular microbiology of very simple organisms was a prophetic vision.[1] The power of these tools to address almost every question of human biology is now widely recognized. Yet until very recently, very little attention was paid to the most basic challenges to parasitic diseases at the molecular genetic level, although there has been a long tradition of morphologic and classical biological and epidemiologic studies. Ken Warren was just getting started in trying to bring basic sciences from other disciplines into the field of tropical disease research. Ken knew that despite the enormous burden of tropical diseases and the urgency of addressing the problems of developing countries, the pool of dedicated scientists and fund of expertise have been very small. It was his vision to draw these resources together through the establishment of collaborative national and international networks. Until 15 years ago, the World Health Organization paid only desultory attention to the cutting edge of biomedical research for most problems in world health. It has been extraordinarily gratifying, as one who has had the privilege of participating in WHO activities, to acknowledge the importance of its Special Programme for Research and Training in Tropical Diseases. This program is the principal means of bringing the cutting edge of science to bear on the problems of tropical diseases in developing countries. The challenge is to make communication possible from the laboratory to the field.

I have enormous faith in the power of the new scientific tools in molecular biology and immunology to address the problems of tropical diseases. There really are going to be one or more malaria vaccines that will work; it should be possible to develop vaccines against leprosy that are effective. There are great opportunities for identifying and cloning targets for antiparasitic drugs and developing new chemotherapeutic agents based on rational structural analysis of the target molecules. But, as in all other aspects of science, we should not count our gratifications and accomplishments too quickly. There are many surprises and disappointments ahead.

Despite the extraordinary tools of modern biological science, we must be humbled by the intricacy of the adaptations of parasites to their vectors and hosts. They show the enormous ingenuity that evolution uses to assure survival, an ingenuity that ranges from something as crude as the development of resistance to an antibiotic by bacteria to such a subtle phenomenon as that evidenced by the filarial worms on two sides of the Indian Ocean that have diurnal parasitemia at strikingly different times of the day. We appreciate the excitement and challenge of evolutionary thinking, no better exemplified than by parasitic diseases; and along with this comes a sense of wonder and mystery at these subtle host-parasite relationships. Furthermore, they provide the most provocative materials for further inquiry in every field of fundamental biology from biochemical adaptation to immunologic networks.[2,3]

The very title of this symposium refers to a volcano, with the implication that volcanos are *out there* someplace in the Third World and are perhaps about to erupt. Yet, the AIDS epidemic is evidence that even the first and second worlds are not exempt from the problems that beset the Third. We should take pride at our sense of moral affiliation with the rest of humanity, the sense of fraternity with mankind. But we can be motivated by self-interest as well, for it is ultimately in our own interest that we take tropical diseases and other diseases of the Third World with greater seriousness. AIDS is a complication of the other circumstances that lead to severe immunodeficiency in populations throughout the world, compounded by problems of nutrition, other infection, migration and war. There is a sense of complacency that as we have produced chemotherapeutic agents against major infectious diseases, we shall be able to do the same now: but not without money, commitment and development of increasing motivation and expertise in young scientists. And, if we have learned anything from the study of evolution and the history of disease, we know that HIV will not be the last new evolved pathogenic infectious agent; and we must appreciate that one of the roles of science, in the area of infectious diseases surveillance, is the anticipation of genetic changes and development of means rapidly to counter them. Parasitic agents and viruses have built-in mechanisms of genetic instability. We would not have the variety of life we see in the biosphere if that had not happened to start with. In the grand time-scale of history, it is absolutely predictable that pandemics like AIDS have occurred in the past and will recur in the future. Above all else then, we must use such motivation for dealing far more aggressively with infectious disease health problems throughout the world. This is one of the rare areas in which self-interest and humanitarian interest converge absolutely and certainly.

It is gratifying to see so many young people and students attending this scientific conference and interested in parasitic and tropical diseases. The challenges are enormous but fascinating. The future is in your hands. In the words of Pasteur, "whether or not your efforts are smiled upon by fate, what really matters in the end is to be able to say, 'I did what I was able to'."

REFERENCES

1. LEDERBERG, J. 1975. DNA splicing: Will fear rob us of its benefits? A.M.A. Prism **3:** 33-37.
2. TRAGER, W. 1986. Living Together: The Biology of Animal Parasitism. Plenum. New York.
3. ENGLAND, P. T. & A. SHER, Eds. 1988. The biology of parasitism: A molecular and immunological approach. *In* MBL Lectures in Biology, 9. Alan R. Liss. New York.

Disease Problems in the Third World

JULIA A. WALSH

Department of Medicine
Division of Infectious Diseases
Harvard Medical School
and
Harvard School of Public Health
Boston, Massachusetts 02115

For those living in the Third World, no matter what their age, the risk of death and disability is always many times higher than for those living in the first world. Despite biomedical advances, illness and death remain common events. These stifle the ability to learn and the capacity to work and raise families, sap one's energy, discourage efforts for advancement, influence attitudes and pervade practically all activities. TABLE 1 shows these higher risks of death.[1,2] The likelihood of dying in the Third World is almost 30 times greater for an infant, 40 to 75 times greater for a child, and more than a 1,000 times greater for a pregnant woman than in any of their counterparts living in an industrialized nation. Even the adolescent and elderly survivors continue to have a greater chance of becoming ill and dying.

One of the first steps in attempting to identify possible methods to prevent this excess ill health and death is to analyze the causes. This paper reviews the available information on the causes of death and outlines the changes that have occurred recently.

HISTORICAL TRENDS

Despite this discouraging picture, health has improved in the last three decades. Infant mortality has declined and the life expectancies have increased in essentially all countries. In 1986, only ten countries had infant mortality rates exceeding 150 per 1,000 live births and none reported a rate greater than 200.[3] TABLE 2 presents this gratifying trend, showing the probability of dying by 5 years of age in various regions. On average, less-developed regions have sustained an annual decline in the risk of dying of 2.5%. The causes of this health improvement are not entirely clear. Improved socioeconomic conditions have undoubtedly played a role. Education, particularly of women, provision of health services and immunizations, and political commitment to health have also contributed.[4]

TABLE 1. Comparison of Extreme Levels of National Age-Specific Mortality Rates

	Highest Levels[a]	Lowest Levels[b]	Ratio of Highest and Lowest Levels
Perinatal	100	12-15	6-8
Infant[a]	185	6-10	18-30
Childhood[b]	40	0.4-1	40-75
Maternal[c]	1,000	0.5-5	1-2,000
Age 5-14 years[b]	5	0.4-0.5	10-15
Age 15-45 years[b]	9-13	0.7-2	5-15
Age 45-65 years[b]	27	8-11	2-3
Age 65-90 years[b]	150	90-100	1.5

SOURCES: United Nations[2] and Preston.[1]
[a] Per 1000 live births.
[b] Per 1000 population.
[c] Per 100,000 live births.

DISEASE PROBLEMS

TABLE 3 presents *estimates* for the causes of death in the developing world ranked according to the number of deaths caused.[5] Some diseases affect primarily the very young, whereas others affect older age groups. For example, circulatory disease occurs among the elderly and is mostly ischemic heart disease, as is the case in the North. Low birthweight affects newborns but has far-reaching effects on the health and development of infants and children.

A more powerful indicator of the relative importance of each of these conditions may be the Years of Potential Life Lost (YPLL). This measures the premature mortality from each condition.[6] For example, if the average age of persons dying from

TABLE 2. Levels and Trends in the Probability of Dying by Age 5 (1950-1985)

Region and Area	Probability of Dying by Age 5 (per 1000 live births) 1950-55	1980-85	Average Annual Rate of Decline (%)
Africa	297	175	1.8
East Africa	286	204	1.1
North Africa	326	152	2.5
South and Latin America	174	78	2.8
South Asia	261	99	2.8
China	266	55	5.3
Southern Asia	327	177	2.0
Oceania	205	64	4.0
Less-developed regions	281	134	2.5

SOURCE: United Nations.[3]

TABLE 3. Causes of Death for Individuals of all Ages in the Developing World

Conditions	Infections[a]	Deaths[a]	Episodes[a]
Respiratory disease (upper and lower)	NA	10,000[b]	15,000,000[c]
Circulatory systems[d]	NA	8,000	No data
(Low Birthweight)[e]	NA	(5,000)	(19,000)
Diarrhea	NA	4,300	2,800,000
Measles[f]	67,000	2,000	67,000
Injuries[g]	NA	2,000	No data
(Malnutrition)[h]	NA	(2,000)	(5-8,000)
Neoplasms[i]	NA	2,000	No data
Malaria	260,000[j]	1,500	150,000
P. falciparum	NA	1,350	120,000
Tetanus	NA	1,200	1,800
Tuberculosis	1,000	900	7,000
Hepatitis[k]	300,000	800	3,700
Whooping cough	55,000	600	51,000
Typhoid	70,000	600	35,000
Maternal mortality	NA	500	NA
Meningitis	NA	350	1,000
Schistosomiasis	200,000	250-500	10,000
Syphilis[l]	15,000	200	250
Amebiasis	500,000	70	40,000
Human immunodeficiency virus (HIV)	4,000	50-70	140
South American trypanosomiasis	24,000	60	1,200
Rheumatic fever and heart disease	NA	52	2,200
Hookworm	800,000	50	1,500
Rabies	35	35	35
Diphtheria	60,000	30	600
Dengue	No data	15	48
Hepatitis A	No data	14	5,000
Yellow Fever	No data	9	82
Japanese B encephalitis	No data	7	28
Ascariasis	700,000	< 10	700
Giardiasis	250,000	< 10	500
Poliomyelitis	150,000	2	220[m]
Leprosy	1,000	1	1,000
Leishmaniasis	1,000	1	1,000
Trichuriasis	500,000	< 1	100
Filariasis	90,000	< 1	1,000
Dracunculiasis	1,000	< 1	1,000
Onchocerciasis[n]	1-5,000	< 1	No data
African trypanosomiasis	No data	< 1	No data
Other[o]	No data	1-2,000	No data

NA = not applicable.

[a] Thousands per year; episodes means yearly occurrence of disease.

[b] Four million of these deaths occur in children under 5 years old.

[c] Twenty-five million episodes of acute lower respiratory tract infectious disease and 15 billion episodes of acute upper respiratory tract infectious disease.

[d] This category includes cardiovascular diseases and certain degenerative diseases (nephritis, cirrhosis of the liver, ulcers of stomach and duodenum, and diabetes).

(Footnotes continued overleaf)

Footnotes to Table 3 (continued)

[e] Low birthweight is the underlying cause of death, although the immediate cause may be respiratory, diarrheal or other disease; therefore, these deaths have also been counted in the other categories.

[f] A small proportion of these deaths may also be counted in the diarrheal disease category.

[g] Occurrences of injury are probably one hundred times more frequent than deaths, but very little reliable data are available on incidence.

[h] Severe malnutrition is the underlying cause of death, although the immediate cause may be respiratory, diarrheal, or other disease; therefore, these deaths have also been counted in other categories.

[i] Includes neoplasms of all types except hepatitis-B-related hepatocellular carcinoma, which is listed separately.

[j] This is the population at risk inhabiting infected areas; 365,000,000 live in highly endemic areas.

[k] The number of infections represent the asymptomatic carriers of hepatitis B surface antigen present in the world. Episodes include acute hepatitis, cirrhosis, and primary hepatocellular carcinoma.

[l] The deaths are primarily excess perinatal deaths among the 10% of seroreactive women giving birth in sub-Saharan Africa. No good information is available on adult deaths from tertiary syphilis or extent of disease in other parts of the world.

[m] Cases of paralysis.

[n] No systematic survey of prevalence and incidence has occurred since the beginning of the onchocerciasis control program in West Africa, which has markedly diminished the occurrence of infection and disease.

[o] Other. Deaths of unclear etiology or diseases with relatively small numbers of cases.

circulatory disease is 60, and the life expectancy is only 65 years, then the YPLL equals 5 years times the disease incidence. YPLL does tend to accord more importance to deaths among the young (for example, a child dying at age 2 may lose decades of life, while an adult may only lose a few years). This system may undervalue lives lost among young adults. They are usually socioeconomically active and the head of young families. Their sickness may affect the well-being of many others. The calculation requires information on causes of death, life expectancy, and age at death for each of these diseases. YPLL from disability may be included if length and degree of disability are known. A few countries have made these calculations (Ghana, Thailand, the United States, and France, among others), but inadequate information is available globally to make these estimations.

The figures in TABLE 3 are aggregated for all the countries of the Third World from the poorest to those emerging into an industrialized economy. The statistics do not represent those of a single nation. The table also ranks the conditions by number of deaths caused, but this tends to minimize the importance of many of the conditions inducing prolonged disability. Enormous societal costs result from diseases such as leprosy and poliomyelitis, which maim rather than kill. The difference between the major causes of death and the major causes of illness becomes evident in comparing TABLE 3 with TABLE 4. TABLE 4 lists the prevalence of illnesses among children in Bangladesh.[7] Upper respiratory infections and diarrheal illnesses top both lists, but the similarity stops there. Skin diseases of various kinds are the next most prevalent illness.

Sources

These estimates derive from World Health Organization studies and expansions of relatively small epidemiologic studies performed in various parts of the world. The data in this table are not based on communicable disease notifications. Case reporting is rarely complete, even in countries with functioning surveillance systems, and becomes sporadic in developing countries. The efforts of the Expanded Programme on Immunization (EPI), UNICEF, and other national and international agencies within the last few years to provide universal immunization have vastly improved the surveillance, monitoring, and reporting system at least for the immunization-preventable illnesses. The bibliography lists some of the references upon which these estimates were based. My recent book *Establishing Health Priorities in the Developing World* provides the full list.[5]

Two of the main problems with many of these global estimates include: (1) generalizability of the small studies, which may only represent a peculiar ecological or epidemiologic niche; and (2) attributability of many deaths that result from an *accumulation* of health insults—for example, children may suffer from low birthweight, malnutrition, measles, and diarrhea. Should such a death be attributed to measles, diarrhea, malnutrition or low birthweight since preventing any one of these may not have averted the death? These all occur most often among the poorest, most deprived in society.

Of all the illnesses listed in TABLE 3, infectious diseases are the most easily prevented and cured with available technology. The decline among these diseases has resulted in the enormous increases in life expectancy that have occurred in the developed countries in the last century.[8] Improved socioeconomic conditions, nutritional status, education, and health services have all contributed. For example, in England in 1881, when life expectancy at birth was only 47 years, the probability of eventually dying from an infectious disease was more than 40 percent, while in 1964, when life expectancy at birth was 70+ years, there was only a 13 percent probability of eventually dying from infections.[1]

In summary, the developing world suffers both from the diseases of poverty (such as an excessive burden of infectious and tropical disease, hazards, and nutritional

TABLE 4. Prevalence of Illnesses in a Cohort of 197 Rural Bangladeshi Children aged 2-60 Months Studied in 1978-1979[7]

Illness	Days	Prevalence (per 100 child-days)
Upper respiratory	37,111	60.3
Diarrhea	7,904	12.8
Impetigo	5,119	8.3
Scabies	4,206	6.8
Other skin infection	2,969	4.8
Chronic otitis	2,457	4.0
Stomatitis	2,449	4.0
Conjunctivitis	1,363	2.2
Asthma	269	0.4
Pneumonia	175	0.3
Measles	138	0.2
Hepatitis	69	0.1
Eczema	55	0.1
Varicella	41	0.1
Tonsillitis	35	0.1
Typhoid fever	20	0.03
Other recorded illnesses	15	0.02
Mumps	14	0.02
Pertussis	7	0.01

deficiencies) and a rising incidence of the diseases of affluence. Infectious diseases are the most easily controlled, and even though they may be decreasing in some areas, they remain the major cause of illness.

DESCRIPTIONS OF THE MAJOR DISEASES

This section describes in detail the current status of the major disorders in the developing world, with regard to epidemiology, importance, and currently available interventions. The conditions are presented in descending order of number of deaths produced annually and the estimates are based on the 1986 population.

Respiratory Infections

This entity heads the list as the major cause of death from infectious disease. With diarrheal disease, it causes half to two-thirds of the morbidity and mortality from communicable diseases in the developing world.[9] Many different organisms can cause respiratory infections. Most episodes resolve on their own. Each of the serious types of cases requires a different drug for treatment and vaccine for prevention. *S. pneumoniae, H. influenzae,* influenza virus, respiratory syncytial virus, parainfluenza and *Staph. aureus* cause 60% of the deaths.

Unlike diarrheal disease, which can be treated by oral rehydration and largely prevented with handwashing and appropriate use of water and sanitation, respiratory infections have no simple, efficacious control measure. Throughout the world, the incidence of acute upper respiratory tract infections appears to be the same: for those under 5 years, 5-6 episodes annually. This decreases to about 2 per year among adults. In developing countries, children suffer from pneumonia and bronchitis more frequently than do children in industrialized nations, and are therefore at much higher risk of death.[9]

Diseases of the Circulatory System

This category includes cardiovascular diseases and certain degenerative diseases such as nephritis, cirrhosis of the liver, ulcers of the stomach and duodenum, and diabetes.[10] These primarily affect adults and the elderly. Few simple efficacious control measures are available. Treatment of hypertension, diet, smoking prevention, and exercise may have some influence on mortality rates, but they require long-term behavioral modification.

The infectious causes of circulatory illness, Chagas' disease, and rheumatic heart disease are considered separately. However, these represent a tiny percentage of global deaths. More deaths from circulatory diseases will certainly occur in the future as people live longer, as diet and exercise patterns change, and as smoking increases.

Low Birthweight

When an infant is born with a birthweight of 2,500 grams or less, it is considered premature or of low birthweight. TABLE 5 lists the proportion of low-birthweight infants born in a sample of countries around the world.[11,12] In many industrialized countries as few as 4% of all infants weigh so little at birth, but in some parts of the developing world almost 50% of babies begin life so disadvantaged. The consequences of low birthweight are myriad: in developing countries few of these infants achieve the normal weight-for-age by even 3 years of age and the majority are malnourished, with all its attendant problems. The risk of dying in infancy and childhood is many times that of a normal-weight baby: for example, in a recent study in the United States, although low-birthweight infants represented only 6% of live births, they accounted for 55% of infant deaths.[13] The risk of having developmental disabilities and retardation in mental and motor skills is high.

TABLE 5. Percentage of Infants with Low Birthweight[a] in Selected Countries (1982-1985)

Country	Percentage
Afghanistan	17
Burkina Faso	21
Guinea	18
Bangladesh	50
India	30
Central African Republic	23
Haiti	17
Sudan	15
Pakistan	27
Guatemala	18
Nicaragua	15
United States of America	7
Sweden	4
Japan	6

SOURCE: UNICEF.[11]
[a] Weighing less than 2,500 grams at birth.

Prematurity results from either pre-term delivery (that is, the fetus grows normally during pregnancy, but the gestation is shorter than 37 weeks) or from slow intrauterine growth but normal gestational duration. A few severely affected infants suffer from both intrauterine growth retardation (IUGR) and short gestation. In industrialized countries, about two-thirds of the low-birthweight babies are pre-term; but in developing countries, most occurrences of low-birthweight appear to result from IUGR, although the data base is inadequate for us to be certain about this. Small improvements in the incidence of low birthweight markedly decrease the infant and child mortality rate. For example, a decrease in incidence of low birthweight from 30% to 15% could result in a decrease in the infant mortality rate of around 25%, for example, from 160 per 1,000 to 120 per 1,000.[13] Few interventions are known to prevent prematurity: malaria chemoprophylaxis or control in areas hyperendemic for *P. falciparum* helps and nutritional supplementation throughout the pregnancy in extremely malnourished mothers will increase birthweights as will the stopping of smoking and alcohol use.[14] Women who have more education, more wealth, and prenatal care, and women who are in their second through fourth pregnancy also have fewer premature babies. However, more research into causes and possible preventive measures is greatly needed. For example, sexually transmitted and gestational infections can precipitate early delivery and affect intrauterine growth rates. Maternal Group B streptococcal infection appears to cause both prematurity and maternal morbidity and mortality. Control of this infection by immunization or targeted treatment could prevent a substantial proportion of this burden.[15] Prematurity is listed in parentheses in TABLE 3 because the infants and children affected by low birthweight usually die from respiratory infection or diarrheal disease and these deaths are counted in these categories.

Diarrheal Disease

A great variety of pathogens produce diarrheal disease: rotavirus, enterotoxigenic *E. coli,* Shigella, *Vibrio cholerae* and Salmonella produce about 60%, a great variety produce a small percentage more, and one-third or more are caused by unknown pathogens.[9] In spite of the multiple etiologic agents, most cases can be treated and deaths averted through the use of oral rehydration. Only those severe cases of bloody diarrhea and dysentery usually caused by ameba, Shigella, and enteropathogenic *E. coli* will not respond to oral rehydration. In developing countries, adults usually suffer from at least one episode of mild diarrhea yearly. In contrast, children under 5 have an incidence of two to ten episodes of diarrhea annually, averaging about four in most poor communities, and this dehydrating illness lasts for several days to a week.

Malnutrition and diarrhea appear to act synergistically. Diarrhea contributes to malnutrition by inducing anorexia and intestinal malabsorption, whereas those who are malnourished are at increased risk of prolonged illness and death when they are stricken with diarrhea.[16] The use of enriched oral rehydration solutions seems to avert many of the nutritional deficits. The standard oral rehydration solution available in packets contains only a small amount of calories from sugar, but the calorie-dense varieties provide nutritional support while still treating the dehydration. Increasing food intake during the recovery period will also help prevent malnutrition.

The provision of and appropriate use of adequate water supplies and sanitation can decrease incidence of and mortality from diarrhea by approximately 20%.[17,18] The development of low-cost handpumps and latrines has increased their installation worldwide. However, presence does not translate automatically into appropriate use. Installations must be accompanied by education and commitment to appropriate use and maintenance.

Measles

Essentially, everyone who is not immunized and who survives beyond the first 6 months of life becomes infected with measles and suffers from this illness. Particularly the very young and the malnourished suffer severe and prolonged disease, with multiple complications including diarrhea, pneumonia, otitis media, and the enormous loss of weight that can lead to malnutrition.[19] Fatality rates in community studies range from

1 to 10%. This preventable infection may cause more than 5% of deaths in all age groups and up to 30% of all infant and child deaths, as illustrated in TABLE 6.[19–21] Immunization of all infants 9 months of age or older will largely eliminate this deadly disease. In the last decade, global immunization coverage has spectacularly increased. Now 43% of infants and children are protected against measles, primarily as a result of enormous international mobilization.[22] Nationwide campaigns by WHO, UNICEF, UNDP and other international agencies, private voluntary organizations, bilateral agencies, and other groups have made universal childhood immunization a major priority. UNICEF and the WHO/Expanded Programme on Immunization (EPI) have been the spearheads for these remarkably successful efforts. The present vaccine costs less than 10 cents a dose purchased through UNICEF suppliers.

TABLE 6. Efficacy of Measles Immunization in Children 10-60 Months of Age in Matlab, Bangladesh (1982-1984)

	%	95% Confidence Intervals
Total mortality reduction	36	21-48
Measles-specific mortality reduction	100	
Diarrhea mortality reduction	59	42-70

SOURCE: Clemens *et al.*[20]

Injuries

Death rates from injuries are remarkably similar in all regions of the world, but few systems gather data about the frequency of their occurrence.[10] Young adults and children have the greatest risk of injuries, usually as a result of exposure to hazardous and unsafe environments in the community, home, and at work. In Chile, after the widespread use of childhood immunization and oral rehydration, injuries became the most common cause of childhood deaths.[23] Burns, motor vehicle accidents, and falls account for the largest number of accidents.[24,25] The loss of these healthy, productive individuals incurs an inordinately great societal cost. Little is known about risk factors or appropriate control measures, but a substantial proportion of these injuries are certainly preventable. Education and improved environmental safety have made a difference in some industrialized countries. The potential exists for a substantial worldwide decline in the incidence of and mortality from injury. Epidemiologic research to identify locally important risk factors and the introduction of appropriate interventions such as education, behavioral change, and improved cooking stoves are prerequisites for such a decline.

Malnutrition

Malnutrition can be defined as a state in which the physical condition of an individual is impaired to the point where she or he can no longer maintain an adequate level of performance at such things as physical work, resisting or recovering from the effects of disease, maintaining an adequate level of growth, or the processes of pregnancy or lactation.[26] This impairment does not result from any other known disease processes. Malnourished individuals can no longer sustain their existence because of their physical disability. For example, to avoid malnutrition a family must be able to do physical work on their land and crops, or sell their labor for cash. The returns must be sufficient not only to secure their immediate food needs, but to sustain productivity over long periods, and to survive through bad years as well as good. They must in addition be able to adjust total production from their resources to keep pace with the number of dependents in the family. If the members of a family cannot maintain these subsistence activities, they become malnourished.

Nutritional status both results from the activities of acquiring, consuming, and utilizing food, and at the same time is crucial to the success of this process. The food an individual eats provides the energy needed to secure food in the future.

Inequality of resources, poverty, and social discrimination remain the foremost causes of malnutrition. Changes in the system of food production and distribution without improvements in resource distribution or alleviation of poverty and social discrimination have little effect on malnutrition. Humans can adapt to a fairly wide range of dietary situations. Only when that adaptive capacity is stretched beyond its limits, does the body fail to maintain its functional capacity, and malnutrition ensues. This means that real malnutrition—that is, physiological states carrying penalties in terms of loss of function as distinct from otherwise benign deviations of growth or body size—occurs much less frequently than previously believed. But such *real* malnutrition is concentrated amongst the most economically and socially deprived sections of the population.

The objective measurements of nutritional status include weight-for-age, skinfold thickness, triceps circumference, weight-for-height, and height-for-age, which are compared to national or international standards. Nutritional surveys primarily assess children. As a result, the estimate for morbidity and mortality in TABLE 3 refers to this age group.

Nutrition and infections are intimately related: infections, particularly diarrheal, exert a negative impact on nutritional status, while malnutrition predisposes the individual to an increased risk of morbidity and mortality from various infections. In Bangladesh, the mortality rate of the children in the lowest decile according to weight-for-age or height-for-age exceeds the rate of those in the top decile by a factor of four.[27] Epidemiologic studies in Guatemala, the Gambia, and Bangladesh have demonstrated a marked relationship between infections and the physical growth and development of the child.[28,29] Diarrhea, measles, and malaria appear to have the greatest impact on nutrition. These diseases probably exert their effect through the mechanisms of decreased food intake, malabsorption, and loss of nutrients in the gastrointestinal tract. Control of these infections should greatly lessen the burden of malnutrition in society. Enough food is produced in the world today to meet the physiological demands of all the individuals inhabiting this planet if only the food were equitably distributed. In spite of this capacity, the number of malnourished children has imperceptibly changed in the last few decades.

How can malnutrition be treated or averted? Many of the more conventional types of nutrition programs—such as promoting the production of specially nutritious foods, special food delivery systems aimed at young children, and projects to educate people about the nutritional value of foods—have had disappointing results.[30] Further attempts are needed to identify more effective alternatives and ways to improve the conventional programs.

Neoplasms

This category includes all the benign and malignant neoplasms affecting humankind.[10] Only a few of the less common types, such as childhood leukemia and Hodgkin's disease, can occasionally be cured. However, one of the most common types of neoplasm in the developing world, hepatitis-B-related hepatocellular carcinoma (listed separately in TABLE 3) will probably be prevented through the immunization of newborn infants. Adults and the elderly are the age group most commonly affected by cancer. Lung cancer is rapidly increasing in incidence in the developing world, following upon the epidemic increase in the use of tobacco. Years of research absorbing more than one billion dollars yearly have not yet resulted in cures or preventions for the most common types of cancer, and prospects for rapid advances remain dim.

TABLE 7. Effect of Malaria Control on Mortality in Kisumu, Kenya (1972-1976)

	Protected Area (per 1,000)	Unprotected Area (per 1,000)
Crude death rate	13.5	23.9
Infant mortality rate	93	157

SOURCE: Payne *et al.*[32]

Malaria

Particularly in sub-Saharan Africa, malaria causes an enormous number of deaths. Distinguishing illness caused by malaria from that of other diseases is difficult since most infected persons living in endemic areas seem to have minimal symptoms. Several studies have shown a decrease of almost one-third in mortality in infants and adults as a result of insecticide spraying.[31] TABLE 7 illustrates the results of a malaria control program in Kisumu, Kenya. The crude death rate declined by almost one-half and the infant mortality rate by one-third![32] These results are probably a better indication of the true burden of illness from this protozoa. However, the epidemiologic studies for the malaria vaccine trials will probably provide the most valid measures of burden of illness.

The current control methods used include:

(1) attack on the parasite in the human host through the use of antimalarial drugs either for treatment or prophylaxis;

(2) development of a malaria vaccine (much effort has been expended on this goal in the last ten years, but an effective vaccine will not be available for probably at least another decade);

(3) reduction of contact between humans and mosquitoes through the use of screening, bed nets, and repellents, for example;

(4) reduction of mosquito breeding sites by environmental alteration such as filling or draining of collections of water, straightening and clearing of streams and rivers, and intermittent drying of irrigated fields;

(5) attack on the larval stages of the mosquito through chemical and biologic methods; and

(6) destruction of the adult mosquito by environmental or household spraying with pesticides.[33] In light of the extensive resistance of protozoa to antimalarial agents and the resistance to pesticides among many mosquito species, source reduction through the use of environmental modification is becoming a more valuable malaria prevention scheme.

Tetanus

About two-thirds of the deaths from tetanus occur in the neonatal period as a result of contamination of the umbilical stump with *Clostridium tetani.* The organism is commonly present in the environment, so that minor soilage can result in infection. Neonatal tetanus can be prevented by immunizing pregnant women against tetanus and by training birth attendants in the use of sanitary techniques for delivery, especially the use of sterile tools for cutting the cord.[34] Non-neonatal tetanus occurs as a result of dirty wounds, and can be prevented by administering tetanus immunization to children followed by booster doses about every 10 years. The underlying cause of these deaths is injuries. When one adds these non-neonatal tetanus deaths to the injury deaths, the enormity of the societal burden from injuries becomes more evident.

Tuberculosis

Despite decades of BCG (bacillus Calmette-Guérin) immunization and drug treatment, the incidence of new cases and deaths from tuberculosis (TB) essentially has not changed. The efficacy of BCG remains questionable, even though it is the mainstay of TB control in many countries.[35] Cure requires multiple drugs and many months of compliance, an extremely difficult task. Practically all adults in developing countries have been infected, as indicated by skin-test reactivity, but fewer than 5% develop clinical disease. Several of the risk factors for the development of clinical disease include age when first exposed, intensity of exposure, presence of other significant illnesses, pregnancy, and recent exposure; however, these factors explain only a small proportion of the clinical cases. Tuberculosis is a disease of young adults (the age group most economically active and most productive in society) and of the impoverished. The challenge for current control programs is to increase and maintain compliance, given the current lengthy course of drugs required for cure. The challenge for biomedical research is the discovery of a better, more efficacious immunization and a successful short-term drug treatment.

Hepatitis B Virus

Among the diseases related to hepatitis B virus, hepatocellular carcinoma and cirrhosis of the liver carry the greatest disability and the highest mortality rates.[36]

These begin to appear in young adulthood, and the incidence peaks between 35 and 40 years of age, at least 20 years after initial exposure to the virus and onset of chronic infection. At present, several studies of the efficacy of vaccines are under way in West Africa and Asia. These will assess the ability to prevent chronic carriage of the virus and ultimately (20-30 years from now) assess the protection from hepatoma and cirrhosis. The vaccine now costs less than $1 per dose (3 doses are needed for immunity) when purchased from the Korean manufacturer. Nevertheless, this price is still many times higher than the few-cents-a-dose cost of the usual childhood vaccines.

Whooping Cough (Pertussis)

Like measles, this disease is highly contagious and affects essentially all children who are not immunized. Three doses induce immunity in more than 80% of children for many years. The disease in nonimmune adults is generally mild. The mortality rate from the cough and the secondary pneumonia exceeds 1%. The prolonged spasmodic cough during the illness frequently interferes with adequate nutritional intake and predisposes to malnutrition. Immunization acceptance has accelerated in the last several years, largely due to UNICEF and the WHO/Expanded Programme on Immunization. The three doses of the vaccine itself cost pennies. Particularly when combined with other vaccines, immunization programs become remarkably cost-effective in terms of cost per death averted.

Typhoid Fever

Approximately 75% of cases of typhoid fever occur among schoolchildren and young adults.[9] The presently available immunization for typhoid gives good protection, but has never been universally administered because (1) it induces side effects in a large proportion of recipients, (2) confidence in its efficacy has been poor, and (3) the short duration of immunity necessitates booster injections every 3 to 4 years. Several newer vaccines are presently undergoing large-scale clinical trials, but the results of these have generally been disappointing.[9] Thus these new vaccines will probably not be available for at least 5 to 7 years. Typhoid transmission occurs most commonly by contamination of food by intestinal carriers of the organism.[37] Provision of adequate water supplies, effective sanitary disposal, and personal hygiene should produce a substantial drop in incidence rates because of the interruption of spread from carriers to susceptible persons. In many endemic areas, such as Lesotho, provision of chlorinated water had no effect on the incidence of disease.[38] However, provision of an adequate quantity of water is a prerequisite for careful personal hygiene. Cleaning of hands prior to handling food is key for the prevention of this disease, and *quantity* of water available in the household is more important than its purity.

Maternal Mortality

Pregnancy carries an enormous risk of death and long-term disability for the mother. According to WHO estimates, about 500,000 women die annually as a result of pregnancy. The public health community has only recently recognized the far-reaching consequences such mortality holds for family health. When a mother dies, usually her newborn dies too. The other living children lose their primary source of love and care. Efficacious and cost-effective control measures are few. The major problems in pregnancy are hemorrhage, severe infection (sepsis), toxemia (or eclampsia), and obstructed labor.[39–42] One-third or more of these deaths occur quite early in pregnancy as a result of primitive attempts at abortion to terminate unwanted pregnancies.[41] Family planning methods available to all women should at least prevent these deaths. Family planning should also promote the woman's ability to time and space her pregnancies so that she can ensure her health at the time pregnancy begins. The World Bank estimates that up to 45% of maternal mortality may be averted through the provision and widespread use of family planning.[41]

Averting complications during delivery requires skilled obstetric care. However, many countries do not have adequate resources for all births to take place in hospitals. If high-risk pregnancies could be easily identified and the women referred for skilled delivery care or if low-cost transport systems could be developed for carrying women to the hospital when complications occur, then maternal health would improve. Skilled care during the birth process may have the additional benefit of decreasing birth trauma, neonatal asphyxia, and low birthweight. Once such cost-effective control measures are developed, then programs can be modified to fit into the social, cultural and economic environment of local areas. However, at this point, the commonly used indicators of high risk are both insensitive and nonspecific so that their application in most developing countries identifies 50% or more of all women as high risk, when only half of the complications may occur among these identified women.[14]

Acquired Immune Deficiency Syndrome

Within the last five years a new infectious disease, the acquired immune deficiency syndrome (AIDS), caused by the human immunodeficiency virus (HIV), has become an important health problem. At present, it causes less disease and death than do the other major public health problems. However, its epidemic proportions and the cost of care throughout the long, devastating illness, may eventually overburden the health system. The loss of these young, productive adults and children make this disease particularly devastating. The extent of the epidemic is still unknown.

RESEARCH PRIORITIES

Persons living in the Third World have substantially excessive risks of dying from a variety of potentially preventable causes. Thus, many deaths could be prevented by providing health services for all. Still, many of the major causes of illness and death have no adequate control measures. The new biotechnology techniques and opportunities that will be described in this symposium should result in rapid progress in finding improved control methods. The U.S. Institute of Medicine analyzed both the burden of illness from a variety of infectious diseases plus the likelihood of vaccine development for each of these. On the basis of these criteria, the Institute identified five vaccines that should be accorded high priority for research.[9] These are vaccines to prevent infection by *S. pneumoniae, Plasmodium* spp., rotavirus, *S. typhi* (Ty2la), and Shigella spp. Efforts to develop these vaccines and other control measures for the diseases discussed above should progressively yield results that will encourage these measures to be used in the villages. An increasing commitment is needed to find better ways to improve health, both in terms of better use of what is known and the discovery of improved measures. Alliances among governments, the private sector, international agencies, and individuals will speed discoveries along the complex journey from the laboratory to the village.

REFERENCES

1. PRESTON, S. H. 1976. Mortality Patterns in National Populations. Academic Press. New York.
2. 1987. Model Life Tables for Developing Countries. United Nations. New York.
3. 1985. Child Mortality in Developing Countries. United Nations. New York.
4. HALSTEAD, S., J. A. WALSH & K. S. WARREN. 1985. Good Health at Low Cost. The Rockefeller Foundation. New York.
5. WALSH, J. A. 1988. Establishing Health Priorities in the Developing World. United Nations Development Programme. New York.
6. 1988. Trends in years of potential life lost due to infant mortality and perinatal conditions, 1980-1983 and 1984-1985. Morbid. Mortal. Wkly. Rep. **37**(16): 249-256.
7. BLACK, R. E., K. H. BROWN, S. BECKER & M. YUNIS. 1982. Longitudinal studies of infectious diseases and physical growth of children in rural Bangladesh. I. Patterns of morbidity. Am. J. Epidemiol. **115**(4): 305-14.
8. SAGAN, L. A. 1987. The Health of Nations. Basic Books. New York.
9. INSTITUTE OF MEDICINE. 1986. New Vaccine Development: Establishing Priorities, Vol. II: Diseases of Importance in the Developing World. National Academy Press. Washington, DC.
10. HAKULINEN, T., H. HANSLUWKA, A. D. LOPEZ & T. NAKADA. 1986. Global and regional mortality patterns by cause of death in 1980. Int. J. Epidemiol. **15**(2): 226-233.
11. 1988. State of the World's Children. UNICEF. New York.
12. WORLD HEALTH ORGANIZATION 1984. The incidence of low birth weight. Wkly. Epidemiol. Rec. **59:** 205-211.
13. ASHWORTH, A. & R. G. FEACHEM. 1985. Interventions for the control of diarrhoeal diseases among young children: Prevention of low birth weight. Bull. WHO **63**(1): 165-184.
14. INSTITUTE OF MEDICINE. 1985. Preventing Low Birth Weight. National Academy Press. Washington, DC.
15. WALSH, J. A. & S. HUTCHINSON. The importance of Group B Streptococcus in the developing world. Ped. Infect. Dis. In press.
16. ROHDE, J. E. 1986. Acute diarrhea. *In* Strategies for Primary Health Care: Technologies Appropriate for the Control of Disease in the Developing World. J. A. Walsh & K. S. Warren, Eds.: 14-29. University of Chicago Press. Chicago, IL.
17. CVJETANOVIC, B. 1986. Health effects and impact of water supply and sanitation. World Health Stat. Q. **39:** 105-117.
18. FEACHEM, R. G. 1984. Interventions for the control of diarrhoeal diseases among young children: Promotion of personal and domestic hygiene. **61**(6): 967-979.
19. WALSH, J. A. 1986. Measles. *In* Strategies for Primary Health Care: Technologies Appropriate for the Control of Disease in the Developing World. J. A. Walsh & K. S. Warren, Eds.: 60-72. University of Chicago Press. Chicago, IL.
20. CLEMENS, J. D., B. F. STANTON, J. CHAKRAABORTY, S. CHOWDHURY, M. R. RAO, M. ALI, S. ZIMICKI & B. WOJTYNIAK. 1988. Measles vaccination and childhood mortality in rural Bangladesh. Submitted for publication.

21. FEACHEM, R. G. & M. A. KOBLINSKY. 1983. Interventions for the control of diarrhoeal diseases among young children: Measles immunization. Bull. WHO. **61**(4): 641-652.
22. WORLD HEALTH ORGANIZATION. 1988. Progress in global coverage. Expanded Programme on Immunization Update (March). United Nations. Geneva.
23. TOUCHER, E. 1981. Chile: Mortalidad de la 4 años de edad: Tendencias y causas; notas de población. Rev. Latinoamericana Demografia. **9**(26): 27-54.
24. MANCIAUX, M. & C. J. ROMER. 1986. Accidents in children, adolescents, and young adults: A major public health problem. World Health Stat. Quart. **39**(3): 227-231.
25. TAKET, A. 1986. Accident mortality in children, adolescents and young adults. World Health Stat. Quart. **39**(3): 232-236.
26. BISWAS, M. & P. PINSTRUP-ANDERSON, Eds. 1985. Nutrition and Development. United Nations University and Oxford University Press. Oxford, England.
27. CHEN, L. C., A. K. M. CHOUDHURY & S. L. HUFFMAN. 1980. Anthropometric assessment of energy-protein malnutrition and subsequent risk of mortality among preschool aged children. Am. J. Clin. Nutr. **33:** 1836-1845.
28. KEUSCH, G. T. & N. S. SCRIMSHAW. 1986. Control of infection to reduce the prevalence of infantile and childhood malnutrition. *In* Strategies for Primary Health Care: Technologies Appropriate for the Control of Disease in the Developing World. J. A. Walsh & K. S. Warren, Eds.: 298-313. University of Chicago Press. Chicago, IL.
29. MARTORELL, R., J. P. HABICHT, C. YARBROUGH, *et al.* 1975. Acute morbidity and physical growth in rural Guatemalan children. Am. J. Dis. Child. **12:** 12.
30. BEATON, G. H. & H. GHASSEMI. 1982. Supplementary feeding programs for young children in developing countries. Am. J. Clin. Nutr. **35:** 864-916.
31. KUZNETZOV, R. L. 1977. Malaria control by the application of indoor spraying of residual insecticides in tropical Africa and its impact on community health. Trop. Doc. **7:** 81-91.
32. PAYNE, D., B. GRAB, R. E. FONTAINE, *et al.* 1976. Impact of control measures on malaria transmission and general mortality. Bull WHO. **54:** 369-77.
33. REBUSH, T. K., III, J. G. BREMAN, R. L. KAISER & M. WARREN. 1986. Malaria. *In* Strategies for Primary Health Care. Technologies Appropriate for the Control of Disease in the Developing World. J. A. Walsh & K. S. Warren, Eds.: 47-60. University of Chicago Press. Chicago, IL.
34. ARNOLD, R. B., T. INDIJATI SOEWARSO & A. KARYADI. 1986. Mortality from neonatal tetanus in Indonesia: Results of two surveys. Bull. WHO **64**(2): 259-262.
35. CLEMENS, J. D., J. J. H. CHUONG & A. R. FEINSTEIN. 1983. The BCG controversy: A methodological and statistical reappraisal. J. Am. Medical Assoc. **249**(17): 2362-2369.
36. SZMUNESS, W., H. J. ALTER & J. Z. MAYNARD, EDS. 1982. Viral Hepatitis. 1981 International Symposium. The Franklin Institute Press. Philadelphia, PA.
37. FEACHEM, R. G., D. J. BRADLEY, H. GARELICK & D. D. MARA. 1983. Sanitation and Disease: Health Aspects of Excreta and Waste Water Management. John Wiley. New York.
38. FEACHEM, R. G., E. BURNS, S. CAIRNCROSS, A. CRONIN, P. CROSS, D. CURTIS, M. K. KHAN, D. LAMB & H. SOUTHALL. 1978. Water, Health and Development. Tri-Med Books, Ltd. London.
39. 1987. Maternal health in Sub-Saharan Africa. Lancet **i:** 255-257.
40. WORLD HEALTH ORGANIZATION. 1985. Prevention of Maternal Mortality. Report of a WHO Interregional Meeting, Geneva, 11-15 November, 1985. FHE/86.1.
41. HERZ, B. & A. R. MEASHAM. 1987. The Safe Motherhood Initiative: Proposals for Actions. The World Bank. Washington, DC.
42. RINEHART, W., A. KOLS & S. H. MOORE. 1984. Healthier mothers and children through family planning. Pop. Rep. **12**(3) Series J. Number 27: J659-J696.

Health Research in Africa: Priorities, Promise, and Performance

ADETOKUNBO O. LUCAS

Carnegie Corporation of New York
New York, New York 10022

I am delighted to participate at this conference because it gives me the opportunity of acknowledging the contributions of individuals, institutions and agencies who have dedicated their skills and resources to the fight against death, disease, and disability in developing countries. I am particularly pleased to join in congratulating Dr. Ken Warren, not only for his direct contributions as a research scientist on tropical diseases, but more importantly for his inspiration and support, which has encouraged and enabled many others to work on these problems.

I have been asked specifically to provide an African perspective and I would like to examine the subject of health research in Africa by reviewing the subject in three historical periods: (*a*) the colonial era, (*b*) the post-independence period, and (*c*) the future.

THE COLONIAL ERA

At some time or other, health and disease have had important effects on the life and fortunes of every nation, but these issues have had their greatest impact in Africa. The political map of Africa was drawn by the ability of early explorers from Europe and elsewhere to survive and settle in various parts of the continent. Subtropical Africa, which is relatively tame, conveniently accommodated Arabs in the north and Europeans in the south. West Africa was inhospitable—the harsh, hostile environment resisted both European penetration from the south as well as Arab invasion from the north. The early explorers in West Africa—the Portuguese, Germans, French and British—suffered high mortality in their attempts to settle in the area which earned and deserved a reputation of being the "white man's grave." East Africa occupied an intermediate position; parts of this region, notably the highlands of Kenya, provided a safe refuge for Europeans settlers. Data in TABLE 1 illustrate the high mortality rates among European visitors to West Africa.

Quite naturally, high priority was given during the colonial era to diseases affecting Europeans in Africa. Their survival depended on it. There was also interest in the diseases that caused devastating epidemic diseases in local populations. This was the golden age of tropical medicine research, when new diseases were encountered, their causes identified, and the life cycles of parasites described, and control measures were devised, tested and applied. Many of these projects were sponsored by colonial governments, but private foundations and medical religious missions also made significant contributions. For example, the Rockefeller Foundation established a laboratory for research on yellow fever in Yaba, Lagos, Nigeria with a branch in Ghana. Christian missionaries were largely responsible for the care of leprosy and research on the subject in many African countries.[1]

One must praise the courage and ingenuity of physicians, parasitologists, entomologists and other scientists who often, at great personal risk, laid the foundations of our knowledge of tropical parasitic and infectious diseases in Africa. There are many heroes and heroines of this era; it would be invidious to single out my personal favorites, but their exploits and adventures have been celebrated in the history books and some have been memorialized in having their names attached to parasites or vectors. Working with minimal equipment and under most difficult conditions, these pioneers made important scientific and clinical observations which have remained as major milestones in our progress towards the conquest of these plagues.

However, two items were missing from the agenda in the colonial era—general health issues and capacity-building.

(*a*) *General Health Issues.* Effort was concentrated on parasitic and infectious diseases, although some nutritional disorders received attention. But not much attention was paid to general health issues and relatively little was known about noncommunicable diseases among Africans. The information gap was filled with a number of popular myths and misconceptions such as "Africans don't suffer from high blood pressure, cancer, peptic ulcer and other diseases of civilization"! It was also tacitly assumed that cosmopolitan diseases would have similar manifestations and trace the same natural history as in other parts of the world.

(*b*) *Capacity-Building.* The colonial powers trained virtually no African medical scientists. Nationals who were employed at research institutes served as bottle-washers or fly-catchers or in other unskilled positions. Few medical professional staffs were trained by the colonial governments. For example, in Nigeria, the British colonial government trained a total of 62 Nigerian doctors at the Yaba Medical School for a population of 35 million! At independence, there were only 500 Nigerian doctors, for most of us had trained abroad under private sponsorship. Other colonial territories under the French, Portuguese, Spaniards, and Belgians had similar experience, mostly having even fewer trained personnel.

THE POST-INDEPENDENCE PERIOD

Important changes occurred in the pattern of medical research after independence. In the former British territories, with the notable exception of a center in The Gambia, which is still being administered directly by the British Medical Research Council, activities in most of the research institutes rapidly declined after the withdrawal of the expatriate staff. The other institutions could not immediately replace the foreign research staff. After varying periods of inactivity, several of these institutions are now being resuscitated under the direction of national scientists.

Similarly in the Francophone countries, research centers—Pasteur Institutes, the Organisation de Coordination et Cooperation pour la Lutte contre les Grandes Epidemies (OCCGE), and Office de la Récherche Scientifique et Technique Outre-Mèr (ORSTOM)—continued to function under the direction of French scientists and only more recently are national scientists and technicians being trained.

New medical schools that had been established close to the time of independence filled some of the gap in research. National and expatriate staff at African universities—Makerere, Ibadan, Lagos, Accra and Nairobi—carried out research in various medical and related disciplines.

In the post-independence era, the priorities for health research, to the extent that they have been clearly enunciated, related more specifically to the health problems of the indigenous population rather than giving priority to the needs of foreigners. The medical faculties included staff from various disciplines who pursued enquiries in their various fields. For many of them, this was the age of discovery. As pioneering specialists in their disciplines, they examined local problems using their expertise in the major medical specialties and in some of the subspecialties to describe and analyze problems affecting the various systems of the body.

Some scientists collected basic data about anatomic, physiological, and biochemical norms of African populations. They recorded the distribution of birthweights,[2] monitored growth patterns,[3] and estimated the frequency of twinning and other multiple births[4]; others explored psychological features and intellectual performance. They identified hemoglobinopathies and other genetic variations and they identified the clinical syndromes associated with them.[5] They collected information about the patterns of cardiac, renal, hepatic and neurologic diseases; about pregnancy and delivery in the local population; and about disorders of the special senses—sight and hearing.

TABLE 1. Early Mortality Rates of Europeans in West Africa[a]

Expedition	Year	No. of Europeans	No. of Deaths
Mungo Park	1805	44	39
Tuckey	1916	44	21
Clapperton	1825-7	5	4
MacGregor-Laird	1832-4	41	32
Trotter	1841	145	42

[a] After Bruce-Chwatt and Bruce-Chwatt.[17]

Cardiologists in Nigeria noted the rare occurrence of ischemic heart disease in the local population; this observation was confirmed by electrocardiographic studies and by autopsy. Comparative studies showed more atherosclerosis and higher concentrations of lipids in the coronary vessels of West Africans than in American blacks.[6] The sequelae of rheumatic heart disease are commonly found, but, as in other tropical countries, the antecedent acute manifestations are usually missed. Much work was done in Nigeria and in Uganda on endomyocardial fibrosis and heart muscle disease, two peculiar heart diseases of the African which are uncommon in other parts of the world. Researchers at Ibadan and Makerere described clinical, pathophysiological, and pathologic features of these two syndromes.[7]

In some parts of Africa, trachoma and onchocerciasis are major causes of eye disease and blindness. In addition to these classical tropical eye infections, African populations suffer from various eye diseases, some of which show important local variations. For example, in the Ibadan area of Nigeria, where neither trachoma nor onchocerciasis are highly endemic, glaucoma was the second commonest cause of blindness next to cataract; hence, it was the most common cause of irreversible blindness in the community.[8] There glaucoma tended to occur at a younger age, with some severe cases presenting in the second decade. The acute congestive form is rarely seen, and response to standard surgical procedures is poor.

Infections such as poliomyelitis and meningitis dominate the neurologic diseases. In Nigeria, doctors identified a chronic ataxic polyneuropathy which is endemic in the southwest of the country. In the severely affected populations one-third to one-half of the adult women walk with a staggering gait. Clinical, epidemiologic, electrophysiological, biochemical, and pathologic studies determined the etiologic role of chronic cyanide intoxication of dietary origin. The important risk factor was a diet based on cassava, *Manioc utilissima;* this tuber contains cyanogens which release cyanide on interaction with stomach acid.[9]

New drugs and vaccines were evaluated in the local population, including some of the earliest studies on the use of measles vaccine. Pyrimethamine in combination with sulfadoxine or with dapsone was evaluated for the chemosuppression of malaria, observations which formed part of the package of data for the registration of two antimalarial drugs, Maloprim (pyrimethamine with dapsone) and Fansidar (pyrimethamine with sulfadoxine).[10] Innovative approaches to therapy included outpatient care of patients with lobar pneumonia and nonsurgical management of spinal tuberculosis. Obstructive uropathy due to *Schistosoma hematobium* generated controversy about its natural history and response to chemotherapy. Workers in Ibadan showed that in children there is a form of reversible obstruction associated with granulomatous processes in the bladder and the lower end of the ureter; these cases usually respond to drug treatment alone.[11] In East Africa, where 8 to 20% of young children showed obstructive uropathy, direct surgical intervention on a mass scale had been advocated, but the recommendation was subsequently withdrawn when the doctors discovered that their own patients similarly responded to chemotherapy.

Epidemiologic surveys established the distribution of goiter, schistosomiasis and various other endemic parasitic infections, the pattern of blood pressure readings in urban and rural populations, and the pattern of psychiatric disorders. New infective agents were discovered including new strains of Salmonellae and a rabies-related virus. *Thermocyclops nigerianicus* was identified as a local vector of guinea worm, *Dracunculus medinensis.* Studies in Nigeria and Uganda showed the association between nephrotic syndrome in childhood with quartan malaria infection.[12] Unusual syndromes were discovered, including the first recognition of rhinophycomycosis due to *Entomophthora coronata.*[13] Clinical and pathologic descriptions of Buruli ulcer owing to *Mycobacterium ulcerans* and African histoplasmosis due to *Histoplasmosis duboisii* were contributed by staff at Makerere and Ibadan.[14] Many of the ancient myths were exploded. A clearer picture of the pattern of health and disease in Africa has emerged from the accumulation of results of these studies.

Pregnancy and its management presented a number of important challenges. Severe anemia of pregnancy in Ibadan was associated with malaria and folate deficiency. Critically ill patients in late pregnancy with hemoglobin levels below 6 grams per 100 ml blood (some levels were below 3 grams!) presented difficult therapeutic problems. Because blood transfusion tended to precipitate heart failure, these severely anemic patients were treated with exchange blood transfusion. Guided by studies on blood volumes, Ibadan obstetricians showed that good results can be achieved by transfusing packed red cells and concomitantly administering ethacrynic acid, a rapidly acting diuretic.[15] Pre-eclamptic toxemia presented unusual clinical features in the Nigerian. The course can be relatively rapid and episodes occur in patients with only modest elevation of blood pressure.[16] Hemoglobinopathy increases the risks associated with pregnancy; these problems were studied and some guidelines for the management of these cases were developed.

In Uganda, Dr. Denis Burkitt drew attention to the lymphoma that bears his name. Studies on this tumor both at Makerere and at Ibadan advanced knowledge on its clinical and epidemiologic features. Clinicians in Ibadan also contributed new information about the diagnosis and management of malignant trophoblastic disease.

These selected examples illustrate the range of research that staff of African medical schools have undertaken in the post-independence era.

Capacity Building

The post-independence era has been characterized by expansion of training opportunities for national scientists. In Nigeria, university enrollment expanded from 5,000 to 150,000 within 25 years of independence. Through national programs and with support from foreign philanthropic foundations and multilateral agencies, national scientists have been trained in a variety of disciplines. For example, the Rockefeller Foundation and the Wellcome Trust have supported the development of indigenous research capabilities through training programs and through support of research in local institutions. The World Health Organization, through both regular and special programs, has trained national scientists and strengthened local institutions. The explosive growth of indigenous expertise has been recently dampened by economic recession in African countries. Many of the newly developed institutions are now struggling to maintain the gains they made in the immediate post-independence period. Some institutions have been severely crippled by a shortage of funds which has affected their ability to subscribe to scientific journals and to buy books and equipment.

International Collaboration

After independence, a mixed pattern of international collaboration has emerged. It includes more traditional patterns, in which expatriate scientists on short or long-term visits have operated with little involvement of national scientists. Other programs have positively involved national institutions. Some innovative programs have involved African scientists and institutions in collaborative research programs. In this way, scientists and institutions in developed countries are sharing skills and expertise with colleagues in African countries.

The post-independence period coincided with a major revolution in the biological sciences. This has given rise to the exciting prospect of using the tools of modern biomedical sciences, such as immunology, molecular biology, biochemistry and genetics, to fashion new drugs, vaccines, and diagnostic tests for the control of malaria, leprosy, schistosomiasis, and other tropical parasitic and infectious diseases.

This revolution has attracted the interest of a new breed of research scientists, chiefly from developed countries, who are basic medical scientists rather than traditional experts in tropical medicine. Their efforts have within the past few decades produced spectacular results and have expanded and deepened our knowledge of tropical parasites and their relationship to the human and other hosts. Even at this early stage, a few new products have become available for disease control and several more are in the pipeline. However, a realistic assessment of the situation indicates that many of these promises will not be fulfilled in the near future. Although antigens have been identified, genes cloned, and biologically active peptides synthesized, a lot more work must be done before these new findings can be converted into protective vaccines. Overoptimistic claims and expectations can lead to frustration and disillusionment. No doubt, these hopes will eventually be fulfilled and efforts must be intensified to accelerate progress.

THE FUTURE

Where do we go from here? How can we best realize the promise of basic biomedical research and translate the results into powerful, effective tools in the control of diseases in Africa? How can we reconcile national and global priorities? Several models have been prescribed:

(1) *North/South Division of Labor.* In this simple model, institutions in developed countries will use their expertise and high technology to develop new products. The role of African scientists and institutions will be to prepare field sites for testing these new products. Such division of labor seems logical at first sight, but would be counterproductive if it becomes established as a permanent goal.

(2) *International Research Institutes.* Another proposal is to develop international centers, on the model of agricultural research institutes, which will assemble a critical mass of investigators to tackle malaria and other tropical diseases. Although this approach was apparently valuable in promoting agriculture in other parts of the world, it has so far had little beneficial effect on African agriculture; this approach could fail even more disastrously in the field of health care.

(3) *National Capability-Strengthening.* The first two models have attractive features, but will not meet the needs of the situation in Africa. Ideally, scientific discoveries should be developed into usable tools and integrated into national programs for disease control. We need to develop a satisfactory model which will facilitate the transition from scientific discovery through development and evaluation of new technologies to their application in national programs for disease control:

Discovery → Development → Deployment

It would be inappropriate to relegate African institutions to a permanent status of field laboratories for use of scientists from developed countries. It is certainly important to have good facilities for testing new drugs, vaccines, and diagnostic tests, but these studies should be carried out in a wider context of peer-level collaboration. African scientists can and must contribute to all stages of the discovery and development of new tools. Their involvement is particularly important in drawing up the specifications of the new tools, optimizing the candidate products, and providing an appropriate interface between scientists and potential users of the products.

I would recommend a different basis for international collaboration for health research. In my view, the top priority for each African nation is to develop and strengthen its epidemiologic and operational research capability so as to be able to assess the major health problems and mobilize available technology to deal with them. Such capability is an absolute minimum and should form the foundation of development of national research programs in Africa. Some mechanism should be developed to combine expertise available in government and private institutions, at research institutes and at universities to create this critical mass for epidemiologic and operational research. The approach needs to be multidisciplinary, involving biologists, physicians, epidemiologists, social scientists, statisticians and other experts. This is the minimal requirement, even for the smallest or least developed countries in Africa.

All governments should recognize this need, which is made more urgent by the present economic crisis, which requires that health resources should be applied to deal with the most important problems and that services should be organized in the most cost-effective manner. Rather than cut spending on such research, African governments should be encouraged to increase their efforts in this area.

In addition, some African scientists and institutions have the capability to contribute to basic biomedical research. How can these capabilities be exploited, especially in the face of severe financial constraints? The best approach would be the sharing of resources among the African institutions and some division of labor. Rather than attempting to develop expertise in many subjects, each African country should selectively concentrate effort on a defined area, share its knowledge with neighboring states, and, in return, utilize their resources. Thus, there would be a network of research centers which will cover a broad range of subjects. There is already a framework for such rational division of labor. Some of the colonial institutes dealt with specific subjects such as African sleeping sickness, leprosy, and malaria. Southeast Asian countries have developed a good model, SEAMEO-TROPMED, which African countries should emulate.

CONCLUSIONS

African governments should restate their commitment to supporting health research, placing initial emphasis on epidemiology and operational research. African scientists and institutions should collaborate to maximize the effectiveness of national institutions in the context of regional needs. They should also work closely with scientists in developed countries, using mechanisms that will at the same time strengthen capabilities in African institutions with the aim of achieving increasing self-reliance.

REFERENCES

1. SCHRAM, R. 1967. The History of Nigerian Medical Services. University of Ibadan Press. Ibadan, Nigeria.
2. ODUNTAN, S. O. & O. AYENI. 1976. Correlates of low birth weights in two Nigerian communities. Trop. Geogr. Med. **28:** 220-223.
3. JANES, M. D. 1974. Physical growth of Nigerian Yoruba children. Trop. Geogr. Med. **26:** 389-398.
4. NYLANDER, P. P. S. 1969. The frequency of twinning in a rural community in Western Nigeria. Ann. Hum. Genet. (London) **33:** 41-44.
5. EDINGTON, G. M. 1963. The abnormal haemoglobins in West Africa Ghana Med. J. **2:** 83-87.
6. WILLIAMS. A. O. *et al.* 1970. Comparative autopsy studies on cerebral atherosclerosis in Nigerian and Senegal Negroes, American Negroes and Caucasians. Atherosclerosis **12:** 401-407.
7. WORLD HEALTH ORGANIZATION. 1965. Cardiomyopathies. Bull. WHO **33:** 257-264.
8. OLURIN, O. 1973. Causes of blindness in Nigeria—a study of 1,000 hospital patients. W. Afr. Med. J. **22:** 97-107.

9. Osuntokun, B. O. 1971. Epidemiology of tropical nutritional neuropathy Trans. Roy. Soc. Trop. Med. Hyg. **65:** 454-479.
10. Lucas, A. O. *et al.* 1969. The suppression of malarial parasitaemia by pyrimethamine in combination with dapsone or sulphormethoxine. Trans. Roy. Soc. Trop. Med. Hyg. **63:** 216-229.
11. Lucas, A. O. *et al.* 1969. Reversibility of the urological lesions of schistosomiasis in children after specific therapy. Ann. N. Y. Acad. Sci. **160:** 629-644.
12. Hendrickse, R. G. *et al.* 1972. Quartan malarial nephrotic syndrome: Collaborative clinicopathological study in Nigerian children. Lancet **i:** 1143-1148.
13. Martinson, F. D. 1963. Rhinophycomycosis J. Laryngol. **77:** 691-705.
14. Cockshott, W. P. & A. O. Lucas. 1964. Histoplasmosis duboisii Q. J. Med. **33:** 223-238.
15. Harrison, K. A. *et al.* 1971. Ethacrynic acid and direct packed blood-cell transfusion in treatment of severe anaemia in pregnancy. Lancet **i:** 11-14.
16. Lawson, J. 1961. Pre-eclampsia and eclampsia in Nigeria. Path. Microbiol. (Basel) **24:** 478-483.
17. Bruce-Chwatt, L. J. & J. M. Bruce-Chwatt. 1971. Malaria and yellow fever. *In* Health in Tropical Africa during the Colonial Period. E. E. Sabben-Clare, D. J. Bradley & K. Kirkwood, Eds. Clarendon Press. Oxford.

Perspectives on Research and Diseases of the Tropics: An Asian View

V. RAMALINGASWAMI

United Nations Children's Fund
New York, New York 10017

In Asia, we are dealing with a region in the developing world which is inhabited by more than 2.5 billion people—more than half of the total population of this planet of ours. In the world of geographical convention, we are used to a flat, distorted projection of our spherical planet, the so-called Mercator projection. Today's geographers depict the world as a global village and give for each country a size, not based on the number of square kilometers it occupies, but on one or another of its socio-economic variables. In such depictions, national boundaries and sizes will change and we get a view of the fate of our planet, impressionistic rather than statistic. I have selected five pictures of the world in this format (FIGS. 1-5) to convey a sense of Asian and global reality of health and disease. The countries are colored from light yellow, which depicts an advantageous situation, through yellow, orange, red, and finally to dark brown, which depicts the opposite—an extremely disadvantageous situation.[1]

ASIAN AND GLOBAL REALITY IN HEALTH AND DISEASE

FIGURE 1 shows the relative sizes of the countries according to the number of illiterate adults. Europe and most of the Americas appear almost nonexistent on this map, whereas Asia and Africa cover the canvas. The coloring scheme is based on the 1985 Gross National Product (GNP) in U.S. dollars, reflecting the amount of resources available at the national level. Countries with a small GNP are identified by dark colors, and those with a higher GNP by progressively lighter colors. The darkest color here represents less than U.S.$1,000 per capita per annum, and the lightest more than U.S.$10,000. The United Arab Emirates has the highest GNP per capita (U.S.$22,870). Kampuchea's GNP is U.S.$80. Seventy percent of the world's illiterate population, of which 60% are women, is in Asia.

FIGURE 2 shows the countries scaled in size according to their economic resources, while the color shading is based on mortality rates of children under five years of age. This picture looks the opposite of FIGURE 1. In terms of economic resources, North America, Europe, and Japan occupy a large part of our planet, whereas Africa and Asia are reduced to a small size. Africa is the size of Italy. In terms of child mortality, the darkest colors are in Africa and Asia, red and brown colors which

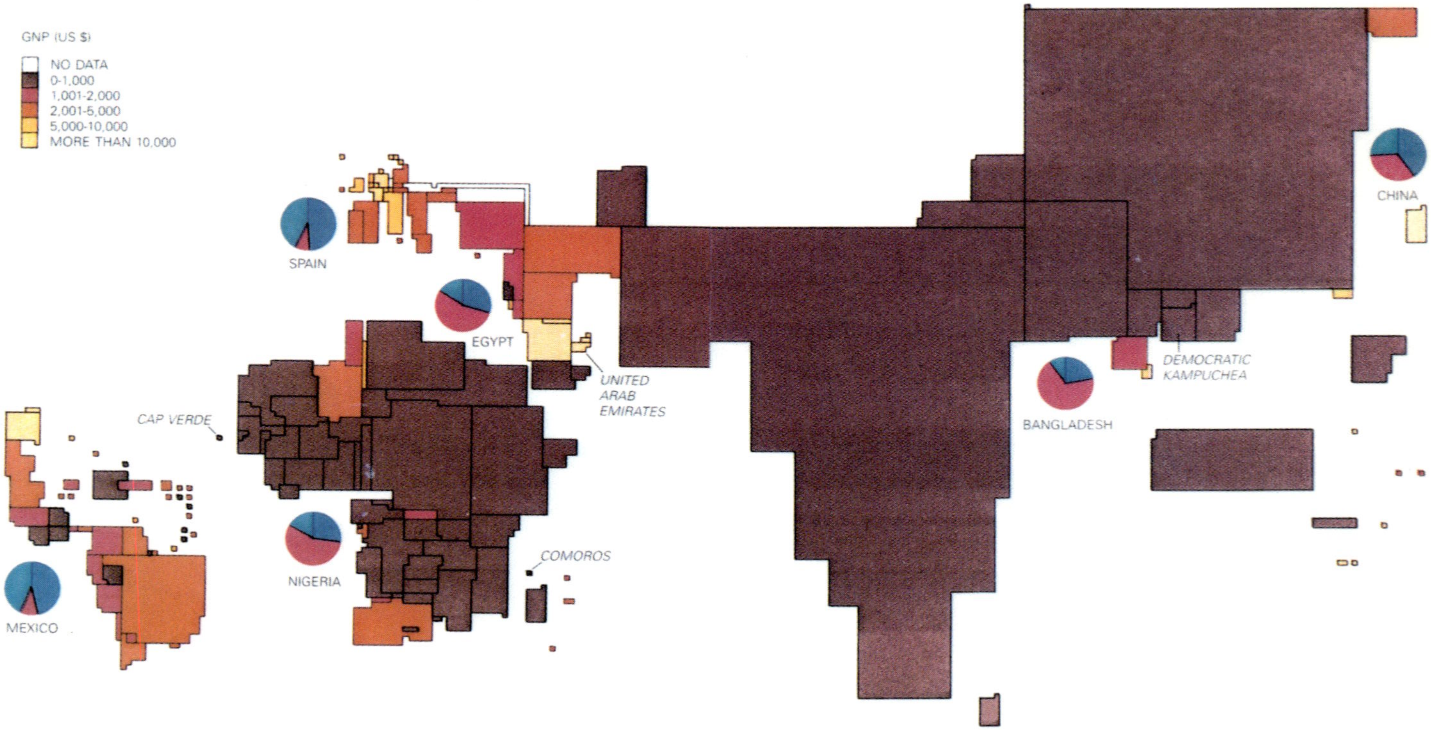

FIGURE 1. The relative sizes of the various countries shows the number of illiterate adults in the world; the colors indicate the amount of money available at the national level.

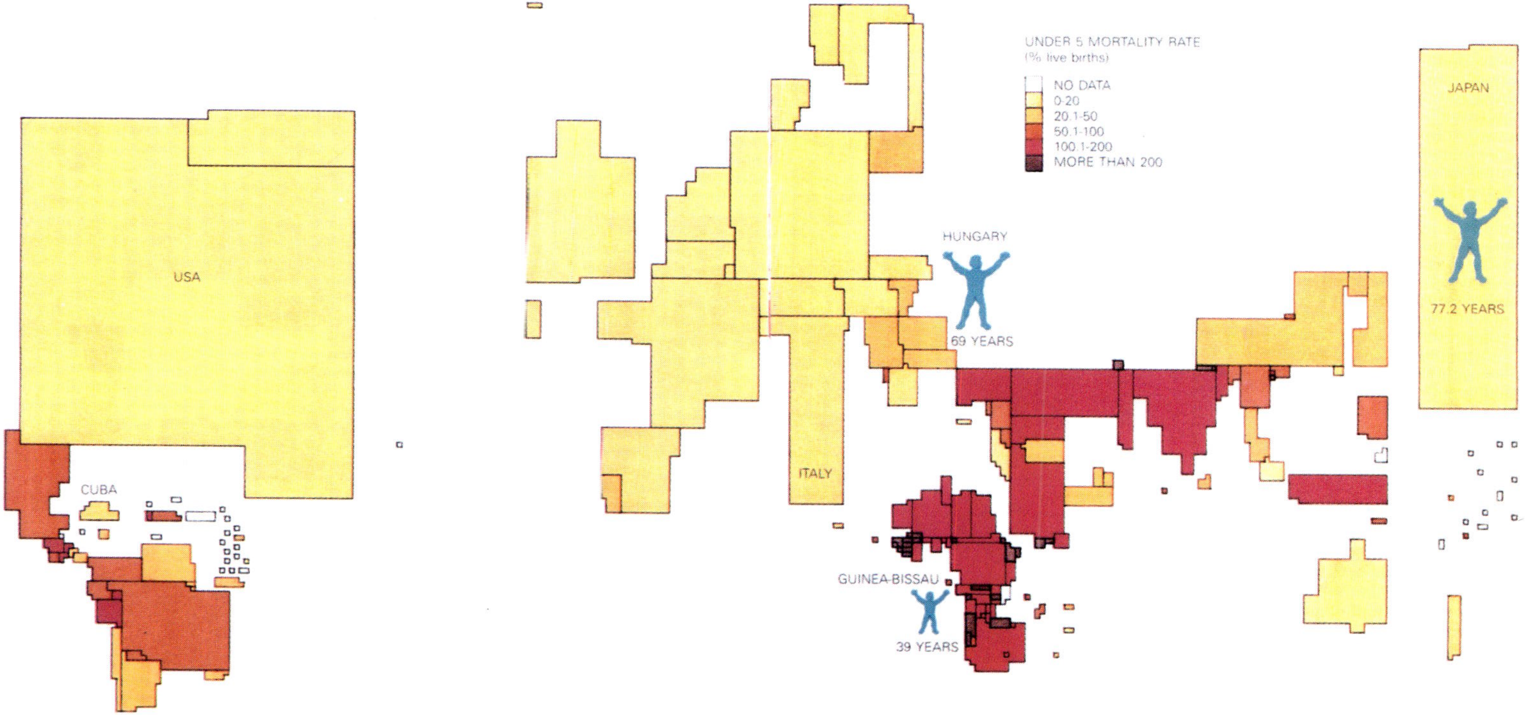

FIGURE 2. Relative economic sources are shown by the sizes of the countries; the colors indicate the mortality rate for children under five years of age.

represent more than 100 and 200 deaths in children under five years per thousand live births, respectively. The figure also shows the life expectancy of Japanese to be 77.2 years, of Hungarians 69.0, and of inhabitants of Guinea-Bissau 39.

FIGURE 3 shows countries scaled according to the number of infants born alive each year. Asia appears larger than its "true size" when compared with others using this criterion. The color indicates the percentage of low-birthweight infants using the cutoff point of 2.5 kilograms. Much of Asia and Africa are represented by the dark colors of red and brown, indicating that more than 20% and 30%, respectively, of live born babies in those areas have low birthweight. Whereas most low-birthweight babies in developed countries are pre-term, a larger proportion of low-birthweight babies in developing countries are full-term infants. Notice that the numbers of children born each year in the United States and Bangladesh are about the same; however, the incidence of low birthweight in the U.S. is 6.8% (yellow), while in Bangladesh it is the highest: 50% (dark brown). Birthweight is reckoned at the start of extrauterine life, so this is the bleak picture in Asia at the start of life. Eleven million low-birthweight babies are born each year in southern Asia alone with all the attendant risks of diminished survival in early infancy and childhood.

FIGURE 4 is sized to express the total population of children under the age of 5 in each country, giving an idea of the worldwide distribution of children in this age group. The colors reflect the prevalence of stunting (height for age) in children in the 1- to 2-year age group which is, in turn, an expression of chronic undernutrition. The countries with the largest surface area are the ones with the most intense colors. The dark-brown-colored countries show that the prevalence of stunting in this age group exceeds 30%, as measured by values below twice the standard deviation of the mean height for age of the reference standard.

FIGURE 5 is scaled to express the estimated number of episodes of diarrhea in children under five across the world. On this basis Europe appears merely as small squares. One episode a year in developed countries, four a year in developing countries, going as high as twelve in some developing countries, is the pattern of diarrhea in children across the world. The colors show the percentage of the population having access to safe water. As would be expected, countries with poor access to clean water are also those with a high incidence of diarrhea. In this figure blue water taps represent urban areas and green taps rural areas. There are two taps for each World Health Organization (WHO) region. The blue taps themselves are smaller for Africa and Asia, and the green taps, by their size, reflect the relative neglect of rural areas in the developing countries of Asia and Africa. This inequity applies even more pointedly to sanitation.

THE DIARRHEA-PNEUMONIA-MALNUTRITION-COMPLEX

Diarrhea, pneumonia, and malnutrition constitute a triad—against a backdrop of rapid population growth—accounting for the bulk of mortality and morbidity in young children in developing countries. All of these factors constitute a challenge to modern biology as well as to the social and behavioral sciences. A historical analysis of health development in the industrialized countries in the eighteenth and nineteenth centuries and continuing into the present reveals the crucial role played by infection control in their transition to healthful conditions. Improvement was first brought about by better nutrition, then by water and sanitation, food and personal hygiene, and joined later by immunization and specific therapies.[2] The Expanded Programme of Immunization

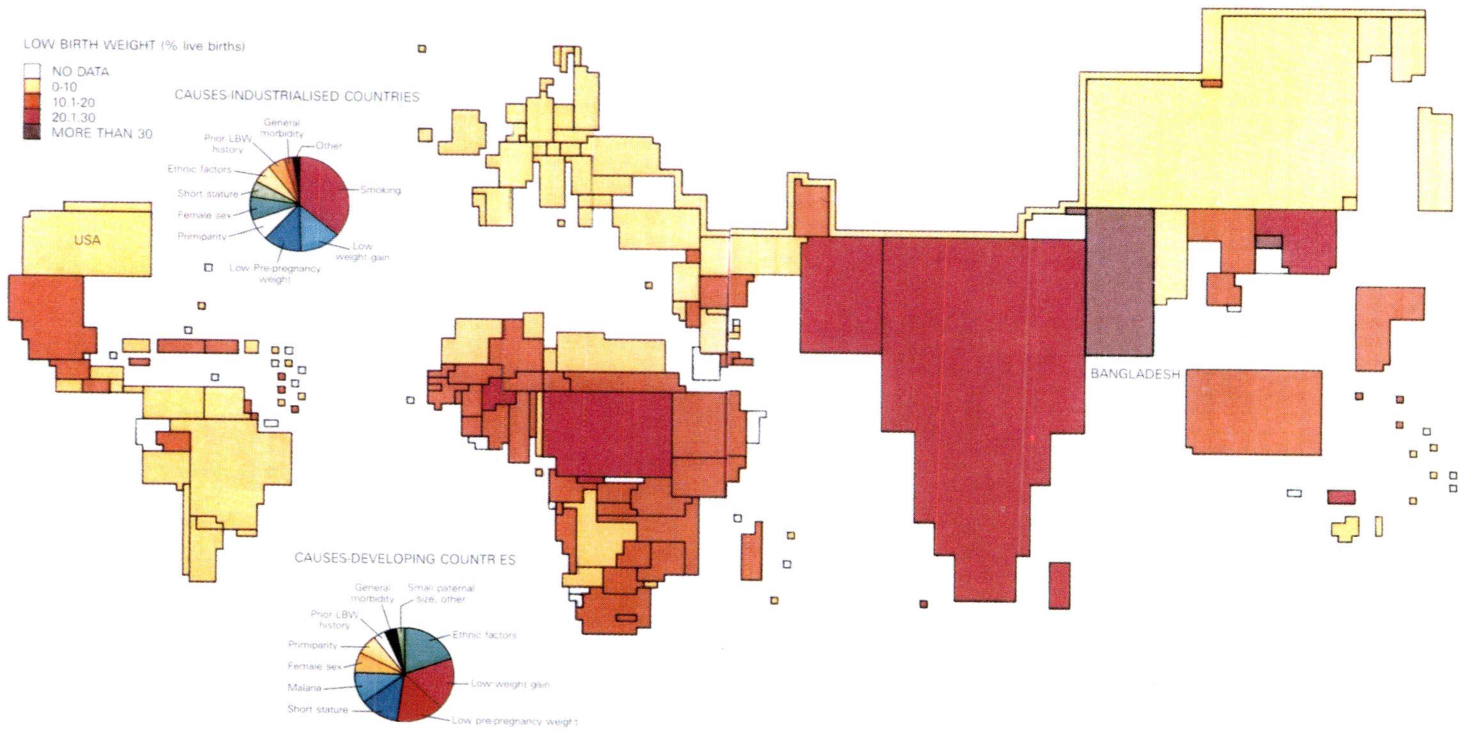

FIGURE 3. Countries are scaled in size according to the number of infants born each year; the colors indicate low birthweight as a percentage of live births.

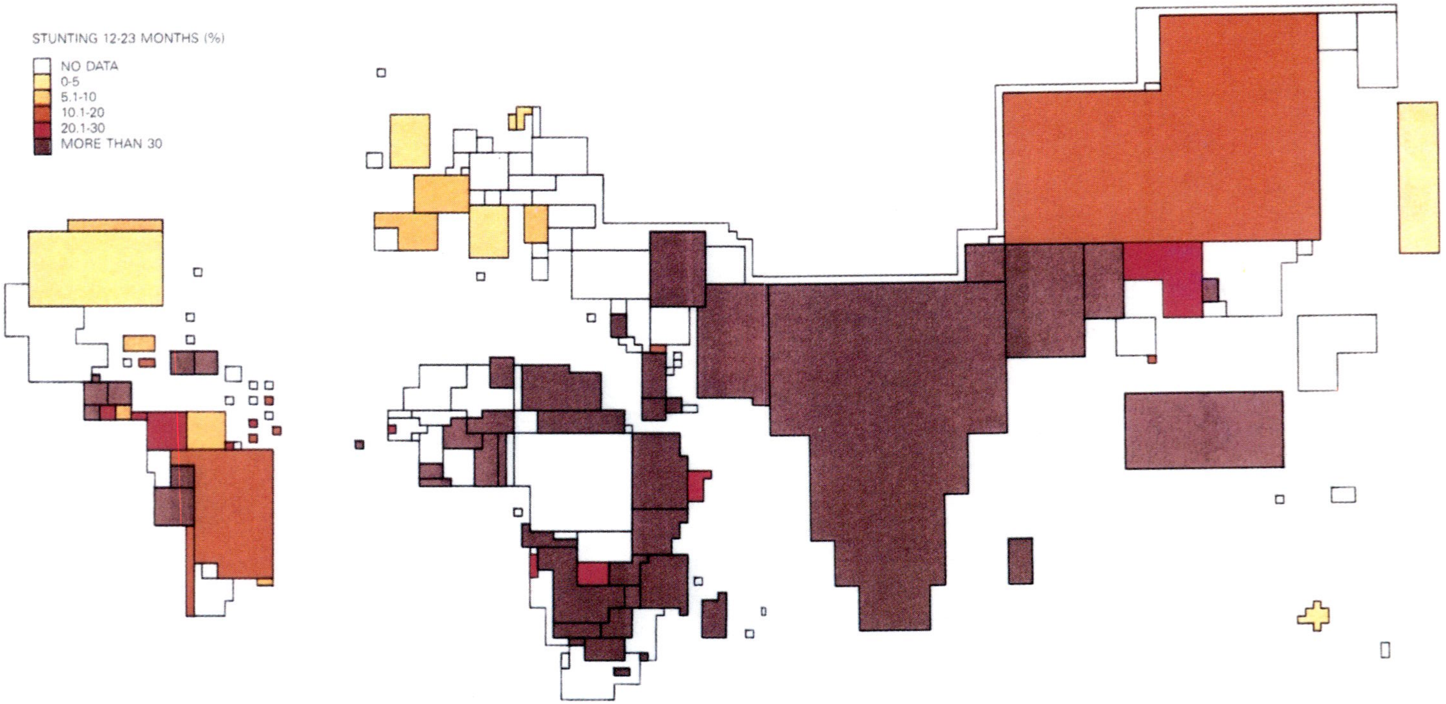

FIGURE 4. Countries are sized to show total population of children under the age of five; the colors show the prevalence of stunting.

(EPI), jointly sponsored by the WHO and UNICEF, is making progress now with more than 50% of children under the age of 1 year receiving vaccination against the six EPI-listed diseases. We envision eradicating poliomyelitis by 2000 A.D. so that a smallpox- and polio-free world could be the gift of the twentieth century to the twenty-first. Prospects of eradicating measles would be brightening as the new century approaches. Oral rehydration therapy along with increasing coverage with safe water supplies and sanitation is cutting down mortality from acute diarrheal diseases, although there is as yet no effective vaccine against any of the major intestinal pathogens to date that can be used in routine immunization. Oral vaccines that stimulate local secretory mucosal immunity are the need of the day. Cholera is still prevalent in Asia, although with rehydration therapy it has now lost much of its old ferocity. Just two months ago, in July-August 1988, an epidemic of cholera broke out in Delhi in India in which several hundreds died. The combined whole cell and toxin-B subunit oral vaccine against cholera currently being tried in Bangladesh[3] has shown a decrease in protection from around 75-80% at the end of six months to around 60% at the end of two years. It is not clear whether this vaccine will be able to provide effective protection over a period of time, but there is no doubt that it is effective in the short run, which itself is a distinct advance. A genetically engineered live oral cholera-typhoid vaccine based on TY21A is in a trial stage as is an oral attenuated antidysentery vaccine consisting of protective antigens of *Shigella* type 1 and other relevant *Shigella* types in the form of a multivalent "cocktail" vaccine. It is anticipated that vaccines against rota-viruses based on rhesus strains might come into control programs in another three years' time. The outlook against typhoid fever, which affects close to 8 million people in Asia, has improved, with the improved formulation of TY21A vaccine and with the new encouraging results obtained with the Vi polysaccharide capsular surface antigen in trials in Nepal.[4]

The importance of acute lower respiratory tract infections in childhood mortality is being increasingly realized. The control of these infections through chemotherapy and immunoprophylaxis within the primary care setting presents both a challenge and an opportunity to biomedical science. Encouraging trials with co-trimoxazole in cutting down child mortality due to these infections at the community level by paramedical personnel hold promise, but getting this technology into operation at the community level is yet to be fully accomplished. Capsular polysaccharide vaccines against pneumococci and *Haemophilus influenzae* type B offer promise of an immunoprophylactic attack on lethal respiratory infections during childhood.

One hundred and three years after the first vaccination against rabies, effective control of rabies in the world as a whole and in Asia in particular is not yet within our grasp. Many developing countries, including India, continue to use the old homogenized animal-brain vaccine, which carries the constant danger of neuroparalytic accidents. The human diploid cell and vero-cell-based vaccines are expensive for routine use in developing countries, and transfer of technology for local manufacture is only just beginning. Ninety-nine percent of rabies cases in humans in Asia are transmitted from rabies in dogs. Recent studies have shown that dog-removal programs are ineffective and expensive. The immunogenicity, safety, and protection rate of three oral antirabies vaccines and the efficacy of oral baits have been recently demonstrated. The social and ecologic factors influencing the size and structure of dog populations and their relationships to man need to be better understood.[5]

Of the insect-vector-borne diseases, malaria has seen, in many countries of Asia, both spectacular successes and equally spectacular resurgences. The waxing and waning promise of malaria control is a part of contemporary history. Chloroquine-resistant *Plasmodium falciparum* is a major problem in many countries of Asia, extending to involve sulfadoxine-pyrimethamine combinations as well. Recent field studies in Thai-

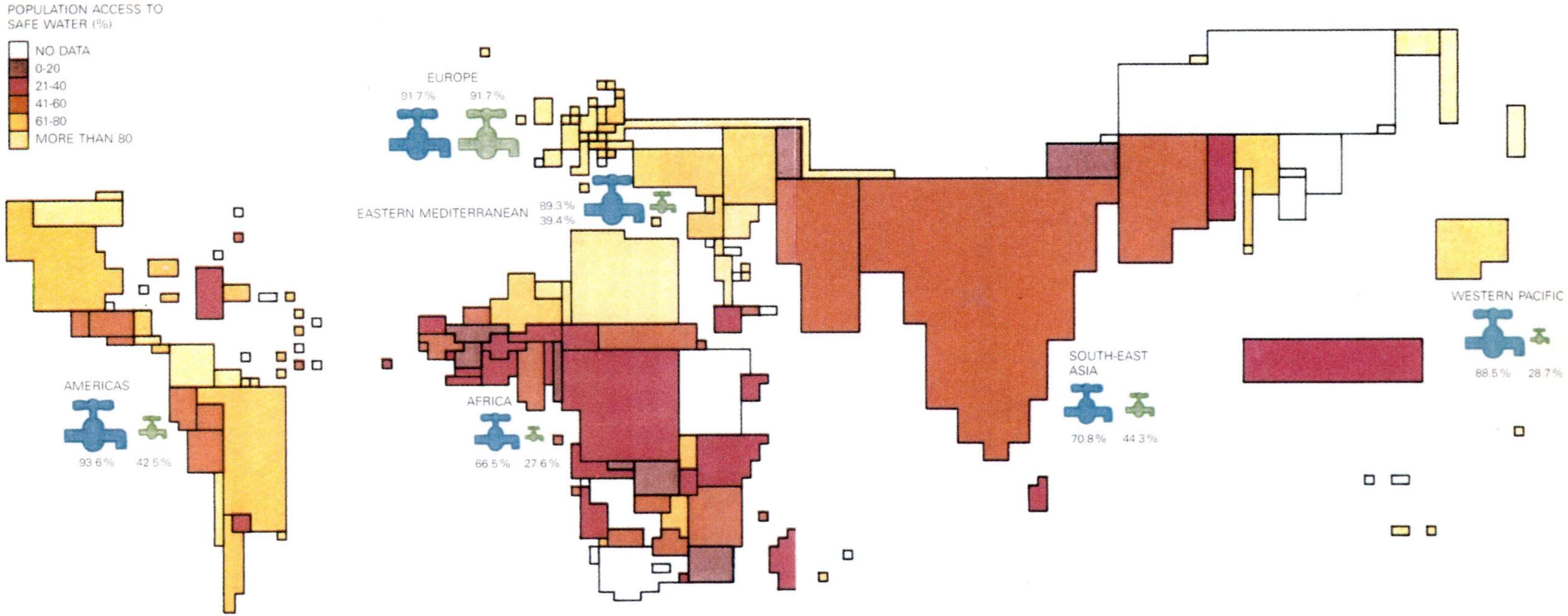

FIGURE 5. Countries are scaled to show estimated number of episodes of diarrhea in children under five; the colors show the percentage of population that has access to safe water.

land yielded excellent results with Mefloquine, although there are concerns about combining this drug with sulfadoxine and pyrimethamine.[6] Forty percent of the total health budget of the central government in India is taken up by malaria control programs. There are some who think we may one day win the war against malaria, but not against mosquitoes. I do not share this view. Despite spectacular advances in antimalarial vaccines, it would seem that at the present time vector control, assisted by chemotherapy, offers great hope. The integrated vector control strategies against malaria and filariasis in India (in Gujarat and Pondicherry) in recent years have been extraordinarily successful by virtue of efforts directed at questions of environmental improvement, source reduction, social aforestation, and use of larvivorous fishes and selective use of formulations of *Bacillus thuringiensis* H14 and *B. sphericus* against immature forms of mosquitoes.[7,8] The use of these microbial control agents has advantages and disadvantages. *B. thuringiensis* is effective against all species of *Aëdes, Anopheles, Culex* and to some extent *Mansonia* and of course against the vector species of *Simulium*. *B. sphericus* is effective against mosquitoes, especially *Culex*, but not against *Simulium*. The duration of effectiveness of these biological control agents in the biotype is an area of deep concern. Molecular biology offers possibilities of improvement in the larvicidal properties of *B. thuringiensis* and *B. sphericus* by enhancing the insecticidal proteins produced by these bacteria and by increasing their residual toxicity.[9]

Lymphatic filariasis is another disease spread by insects. It is expressed clinically as elephantiasis, which is endemic over wide areas in the developing world. About 905 million people are exposed to the risk of filarial infection and more than 90 million are believed to be infected. The Indian subcontinent constitutes a vast laboratory where lymphatic filariasis is well established and is spreading to fresh territories. Some of the advances made toward countering lymphatic filariasis under the WHO Tropical Diseases Research program include the development of a safe, highly effective microfilaricide (ivermectin), as well as vector diagnostic probes, the discovery of diethylcarbamazine's virtues in chemoprophylaxis and treatment, the use of immunodiagnostic tests to supplant night blood films, the development of animal models of lymphatic filariasis, and the recognition of *B. sphericus* as an excellent biological control agent for *Culex quinquefasciatus*. At the Madras Centre for clinical trials of lymphatic filariasis for Phase I, II and III, a single dose of ivermectin was shown to be microfilaricidal in lymphatic filariasis. And, while its adverse reactions are no different from those observed with diethylcarbamazine (DEC), ivermectin possesses a great advantage in that only a single dose is required as compared with the 12-day period of therapy needed with DEC. Ivermectin in a single dose as low as 25 μg/kg of bodyweight is effective. Clearly a new phase in the control of lymphatic filariasis is emerging.

Visceral leishmaniasis, kala-azar, virtually disappeared as a clinical entity from the Indian subcontinent as a side benefit from malaria control operations using residual indoor DDT spraying. For years I was unable to demonstrate *Leishmania donovani* bodies to medical students in bone marrow and splenic smears. But alas, with the return of malaria, kala-azar too came back in the form of explosive outbreaks from the mid-1970s onwards in the eastern states of Bihar, Bengal, and adjoining Assam in India. The fires of kala-azar have not yet been extinguished. Case fatality rates are high despite the fact that the vector, *Phlebotomus argentipes*, remains susceptible to DDT and the parasite also remains susceptible to antimonial agents, first discovered by Upendranath Brahmachari in Calcutta in the early 1920s. Serious deficiencies in our knowledge of the epidemiology of kala-azar and of sandfly biology are hindering the successful deployment of effective tools today. Allopurinol riboside, which blocks a biochemical pathway and leads to cessation of protein synthesis and death of the parasite, is an addition to the therapeutic armamentarium against kala-azar discovered under the tropical disease research program of the World Health Organization.

Leprosy and tuberculosis continue to be major health problems in Asia despite the availability of effective multiple drug therapies. Early case detection and problems in patients' compliance in protracted courses of therapy have remained as obstacles to progress, but of late, in the case of leprosy, the tide has turned. Astonishingly high compliance rates are being achieved, and practically no relapses have been reported to date.[11] It is to be hoped that the short-course chemotherapy for tuberculosis, again using multiple drug therapy, will bring about a similar transformation in the control of tuberculosis, which otherwise presents a picture of slow regression. Because of overconfidence in the multi-drug technology, interest in research in tuberculosis has diminished over the years. Now it is time to apply the new biology to develop rapid and early diagnostic tests, new vaccines, and drugs effective in the short run.[12]

In this rather cursory review of the Asian drama, I should not omit to mention two not so new problems that have emerged in Asia in recent years: Japanese B encephalitis and dengue fever. These diseases—which are causing much mortality and morbidity—pose a direct challenge to biomedical science. The status of Japanese B encephalitis has now changed from a sporadic endemic problem to one of major outbreaks that is possibly related to ecologic changes. There is no specific treatment for Japanese B encephalitis, the case fatality rate is high, and the affected countries are forced to manufacture the old mouse-brain vaccine. We hope to control the other phenomenon, epidemics of dengue hemorrhagic fever occurring in Southeast Asia, with a live attenuated polyvalent vaccine. This vaccine, which will protect against all four types of the dengue virus, is now being developed in Thailand. Both diseases are awaiting the use of molecular biological approaches to develop subunit vaccines which confer a high level of protection without pathogenicity.

Developments in molecular biology and immunology have led to visions of making immunizing agents against some of the common cancers of the tropics, such as hepatitis B and primary carcinoma of the liver, the human papilloma virus and cancer of the uterine cervix, the Epstein-Barr virus and Burkitt's lymphoma, and nasopharyngeal carcinoma. Two hundred and fifty thousand new cases of liver cancer arise each year, most of which occur in China, Southeast Asia, and Africa. Five hundred thousand new cases of cervical cancer occur each year, the bulk of them in the Third World. Fifty thousand new cases of nasopharyngeal carcinoma occur each year, mostly in southern China and Southeast Asia. Five to ten thousand fresh cases of Burkitt's lymphoma occur mainly in the malarial areas of Africa. There are providential gaps in cancer progression that can be exploited in cancer control programs. For example, there is a gap of two to three months from perinatal infection to persistence of hepatitis B virus infection in blood, providing an opportunity to use a vaccine to prevent the carrier state.

A new form of epidemic water-borne non-A, non-B hepatitis with a particular predilection for young adults is coming to light in many parts of the developing world—Asia, Africa, and possibly even Latin America. The disease is usually mild, except in pregnant women, who have a high fatality rate from fulminant hepatic failure.[13] There is as yet no vaccine against this disease.

CONCLUSION

The discovery of new tools to fight the persistent problems of the tropics is essential but not sufficient in itself to solve these problems. Having a tool, whether a vaccine or a drug, and having an effective control program are not one and the same thing. In addition to the technology, socioeconomic, cultural and behavioral factors must be studied and the knowledge so acquired utilized in program implementation. This indeed is the Achilles heel of the health problems in the Third World. Biomedicine's greatest challenge lies in prevention. This is what I suspect lies "under the volcano."

REFERENCES

1. WORLD HEALTH ORGANIZATION. 1988. A Health and Nutrition Atlas.: 2-31. WHO. Geneva.
2. ADVISORY COMMITTEE ON HEALTH RESEARCH. 1986. Health Research Strategy.: 1-89. World Health Organization. Geneva.
3. CLEMENS, J. D., J. R. HARRIS, M. R. KHAN, B. A. KAY, M. D. YURRUS, A. M. SVENNERHOLUR, D. A. SALK, J. CHAKRABORTY, B. F. STANTON, M. V. KHAN, W. ATKINSON & J. HOLMGREN. 1986. Field trial of oral cholera vaccines in Bangladesh. Lancet **ii:** 124-127.
4. ACHARYA, I. L., C. U. LOWE, R. THAPA, V. L. GURUBACHARYA, M. B. SHRESTHA, M. CADOZ, D. SCHULZ, J. ARMAN, D. A. BRYLA, B. TROLLFORS, T. CRAMTON, R. SCHNEFFERSON & J. B. ROBBINS. 1987. Prevention of typhoid fever in Nepal with Vi capsuler polysaccharide of Salmonella typhi. N. Engl. J. Med. **317:** 1101-1104.
5. Weekly Epidemiological Record. Aug. 19, 1988: 257-258.
6. PIMICHPONGSE, S. 1988. The operational introduction of Mefloquine, a new anti-malarial drug, by the Anti-Malaria Programme of Thailand. Presentation to the Scientific and Technical Advisory Committee of the Tropical Disease Research Programme of the World Health Organization. Geneva.
7. RAJAGOPALAN, P. K. & P. K. DOS. 1987. Project report on control of Bancroftian filariasis in Pondicherry urban agglomeration by controlling the vector *Culex quinquefasciatus* (1981-1985).: 164. Indian Council of Medical Research.
8. SHARMA, V. P. 1987. Bioenvironmental control of malaria in Nadiad, Kheda district, Gujarat. Ind. J. Malariology. **23**(2): 95-118.
9. WORLD HEALTH ORGANIZATION. 1987. Report of an Informal Consultation on the Role of Molecular Biology and Genetic Engineering in the biocontrol of Disease Vectors.: 15. WHO. Geneva.
10. KUMARASWAMI, V., E. A. OTTESEN, V. VIJAYASEKHARAN, S. UMA DEVI, M. SWAMINATHAN, M. A. AZIZ, G. R. SHARMA, R. PRABHAKARAN & S. P. TRIPATHY. 1988. Ivermectin for the treatment of *W. bancroft* filariasis. JAMA **259:** 3150-3153.
11. RAMALINGASWAMI, V. & R. H. PURCELL. 1988. Water-borne non-A non-B hepatitis. Lancet **i:** 571-573.

Biomedical Research in Latin America: Old and New Challenges

A. MARTÍNEZ-PALOMO[a] AND J. SEPÚLVEDA[b]

[a] *Center for Research and Advanced Studies,*
and
[b] *General Directorate of Epidemiology*
Ministry of Health
Mexico City, Mexico

A SOLID TRADITION IN BIOMEDICINE

Latin America has a long-standing tradition in biomedical research. Several of the most important tropical diseases prevalent in the region were discovered by local scientists. The best examples are the exceptional studies carried out at the turn of this century by Carlos Chagas[1] of Brazil, who discovered the parasite, the transmitter, and the disease that now bears his name, and by Rodolfo Robles[2,3] of Guatemala, who defined the principal characteristics of human onchocerciasis (among them blindness), when scientists in the developed world were of the opinion that this was merely a dermatological disease of little medical interest. Older landmarks include Daniel Carrion's experiment in Peru, which cost him his life, to elucidate bartonellosis,[4] and the fundamental contribution of Carlos Finlay of Cuba on the role of the mosquito in transmitting yellow fever.[5]

This solid tradition of excellence in tropical medicine research is still alive in Latin America. Recent examples include, among others, the malaria vaccine devised by Patarroyo's group in Colombia,[6] and the immunotherapy for leprosy and leishmaniasis described by Convit in Venezuela.[7]

In addition to tropical medicine, basic biomedical sciences have also held a prominent place in the history of Latin American science. The best known example is the Nobel prize-winning study of Bernardo Houssay in Argentina on the physiology of the pituitary.[8] These and other contributions have paved the road—still defective, but full of hopes—of Latin American biomedicine. However, we should note that these examples are a confirmation that scientific endeavor in Latin America still relies on exceptional individuals, rather than being an integral part of the society as a whole.

THE FALTERING SUPPORT OF SCIENCE IN LATIN AMERICA

Latin America includes 8% of the world's population and produces 5% of the gross global product. However, the relative percentage dedicated to research and development is disproportionately smaller: a mere 1.8%. At the beginning of this decade, the total number of scientists and engineers in the region was only 2.4% of the world's total. Furthermore, the average percentage of gross national products dedicated to research and development was less than 0.7%. In fact, in all Latin American countries during the present decade, these percentages have been under the minimum 1% recommended by UNESCO. The result is that the region has produced only 1.3% of the world's scientific publications.[9,10] In the words of the eminent physicist and Nobel Prize winner Abdus Salam: "We in the Third World are just not serious about science and technology".[11]

The percentage of research and development budgets devoted to health in the region shows, in turn, striking differences. For example, between 1980 and 1984, health only received 5.2% in Brazil, while it reached 22.5% in Venezuela.[10]

In spite of these limitations, significant efforts were carried out to strengthen science in Latin America during the early 1980s. This was rapidly reflected in a remarkable increase in productivity. A comparison of the total number of published scientific articles shows that Brazil, Argentina, Mexico, Venezuela, and Cuba roughly doubled their scientific output between 1976 and 1983.[10] More recently, however, in most Latin American countries, a deepening economic crisis, accentuated by a huge foreign debt, has slowed down this promising upward trend towards scientific advancement. Brazil may be the only country in the region that is advancing its scientific and technological infrastructure as an alternative to overcome that crisis.

OLD CHALLENGES: INTESTINAL AND RESPIRATORY INFECTIONS

The most recent indicators of mortality in the region were published in 1986 by the Pan American Health Organization in a monograph entitled *Health Conditions in the Americas, 1981-1984.*[12] In spite of the limitations of the data, it is clear that the overall mortality in Latin America is no longer dominated by infectious diseases. In part as a consequence of improvements in life expectancy, economic development, and control activities, infections have been replaced as the main cause of death by chronic degenerative diseases in the elderly, by violent deaths in children and young adults, and by adverse environmental and lifestyle effects.

Nevertheless, between 1981 and 1984, intestinal and respiratory infections were still among the five leading causes of death for all ages in ten of fifteen Latin American countries analyzed by the Pan American Health Organization.[12] When mortality in children between 1 to 4 years of age is taken into consideration as an accepted indicator of health conditions, gastrointestinal and acute respiratory infections continue to lead the list in Latin America.

Mortality from acute respiratory infections for all ages is higher in Central America than in any other part of the world, and for children below the age of 14 this rate is 10 to 15 times higher than in North America.[13]

The present economic recession may have a significantly negative impact on morbidity and mortality due to respiratory and diarrheal diseases, because the crisis strikes progressively harder at the poorest population groups, particularly the most vulnerable group of all, mothers and their young children. In Latin America, per capita incomes fell in 17 of 19 countries during 1983 and the gross national product as a whole dropped by more than 5%. Probably as a consequence, infant mortality is rising rapidly in the poorer states of Brazil, child malnutrition has increased steeply in the drought areas in Bolivia, and outbreaks of tuberculosis, malaria and other infections in Peru are increasingly common in children.[14]

Epidemiologic research, health services, behavioral investigations, and applied studies to establish and evaluate treatment norms for use in primary care settings are urgently required. However, basic biomedical research on the etiologic agents of those infections is also essential to improve diagnosis, treatment, and to evaluate perspectives of vaccine development. It has already been shown that morbidity and mortality from the diarrheal diseases may be reduced with appropriate technology produced by basic research. Therefore, solid scientific and technological efforts should be carried out in the region to reduce the burden of diarrheal and acute respiratory diseases. The relationship between these infections and malnutrition should also be further explored.[15]

MORE OLD CHALLENGES: TROPICAL DISEASES

Tropical diseases are still a major health problem in Latin America, as shown in TABLE 1, where recent estimates for eight important diseases are shown. These include seven parasitic diseases: malaria, schistosomiasis, invasive amebiasis, Chagas' diseases, onchocerciasis, leishmaniasis, and cysticercosis and one bacterial infection, leprosy. If we recall that most tropical diseases are more related to socioeconomic deprivation of the population rather than to the climatic environment, we can also include in this list another bacterial infection, tuberculosis, of which an estimated 230,000 new cases appear every year in Latin America.[12]

TABLE 1. Common Tropical Diseases in Latin America

Disease	No. of Cases	Reference
Chagas' disease	10-20,000,000	TDR, 1987[17]
Schistosomiasis	8-10,000,000	PAHO, 1986[12]
Amebiasis (invasive)	10,000,000	Walsh, 1988[18]
Malaria	4,500,000	PAHO, 1986[19]
Leprosy	400,000	OTA, 1985[20]
Cysticercosis	350,000	Schenone, 1982[21]
Onchocerciasis	105,000	PAHO, 1986[12]
Leishmaniasis	16,000	PAHO, 1986[12]

Malaria increased 30.5% between 1981 and 1984 in Latin America, as a complex series of problems that include vector resistance to insecticides, resistance of *Plasmodium falciparum* to chloroquine in some countries, migratory movements caused by local political conflicts, insufficient economic resources, and last, but not least, the weakening of the political and administrative structures overseeing malaria control campaigns. More information concerning the extent of schistosomiasis as a medical and social problem in Latin America is required, particularly because of the possibility of increased spreading of the infection upon completion of new irrigation projects and the construction of hydroelectric dams in South America.

Biomedical research on malaria and schistosomiasis in Latin America clearly needs strengthening; at present the number of productive research groups is too low in comparison to the importance of these infections.

In contrast to the paucity of recent investigations on malaria and schistosomiasis, research on Chagas' disease, amebiasis, cysticercosis, leprosy, and leishmaniasis has produced significant achievements that represent good examples of the high potential of biomedical research in Latin America. It is obviously too early for the products of this young science to have had a significant impact on the morbidity and mortality of the infections under study. We hope that this will be achieved in the near future, provided the pace is accelerated to obtain better diagnostic methods, more useful drugs, effective vaccines, and also to achieve a deeper insight into the mechanisms of disease.

Biomedical research in Latin America will have to continue addressing the problem of infections for many years. The reactivation of malaria, the reappearance of dengue, and the emergence of AIDS are clear warnings of the need to strengthen the regional capacity to analyze and to find new ways to control infectious diseases. As a local example, the annual patterns of incidence of dengue, malaria and AIDS in Mexico are shown in FIGURE 1.

NEW CHALLENGES: THE TRANSITION PROCESS

The promotion of better health in Latin America not only implies the continued fight against infections and malnutrition; the negative health effects of industrialization and urbanization must also be taken into consideration. This epidemiologic transition refers to complex long-term changes in the patterns of health and disease as communities transform their social, economic, and demographic structures. The process, taking place in many Latin American countries, is characterized by a decline in the incidence of infectious diseases and a rapid increase in the importance of chronic degenerative illness and accidents.[16]

As an example, FIGURE 2 illustrates the dramatic decrease of malaria, whooping cough, and dysentery as causes of death in Mexico over a period of 30 years. In contrast, the equally striking increase of ischemic heart disease, diabetes, and motor vehicle accidents for the same period and country is shown in FIGURE 3. A more thorough list, comparing the proportions of selected causes of death in Mexico in 1950 with those in 1984, is presented in FIGURE 4. The decreased proportion of infections, together with the increase in deaths attributed to cerebrovascular illness, accidents, liver cirrhosis, and diabetes represent a distinct example of epidemiologic transition. This is reflected in the five main causes of death for all ages in Mexico at present, which in order of magnitude are: (1) heart diseases, (2) accidents, (3) malignant neoplasms, (4) intestinal infections, and (5) respiratory infections (TABLE 2).

The epidemiologic transition may not follow the same pattern in developing countries as it does in developed nations. As Soberón *et al.* have stated,[16] a "protracted transition" may result in persistence of both infectious and chronic diseases, leading to an "epidemiologic polarization" whereby the better-off members of the society would have completed the transition, while the poorer groups would continue to suffer from the pretransitional pathology.[16] Latin America may be entering, thus, an era in which health problems will be characterized by the "worst of both worlds." A final consideration should be given to the unevenness of the transition process, not only

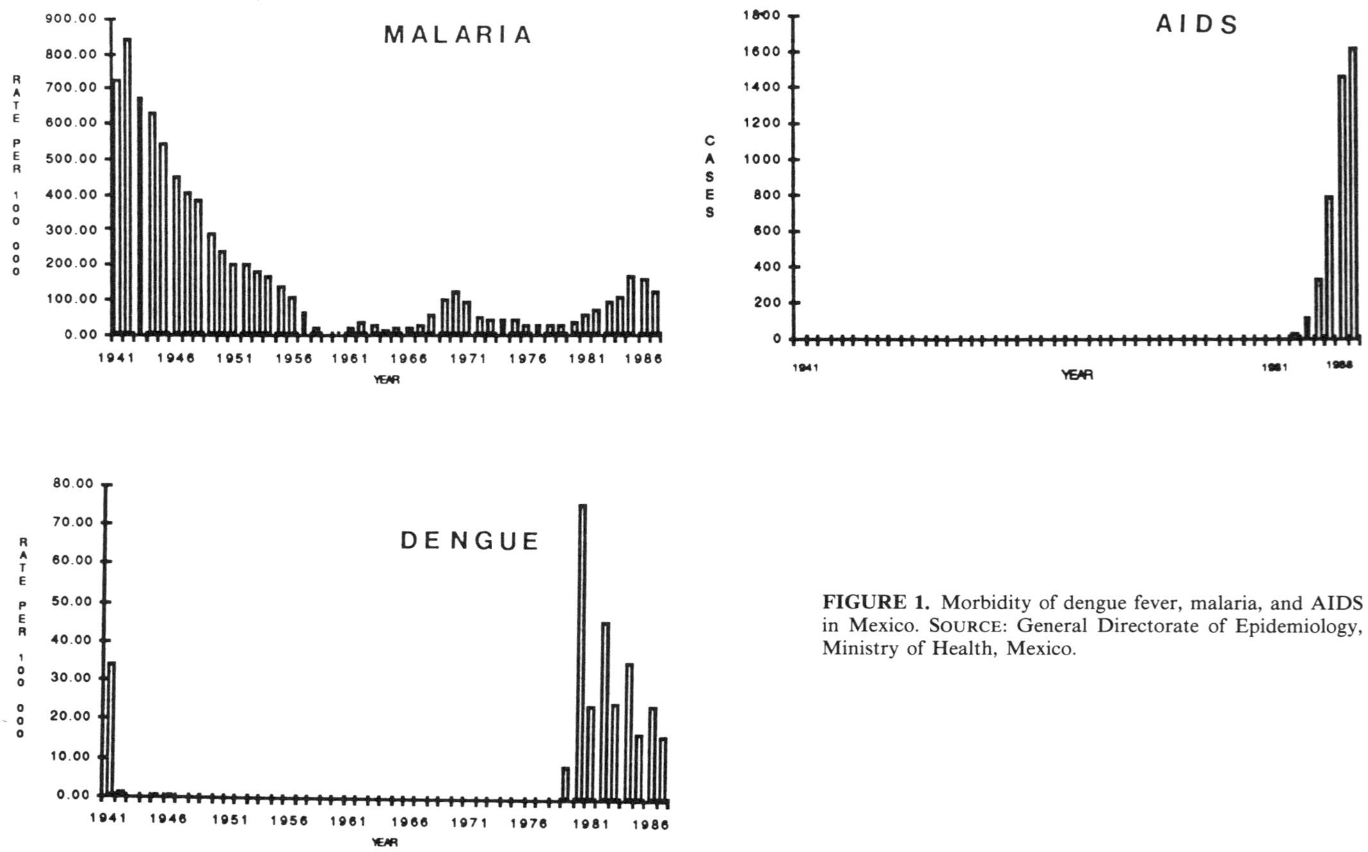

FIGURE 1. Morbidity of dengue fever, malaria, and AIDS in Mexico. SOURCE: General Directorate of Epidemiology, Ministry of Health, Mexico.

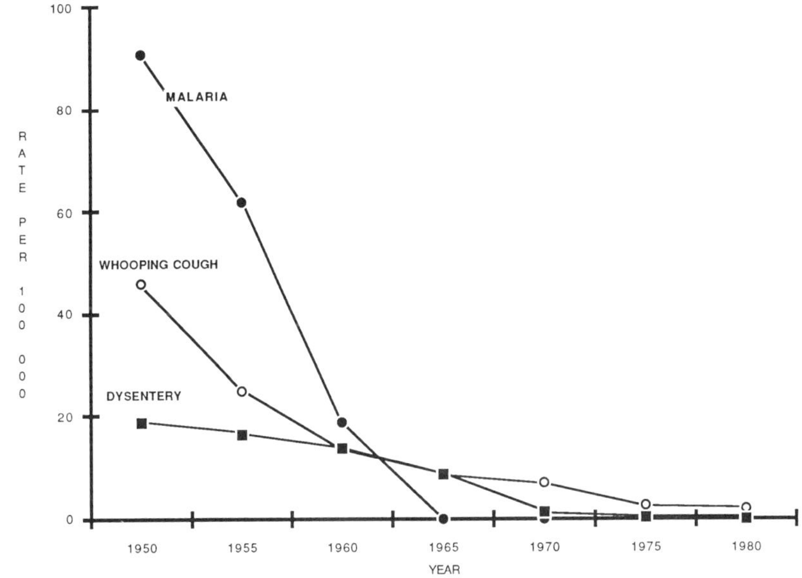

FIGURE 2. Main causes of death with a downward trend during the period 1950 to 1980 in Mexico. SOURCE: General Directorate of Epidemiology. Ministry of Health, Mexico.

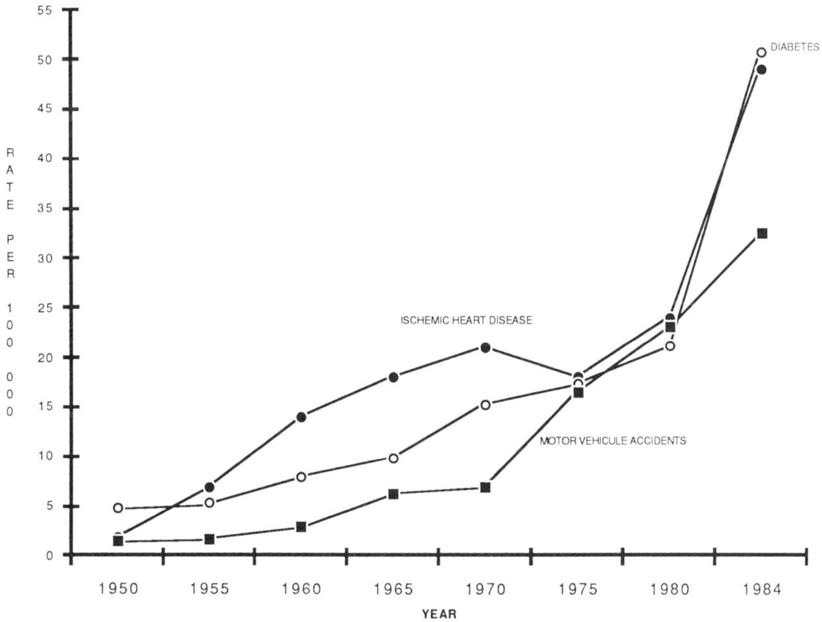

FIGURE 3. Main causes of death with an upwards trend during the period 1950 to 1984 in Mexico. SOURCE: General Directorate of Epidemiology. Ministry of Health, Mexico.

between countries in Latin America, but also within a given country. FIGURE 5 illustrates the pronounced regional differences in Mexico in mortality rates due to heart diseases—rates that are clearly related to socioeconomic inequalities.

RESEARCH PRIORITIES vs. RESEARCH AS A PRIORITY

Taking into account the aforementioned considerations, biomedical researchers in Latin America are confronted with a bewilderingly complex mosaic of health problems, with very few resources but very high expectations from the society that supports

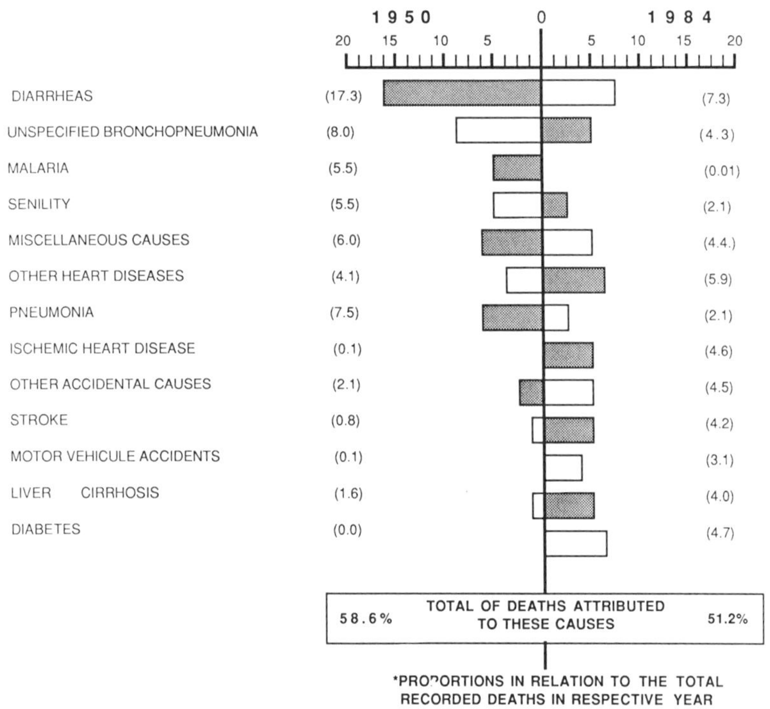

FIGURE 4. Comparison of the proportions of selected causes of death in Mexico in 1950 and in 1984. Figures refer to proportions in relation to the total recorded deaths in respective years. SOURCE: General Directorate of Epidemiology. Ministry of Health, Mexico.

them. When the slippery zone of priority-setting of biomedical investigations in Latin America is approached, the main priority has to be only this—scientific quality, relevance, and productivity. In addition, experience has demonstrated that multidisciplinary projects and those related to the most pressing health needs are more likely to get adequate support. The demands are obviously too vast for resources that are

TABLE 2. Five Main Causes of Death in Mexico in 1984 (All Ages)

Causes of Death	Deaths	Rate per 100,000
Heart diseases	51,328	67.2
Accidents	46,242	60.6
Malignant neoplasms	31,885	41.8
Intestinal infections	29,806	39.1
Influenza and pneumonia	27,249	35.7

SOURCE: General Directorate of Epidemiology, Ministry of Health, Mexico City, Mexico.

evidently too scarce. Regional cooperation in biomedical research barely exists in Latin America and should therefore be strongly supported by international agencies. Two important assets of the region favor an optimistic attitude: a common and rich cultural heritage and a tradition of high levels of excellence in medical practice and research.

It is clear, however, that the major responsibility of supporting biomedical investigations and improving health conditions lies with local government. There is an urgent need for a stronger political commitment to health research. Governments ought to start being serious about science and technology for health. Both in terms of the scarcity of human resources and the lack of economic support, the problem is more qualitative than quantitative in nature. The amount of money disbursed is less important than the knowledge of how to spend it well and distribute it wisely. Some governments spend valuable resources setting priorities for research without realizing that, in fact, research is not by itself an important priority. Thus, continued and solid policies in the area of social development that include science and technology as tools

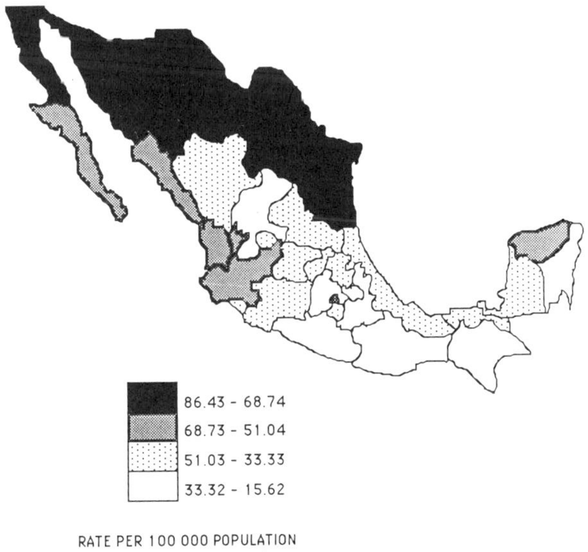

FIGURE 5. Mortality of heart diseases by state in Mexico for 1984. SOURCE: General Directorate of Epidemiology. Ministry of Health, Mexico.

of this development are also needed. In turn, scientists have to redouble their enthusiasm, knowledge, and activity.[22] Probably then, the balance of the future of Latin America will lean towards a positive outcome, helped by the amelioration of health conditions in the region.

REFERENCES

1. Chagas, C. 1909. New human trypanosomiasis. 1978. *Reprinted in* Tropical Medicine and Parasitology. Classic Investigations. B. H. Kean, K. E. Mott & A. J. Russell, Eds. Vol. **1:** 214-220. Cornell University Press. Ithaca, NY.
2. Figueroa Marroquín, H. 1963. Historia de la Enfermedad de Robles en América y de su descubrimiento en Guatemala. *In* Enfermedad de Robles.: 3-82. Editorial Universitaria. Guatemala.
3. Robles, R. 1917. A new disease in Guatemala 1963. *Reprinted in* Tropical Medicine and Parasitology. Classic Investigations. B. H. Kean, K. E. Mott & A. J. Russell, Eds. Vol. **2:** 446-450. Cornell University Press. Ithaca, NY.
4. Schultz, M. G. 1968. Daniel Carrion's experiment. N. Engl. J. Med. **278:** 1323-1325.
5. Rodríguez Espósito, C. 1951. Finlay. Librería Selecta. Havana, Cuba.
6. Patarroyo, M. E., R. Amador, P. Clavijo, A. Moreno, F. Guzmán, P. Romero, R. Tascon, A. Franco, L. A. Murillo, G. Pontón & G. Trujillo. 1988. A synthetic vaccine protects humans against challenge with asexual blood stages of *Plasmodium falciparum* malaria. Nature **332:** 158-161.
7. Convit, J., P. L. Castellanos, A. Rondón, M. E. Pinardi, M. Ulrich, M. Castes, B. Bloom & L. García. 1987. Immunotherapy versus chemotherapy in localised cutaneous leishmaniasis. Lancet **i:** 401-404.
8. Foglia, V. G. & V. Deulofeu. 1981. Bernardo A. Houssay. Su Vida y Su Obra. Academia Nacional de Ciencias Exactas, Físicas y Naturales. Buenos Aires, Argentina.
9. Sagasti, F. R. 1981. Ciencia, Tecnología y Desarrollo Latinoamericano. Fondo de Cultura Económica. Mexico City, Mexico.
10. Sagasti, F. R. & C. Cook. 1985. Tiempos Difíciles: Ciencia y Tecnología en America Latina Durante el Decenio de 1980. Lima, Peru.
11. Salam, A. 1988. Notes on Science Technology and Science Education in the Development of the South. Third World Academy of Sciences: 27. Trieste, Italy.
12. Pan American Health Organization. 1986. Health Conditions in the Americas: 1981-1984. PAHO Scientific Publication No. 500.
13. Pan American Health Organization. 1983. Acute Respiratory Infections in Children. RD/21/3.
14. United Nations Children's Fund. 1985. The State of the World's Children 1985: 18. Oxford University Press. Oxford, England.
15. Sepúlveda, J., W. Willett & A. Muñoz. 1988. Malnutrition and diarrhea. A longitudinal study among urban Mexican children. Am. J. Epidemiol. **12:** 365-376.
16. Soberón, G., J. Frenk & J. Sepúlveda. 1986. The health care reform in Mexico: Before and after the 1985 earthquakes. Am. J. Pub. Health **76:** 673-680.
17. World Health Organization. 1987. Tropical Disease Research: A Global Partnership. World Health Organization. Geneva.
18. Walsh, J. 1988. Prevalence of *Entamoeba histolytica* infection. *In* Amebiasis. Human Infection by *Entamoeba histolytica.* J. R. Ravdin, Ed.: 93-105. Wiley. New York.
19. Organización Panamericana de la Salud. 1986. Biotecnología: su importancia potencial para la salud en América Latina y el Caribe. Bol. Epidemiol. **7:** 10-12.
20. Office of Technology Assessment. 1985. Status of Biomedical Research and Related Technology for Tropical Diseases.:82. Washington, DC.
21. Schenone, H., F. Villarroel, A. Rojas & R. Ramírez. 1982. *In* Cysticercosis: Present State of Knowledge and Perspectives. A. Flisser, K. Willms, J. P. Laclette, C. Larralde, C. Ridaura & F. Beltrán, Eds.: 25-38. Academic Press. New York.
22. Martínez-Palomo, A. 1987. Science for the Third World: An inside view. Perspect. Biol. Med. **30:** 546-557.

World Health Organization Expanded Programme on Immunization: Progress and Evaluation Report[a]

R. H. HENDERSON

Director, Expanded Programme on Immunization
World Health Organization
1211 Geneva 27, Switzerland

INTRODUCTION

During the past 15 years a public health revolution has quietly taken place. Immunization services, which were virtually nonexistent in developing countries in 1974, now administer the single dose of measles vaccine to half the children of the world (generally by early in their second year of life), the third dose of polio or DPT vaccines to more than 60% of children reaching their first birthday, and BCG vaccination to more than 60% (TABLE 1 and FIGS. 1 and 2). The Expanded Programme on Immunization (EPI) thus now prevents some 1.9 million deaths from measles, pertussis and neonatal tetanus and some 240,000 cases of poliomyelitis annually (TABLE 2).

Yet the daily tragedy of vaccine-preventable death and disability continues. Each year nearly three million children die, more than 200,000 are paralyzed and some 150,000 are blinded by these diseases (TABLE 3). Immunization levels must be raised

[a] EDITOR'S NOTE: Although the next two papers in this volume were not presented at the conference we believe them to be of sufficient interest to warrant inclusion in this book. They are published with the permission of the World Health Organization and are only slightly modified from their original form. The reports began with the following note:

Following consideration by the Executive Board of the World Health Organization at its eighty-third session in January 1989, this report, which complements the information provided to the Thirty-ninth World Health Assembly (Document WHA39/1986/REC/1, Annex 8), has been brought up to date for presentation to the Forty-second World Health Assembly. The Programme's Global Advisory Group reviewed the report in its original form in October 1988 and recommended endorsement of the activities proposed for the 1990s, including the Plan of Action for Global Eradication of Poliomyelitis by the Year 2000 [the subsequent paper in this volume. **Ed.**].

Tables showing immunization coverage and estimates of prevented and actual mortality and morbidity are included herein.

A resolution recommended for consideration by the Health Assembly forms part of resolution EB83.R2 adopted by the Board at its January session.

[b] See document WHA41/1988/REC/1, Annex 6.

to at least 80% for all children of the world by 1990 and at least 90%—in the context of comprehensive maternal and child health services—by the year 2000. This will require continued efforts, particularly in sustaining resources and in improving the management of immunization services.

The Expanded Programme on Immunization (EPI), like the global smallpox eradication program before it, provides a compelling demonstration of what can be accomplished when there is unity of purpose. Few believed when the EPI was created that the 1990 goal was anything but wishful thinking. But now the dream is being realized. This is because public health and political and community leaders have combined their efforts to make this worldwide program succeed, and they have done so because it is inexpensive, easily implemented and easily understood, and because it brings immediate, evident benefits.

This progress and evaluation report reviews the EPI's experience to date, assesses the prospects for attaining its goal of providing immunization services for all children of the world by 1990, and presents new goals and challenges for the coming decade.

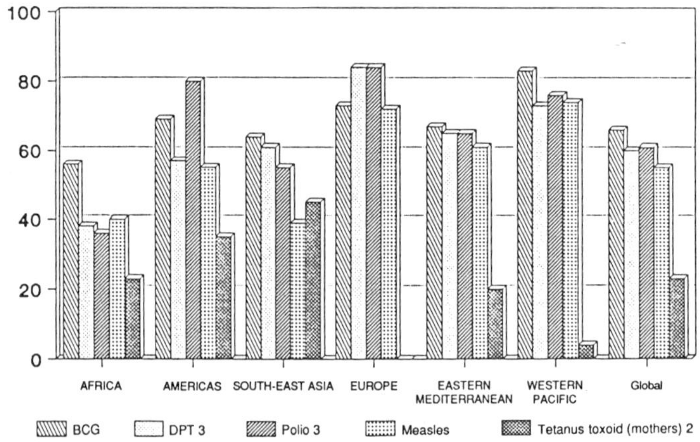

FIGURE 1. Estimated percentage of children immunized in the first year of life (BCG, DPT, polio, and measles [children up to 60 months of age] vaccines) and percentage of pregnant women immunized against tetanus (December 1988). *Horizontal axis:* WHO region; *vertical axis:* percentage of coverage.

Background

The Expanded Programme on Immunization has its basis in resolution WHA27.57, adopted by the World Health Assembly in May 1974. General program policies, including the EPI goal of providing immunization for all children of the world by 1990, were approved in resolution WHA30.53, adopted in May 1977. The importance of the EPI as an essential component of maternal and child health and primary health care was emphasized in resolution WHA31.53, adopted in May 1978, and in the Declaration of Alma-Ata in September 1978. In 1982, the Health Assembly warned

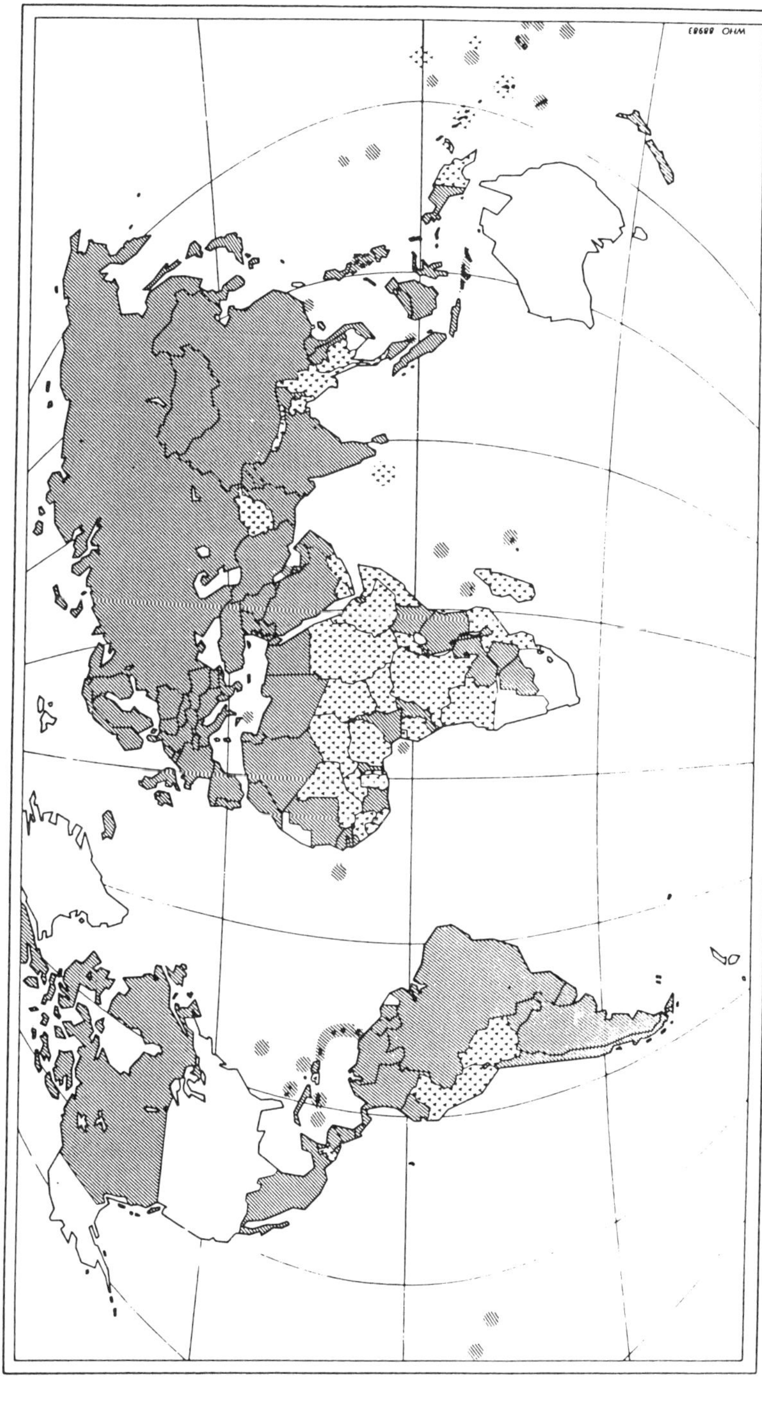

FIGURE 2. Countries/areas with immunization coverage above and below 50%: Third dose of polio or DPT vaccines for children reaching 12 months of age. Areas represented by crosshatching: 50% and over; areas represented by stippling: less than 50%; areas represented by white space, no information.

TABLE 1. Estimated Immunization Coverage with BCG, DPT, Polio, Measles, and Tetanus Vaccines (December 1988)

				Immunization Coverage (%)				
				Children Less than 1 Year of Age				Pregnant Women
	Country[a]	Newborns Surviving to 1 Year of Age (millions)	Cumulative Percentage of Infants (%)	BCG (%)	DPT 3 (%)	Polio 3 (%)	Measles[b] (%)	Tetanus 2 (%)
1.	India (*a*)	22.56	25	72	73	64	44	58
2.	Indonesia (*a*)	5.15	31	74	61	62	55	29
3.	Nigeria (*b,c*)	4.59	36	37	21	21	24	17
4.	Bangladesh (*b*)	4.15	40	14	9	8	6	7
5.	Brazil (*b*)	4.07	45	68	57	90	55	62
6.	Pakistan (*b*)	4.03	49	72	62	62	53	27
7.	Mexico (*b*)	2.68	52	71	62	97	54	42
8.	Ethiopia (*b,c*)	1.99	55	27	16	6	13	7
9.	Islamic Republic of Iran (*b*)	1.98	57	56	74	74	76	12
10.	Philippines (*b,c*)	1.83	59	92	73	73	68	49
11.	Viet Nam (*b*	1.78	61	68	61	75	60	*c*
12.	Egypt (*b*)	1.78	63	72	81	81	86	12
13.	Thailand (*b*)	1.44	64	61	48	47	34	38
14.	Turkey (*b*)	1.41	66	34	71	70	50	*c*
15.	Zaire (*b*)	1.29	67	54	36	36	39	25
16.	South Africa	1.28	69	*c*	*c*	*c*	*c*	*c*

TABLE 1.—*Continued*

17.	Burma (*b*)	1.17	70		45	23	13	14	24
18.	Kenya (*b,s*)	1.13	71		86	75	75	60	37
19.	United Republic of Tanzania (*b,d*)	1.07	73		94	81	65	88	54
20.	Republic of Korea (*b*)	0.95	74		95	85	93	95	[c]
21.	Sudan (*b*)	0.94	75		46	29	29	22	12
22.	Algeria (*b,s*)	0.90	76		95	66	66	59	[c]
23.	Colombia (*b*)	0.88	77		80	58	82	59	6
24.	Morocco (*b*)	0.85	78		87	78	78	76	33
25.	Argentina (*b,c*)	0.75	78		91	75	85	81	[c]
	Total 25 countries	70.63	78		63	58	58	46	35
	Other developing countries	19.46	22		61	48	48	46	25
	Subtotal, developing countries (excluding China)	90.09	100	82	63	55	56	46	33
	China (*b,s*)	19.94		18	85	75	77	77	[c]
	Total, developing countries (including China)	110.03		100	67	60	60	52	27
	Total, industrialized countries	18.11			59	66	68	76	[c]
	Global total	128.14			66	60	61	55	23

[a] Developing countries ranked by number of surviving infants: (*a*) = 1988 coverage data; (*b*) = 1987 coverage data; (*c*) = 1986 coverage data; (*d*) = 1985 coverage data; (*s*) = survey data.

[b] Children up to 60 months of age.

[c] No information available.

that progress would have to be accelerated to meet the 1990 goal and urged member states to take action on a five-point programme (resolution WHA35.31).

In 1986, the Health Assembly again warned that continuing acceleration of national programs would be needed to meet the goal and urged member states to pursue vigorously three general and four specific recommendations by the Director-General for action (resolution WHA39.30). In 1988, in light of the EPI's progress, the Health Assembly declared the commitment of the WHO to the global eradication of poliomyelitis by the year 2000, emphasizing that eradication should be pursued in ways that strengthen the development of the EPI as a whole, fostering its contribution in turn to the development of primary health care (resolution WHA41.28).

Programme Origins: Building the Coalition

Begun as a collectively sponsored WHO initiative, the EPI has now grown to be an operational program of member states working with a broad-based network of organizations of the United Nations system, multilateral and bilateral development agencies, and private and voluntary groups. The past years have seen the progressive formation of a global immunization coalition, uniting financial support and managerial expertise at international level to meet the needs of country programs.

Countries have strongly supported the EPI from the beginning. This has been reflected in resolutions adopted by World Health Assemblies over the past decade. More important, countries have taken action resulting in spectacular increases in immunization coverage in recent years.

International support has been essential for national progress and has grown at an increasing rate with the success of the Programme.

Some of this support has been used to finance, *inter alia,* vaccines, injection and sterilization equipment, cold-chain equipment and supplies, and, in some of the least-developed countries, subsidies for staff salaries and operating expenses.

A comprehensive list of all sources of external funding for the Programme would be long indeed; UNICEF is the major provider of vaccines, supplies and equipment. The majority of multilateral and bilateral development agencies and several other organizations of the United Nations system (including the World Bank and UNDP) support the Programme through contributions to WHO and UNICEF, through bilateral contributions specifically for EPI, or through cooperation in broader development initiatives.

A wide array of other private and voluntary groups (including the Rockefeller Foundation and the "Save the Children" Funds of the Netherlands, the United Kingdom of Great Britain and Northern Ireland and the United States of America) also support the Programme. Rotary International, through its "Polio Plus" initiative, has raised over 200 million US$ for EPI, mainly for the purchase of poliovirus vaccine. Even more important than the funds, however, is the impact which thousands of individual Rotarians are having through their personal commitment to the immunization cause, lobbying in industrialized countries for more resources for immunization and working with ministries of health in a number of developing countries to promote immunization.

Technical support from the international community has rivalled financial support in importance. In addition to providing international direction and coordination, WHO has served as the technical authority for EPI. It developed an operations manual and, from it, produced prototype training materials which have been intensively used in

TABLE 2. Estimated Annual Number (in thousands) of Prevented Neonatal Tetanus Deaths, Prevented Pertussis and Measles Cases and Deaths, and Prevented Poliomyelitis Cases in 25 Developing Countries, Excluding China (December 1988)

	Newborns[a]	Surviving Infants[b]	Prevented Neonatal Tetanus Deaths[c]	Prevented Pertussis Cases[d]	Prevented Pertussis Deaths[e]	Prevented Measles Cases[f]	Prevented Measles Deaths[g]	Prevented Poliomyelitis Cases[h]
Twenty-five largest developing countries	77,176	70,633	274	28,357	325	30,803	918	195
Other developing countries	21,464	19,558	51	6,594	75	8,546	256	45
Total, developing countries	98,640	90,191	325	34,950	400	39,349	1,174	239

[a] Based on 1987 estimated population and crude birth rates.

[b] Based on estimated number of newborns and infant mortality rate.

[c] Based on mortality estimates from surveys or reports, a vaccine efficacy of 0.95 and immunization coverage reported as of December 1988. Countries without data were arbitrarily placed in one of three neonatal tetanus mortality classes: 5, 10 or 15 per thousand live births.

[d] Based on an estimated incidence of 80% of newborns in the absence of an immunization program, a vaccine efficacy of 0.8 for three doses, and immunization coverage reported as of December 1988.

[e] Based on mortality estimates of one-third of measles deaths, a vaccine efficacy of 0.8 for three doses, and immunization coverage reported as of December 1988.

[f] Based on an incidence estimation of 100% surviving newborns in absence of an immunization program, a vaccine efficacy of 0.95, and immunization coverage reported as of December 1988.

[g] Based on arbitrary case fatality rates ranging from 2% to 4%, a vaccine efficacy of 0.95 and immunization coverage reported as of December 1988.

[h] Based on an estimated incidence of 5 per 1000 newborns in the absence of an immunization program, a vaccine efficacy of 0.95 and immunization coverage reported as of December 1988.

national programs and are revised and extended to cover other forms of primary health care intervention (e.g., in child spacing and vitamin A supplementation). WHO established the basic EPI information system, which permits global estimates of immunization coverage and disease incidence. WHO periodically issues technical papers and publishes approximately quarterly an "EPI Update," each issue of which summarizes technical information in a particular area.

WHO has been the leader in introducing improved methods and materials to maintain the "cold chain," the system required to keep vaccines potent in transport between the place of manufacture and the place of use, and in storage. The Organization has collaborated closely with UNICEF in these efforts. During the past decade, this partnership has resulted in a whole new generation of cold-chain equipment's becoming available which is specifically designed to meet the needs of immunization programs in developing countries.

UNICEF has also collaborated with WHO to strengthen national managerial capacities in immunization, particularly by supporting training activities and by reviewing national programs with WHO and other collaborators. WHO and UNICEF issue joint statements on technical issues pertaining to a number of primary health care interventions. Recent immunization statements include: "Planning Principles for Accelerated Immunization Activities" (1985), "Selection of Injection Equipment" (1986), "Immunization and AIDS" (1987), and "Vitamin A for Measles" (1987). During 1987 and 1988, UNICEF and WHO collaborated in producing material for briefing on accelerating and sustaining national immunization programs in developing countries, especially for their staff and national program managers.

UNICEF has been particularly effective in social mobilization and in eliciting increased financial support for the Programme. The annual publication of *The State of the World's Children* has brought to the attention of world leaders the problems afflicting children in developing countries and the impact that low-cost interventions—including immunization—can have in promoting child survival and development. UNICEF has helped to publicize the dramatic success of Colombia's national immunization days in 1984 and to spread the philosophy and techniques worldwide; national days have become an important element in recent program acceleration. In 1986, UNICEF initiated the pledge: "We the peoples . . . ," renewing commitment to the 1990 immunization goal and commemorating the fortieth anniversary of the United Nations (1986). The many signatures obtained from heads of state and other eminent persons attest to the renown and popularity of the program.

In 1984 WHO, UNICEF, the World Bank, UNDP and the Rockefeller Foundation together formed the Task Force for Child Survival. This followed a meeting on the global immunization initiative involving these agencies and leaders in the field of health and development at the Rockefeller facilities in Bellagio, Italy. Follow-up meetings have been held in 1985 in Cartagena, Colombia and in 1988 in Talloires, France, each devoted primarily to immunization, but laying increasing emphasis on other aspects of primary health care. The most recent meeting, entitled "Protecting the World's Children—An Agenda for the 1990s" resulted in the "Declaration of Talloires," which proposed a number of health and development targets, primarily relating to the health of women and children, for the coming decade.[b] These targets are reflected in the proposals being made for EPI to be discussed later in this paper.

Immunization is one of the essential elements of primary health care defined by the International Conference on Primary Health Care held in Alma-Ata (USSR) in 1978. EPI itself is a building-block for primary health care: immunization services, because of their basic simplicity, provide an excellent means for strengthening the health infrastructure to deliver other services at the same time so as to ensure maximum combined benefits for women and children. When children thrive, parents gain the

TABLE 3. Estimated Annual Number of Deaths (in Thousands) from Neonatal Tetanus, Measles and Pertussis, and Annual Number of Cases of Poliomyelitis in Developing Countries, Excluding China (December 1988)

	Deaths from Neonatal Tetanus[a]	Deaths from Measles[b]	Deaths from Pertussis[c]	Total Deaths	Cumulative Percentage of Total Deaths (%)	Poliomyelitis Cases[d]	Cumulative Percentage of Cases (%)
25 largest developing countries	590	1,263	402	2,256	79	159	75
Other developing countries	164	330	121	615	21	53	25
Total, developing countries	754	1,593	523	2,871	100	212	100

NOTE: Using the immunization coverage data in TABLE 1, the following assumptions were made:

[a] *Neonatal tetanus:* based on survey data or, in the absence of survey, extrapolated from countries with similar socioeconomic conditions.

[b] *Measles:* it is assumed that the vaccine efficacy is 95% and that all unimmunized children will contract measles. Coverage is assumed to be "zero" in countries for which data are not available.

[c] *Pertussis:* it is assumed that the vaccine efficacy is 80% and that 80% of unimmunized children will contact pertussis. Coverage is assumed to be "zero" in countries for which data are not available.

[d] *Poliomyelitis:* in view of the narrow limits of variation of results of poliomyelitis surveys, and in the absence of an immunization program, a fixed incidence rate of 5 cases per thousand newborns is used. A vaccine efficacy of 95% is assumed. Coverage is assumed to be "zero" in countries for which data are not available.

confidence to limit the number of births to the number of children they desire, and this, in turn, provides further health benefits for mother and child.

EPI has been working in close collaboration with the WHO Diarrheal Diseases Control Programme, integrating training materials for combined courses. The two programs have also developed, in collaboration with the WHO Division of Family Health, a teaching module on child-spacing suitable for inclusion in EPI and/or diarrheal disease control courses. During the past year, in collaboration with the Nutrition unit, EPI has worked to introduce vitamin A and iodine supplementation in immunization programs serving populations at risk from deficiencies in those substances. These activities ensure that EPI serves as a promoter of various interventions while convincing other programs of the priority of immunization.

The coalition that has resulted from these many activities reflects a remarkable consensus in a world where so many things go wrong: children *should be* immunized, children *can be* immunized, children *will be* immunized. But the task of the coalition is not yet finished, for universal childhood immunization has yet to be achieved.

PROGRESS AT THE REGIONAL LEVEL

All WHO regions have made substantial progress since the last report to the Executive Board in 1986. But now, as then, the rate of progress and the levels of immunization largely reflect underlying socioeconomic conditions. Europe and the Americas, the most economically advanced regions, continue to have the strongest immunization programs, while Africa, economically the poorest region, continues to have the largest proportion of infants below the 50% level of coverage for the EPI antigens (FIGS. 1 and 2).

The African Region

In the African Region, immunization coverage with the EPI antigens, with the exception of measles and BCG, lags behind that of other regions (FIGS. 1 and 2). As just noted this reflects its level of socioeconomic development and the level of development of the health infrastructure. Coverage has been increasingly rapid, however, partly as a result of initiatives taken during 1986, designated by the Regional Committee for Africa as "African Immunization Year." According to routine reports and national surveys on coverage, the majority of African countries have surpassed 50% coverage for several EPI antigens, but coverage remains low in some; coverage for a third dose of DPT vaccine is less than 20% in Angola, Chad, Equatorial Guinea, Ethiopia, Guinea, Guinea Bissau, Liberia, Mali, and Niger.

Most countries routinely employ a mixed strategy for vaccine delivery using fixed centers supplemented by scheduled "outreach" activities; less frequently, in more remote areas, mobile teams are employed. In addition, 41 (89%) of the 46 countries in the African region have accelerated their national immunization programs. Some have also embarked on urban immunization campaigns.

Social mobilization and community participation in EPI have been ensured by the involvement of political and religious leaders, and this seems to be particularly effective in the African setting. Rapid progress has been noted in the district health development approach being promoted by the Regional Office; 54% of the 3217 districts in the region now have district health development committees, plans of action and one or more primary health care program elements, often including EPI.

A number of different policies have been adopted by countries to encourage self-reliance in the delivery of immunization services: establishment of a special EPI budget, sharing EPI costs with nongovernmental organizations, and the promotion of community cost-recovery schemes, such as those described in the Bamako Initiative. However, some African countries still depend heavily on external financial support and are likely to require such support well into the future. For all countries, efficient management of scarce financial resources remains a priority.

Since 1979, an estimated 50,000 people in the African region have received EPI training. Many national programs have produced their own training manuals. In more than half of the countries EPI materials have been incorporated in the curricula of health training institutions.

Regional EPI activities were evaluated in 1982 to identify initial problems, in 1985 to define acceleration strategies, and in 1987 to elaborate measures for sustaining the program. Since 1977, a total of 88 national program evaluations and 721 immunization coverage surveys have been carried out.

Considerable efforts have been made to improve the collection and analysis of data for disease surveillance and on immunization coverage at local, national, and regional levels. Until recently there was no standard reporting procedure and the regional collection of national data and comparison was extremely difficult. In 1988, a standardized biannual reporting form, to include information on disease incidence as well as on immunization coverage and vaccine delivery, was approved by the Regional Directors of UNICEF and WHO. Each national EPI program manager will submit the same standardized report biannually to the ministry of health, the WHO representative and the UNICEF representative. A second achievement of 1988 was the establishment of an EPI computer information system at the Regional Office. The system is compatible with the headquarters system and it will be extended gradually to countries in the region.

Countries have been encouraged to formulate targets in terms of reduction in numbers of cases of diseases, and several countries with well-established national programs and more developed surveillance systems have begun to document such reductions.

A number of preparatory activities have been undertaken in the region for the eradication of poliomyelitis; the situation has been assessed in 20 countries; laboratory services have been reviewed in seven countries; a "round table" discussion was held from 8 to 10 August 1988 at the Regional Office to review available information and to determine priorities for poliomyelitis eradication. The recommendations of the "round table" were endorsed by the joint WHO/UNICEF Technical Group on Immunization, which met from 20 to 23 August 1988 in Nairobi. The Group agreed to serve as a review body to monitor progress and promote inter-agency cooperation in support of the poliomyelitis eradication initiative. If the momentum generated by African Immunization Year is sustained, the eradication of poliomyelitis in the region will be possible.

The thirty-eighth session of the Regional Committee, in September 1988, unanimously adopted a resolution on the elimination of neonatal tetanus from the region by 1995. In collaboration with the Canadian Public Health Association, the "Combating Childhood Communicable Diseases" and "Resources for Child Health" (REACH) projects (United States of America), and UNICEF, the Regional Office organized two workshops in which countries assessed strategies for neonatal tetanus control and drafted plans of action for its elimination. Technical assistance was also provided by the Organization for Coordination and Cooperation in the Control of

Major Endemic Diseases (OCCGE) and the Organization for Coordination in the Control of Endemic Diseases in Central Africa (OCEAC). Three more such workshops are planned during the coming months.

At its meeting in August 1988 the joint UNICEF/WHO Technical Group on Immunization reviewed the yellow fever situation in the region, including data from recent outbreaks in Nigeria and in Mali. The Group urged yellow-fever-endemic countries to consider incorporating yellow fever vaccine into their EPI schedules on a routine basis.

The Regional Office collaborates with EPI at WHO headquarters in coordinating studies for the "cold chain," trials of new vaccines and equipment, and operational studies such as "missed opportunity" surveys. The initiatives for poliomyelitis eradication and neonatal tetanus elimination are expected to lead to increased operational research in the region.

Region of the Americas

In the region of the Americas, EPI continues to make progress towards the 1990 targets of immunizing all children and eradicating the indigenous transmission of wild poliovirus from the Western Hemisphere.

Coordination among the agencies supporting the program in the Americas, namely PAHO, UNICEF, USAID, the Inter-American Development Bank, Rotary International and—since the end of 1987—the Canadian Public Health Association, has ensured smooth implementation of the program at regional and country levels. More than 90 million US$ have been committed for the period 1987-1991. Intensive national efforts in program planning and financial analysis produced work plans for the five-year period 1987-1991 for every country in the region. The work plans are now the framework for program implementation and inter-agency coordination in support of the country programs.

In general, the countries of the region are improving vaccination coverage as a result of EPI acceleration and the implementation of national vaccination days. In 1988, on the advice of the EPI Technical Advisory Group, the 14 countries in which poliomyelitis is endemic elected to conduct national immunization days at least twice a year. Each of the 14 countries (except Brazil) is including the other EPI antigens in the national days. National vaccination days should be considered a complement to and not a replacement for immunization services offered as part of the basic health services. Positive effects have been observed in several countries, where coverage for measles and DPT vaccines has increased and drop-out rates have declined.

Surveillance has evolved rapidly and many countries have improved the quality of their information systems. Focus on the district as the primary reporting unit has been an important step forward. Poliomyelitis is now reported weekly by district, including reports of no cases; those of the 14,636 districts at highest risk in the region are thus readily identified, so that resources may be mobilized to assist them.

Despite fuller reporting as a result of closer surveillance, the total number of confirmed cases of paralytic poliomyelitis reported decreased in 1987 (635 compared with 907 in 1986), and even further in the first 39 weeks of 1988 (306 cases compared with 464 cases in the first 39 weeks of 1986). The decline in measles and pertussis has continued since 1984, although the data must be interpreted cautiously since surveillance for these diseases is not as well developed as for poliomyelitis. However, the decline of cases in all the subregions is consistent with the respective increase in vaccination coverage.

The English-speaking countries of the Caribbean reported 9000 cases of measles in 1982 and only 1300 cases in 1987. In September 1988 the Ministries of Health of the English-speaking Carribean countries set a target for measles elimination from that subregion by 1995.

There are 1000-2500 cases of neonatal tetanus reported annually in the region (excluding Brazil). The district focus will allow neonatal tetanus control efforts to be directed to those districts reporting cases, while simultaneously strengthening surveillance.

The Southeast Asia Region

In the Southeast Asia Region, progress is being monitored through the regional computerized EPI information system, which collects information on reported numbers of cases and deaths from EPI target diseases; reported numbers of children immunized with BCG, DPT, oral poliovirus and measles vaccines; reported numbers of pregnant women or women of child-bearing age immunized with tetanus toxoid; results of immunization coverage surveys; EPI-related training activities; EPI funds; and population denominators. Further exchange of information occurs during yearly or biennial inter-country consultative meetings of EPI managers.

In national EPI program reviews, participants are strongly encouraged to identify program strengths and weaknesses, to recommend ways to improve performance, and to refine strategies for program acceleration. Most countries have held such reviews and are now beginning to conduct follow-up reviews, often combined with other primary health care programs such as those for diarrheal disease control. Increased emphasis is being placed on the assessment of immunization coverage in urban areas and on the development of specific plans for program acceleration in urban areas. Recent EPI reviews have looked specifically at coverage in Jakarta, Bangkok, and Rangoon City.

It is important to involve those providing curative facilities more in the implementation of EPI if opportunities for immunization are not to be missed. This has been emphasized by studies in six countries.

If personnel are inadequately trained in EPI activities the effects are felt at almost all levels. Management skills, including field supervision, particularly need strengthening. In order to improve performance in other primary health care activities, training in both management and technical aspects of EPI has been given high priority in the region.

Data from the EPI information system indicate that since 1985 there has been an increase in contributions from governments as well as from external resources. Available funds totalled 19 million US$ in 1985, 30 million US$ in 1986, and 60 million US$ in 1987. A breakdown of 1987 funds by source shows 34.5 million US$ from governments, 1.6 million US$ from WHO, 21 million US$ from UNICEF, 1.1 million US$ from the World Bank, 0.8 million US$ from bilateral agencies, and 1.3 million US$ from private agencies (Rotary International and others).

In the Democratic People's Republic of Korea, Mongolia, Sri Lanka and Thailand, an overall reduction in morbidity from some target diseases has already demonstrated the impact of EPI. Although measles morbidity is often a good indicator of program impact, measles immunization coverage in the region was so low until 1986 that morbidity has not yet been significantly affected by immunization.

The European Region

In the European Region, data from 29 member states presented at the national EPI program managers' meeting in Budapest in April 1988 showed large variations in the quality and efficiency of national immunization programs. Because of reported or suspected problems with the "cold chain," formal comprehensive evaluations of "cold chains" have been initiated in 14 countries.

For most of the target diseases, regional incidence decreased in 1987 compared with 1986: poliomyelitis declined by 6%, diphtheria by 9%, pertussis by 7%, tetanus (total) by 8%. But between 1986 and 1987 the regional incidence of measles increased by 6%.

Sixteen member states have already introduced or made plans to introduce measles, mumps and rubella (MMR) vaccine in their national programs. Procurement problems with rubella vaccine and/or mumps vaccine has made it difficult to implement MMR vaccination in some countries. Although it is too early to demonstrate an impact of this policy on the incidence of measles, mumps, and rubella in the region as a whole, reduction in the incidence of these diseases has been successfully demonstrated in Norway and Sweden.

Increased regional support is needed now and in the medium term to further strengthen national programs including: development of regional immunization policies; improvement of surveillance and information systems; training of national EPI managers; laboratory support; mobilization of public demand for immunization; program evaluation; and provision of expert advice, especially in emergency situations.

Such support will be particularly important in view of the plan of action for the eradication of poliomyelitis from the region by 1990. Immediate acceleration of national immunization programs will be necessary if this goal is to be achieved and will provide the opportunity simultaneously to increase immunization with all EPI antigens. Currently 15 member states with a total population of 94 million (11% of the regional population) are considered free from poliomyelitis caused by wild poliovirus. However, the recent outbreak of poliomyelitis in Israel shows that there is no room for complacency.

Eastern Mediterranean Region

In the Eastern Mediterranean Region coverage has increased over the past 12 months. Some countries continue to accelerate their EPI activities either through campaign approaches or by strengthening existing delivery services. In almost all countries, EPI has been integrated within primary health care. There is increasing evidence that immunization services are being offered in most health facilities, in both the private and public sectors.

Acceleration in the region has been achieved through better inter-sectoral collaboration and effective social mobilization. Commitments from political, religious and other leaders have been important. Public awareness has been increased, resulting in an enthusiastic reception of services offered. Improvements in immunization coverage suggest that a sustained increase of the order seen during the previous 12 months, if extended to areas or populations where basic services are still inadequate, could put the universal immunization of children by 1990 within reach in most countries of the region.

Political unrest, armed conflict, economic depression and lack of manpower have accounted for many of the problems in the five countries where progress was the slowest (Afghanistan, Democratic Yemen, Somalia, Sudan and Yemen). The Regional Office is giving them special attention. A special meeting was convened in Khartoum in February 1988, and necessary technical support has been made available to four of them through the reassignment of WHO staff members.

During the fifth inter-country meeting for EPI program managers in Cairo in July 1988, progress in the prevention of neonatal tetanus was discussed, problems were identified, and solutions were recommended. Participants confirmed that neonatal tetanus is still common in most countries of the region and that the magnitude of the problem is not sufficiently appreciated by those responsible for health planning and finance. It is estimated that 27,000 deaths from neonatal tetanus were prevented in the region in 1987; more than 100,000 deaths still occurred unnecessarily. All participants in the meeting reaffirmed their commitment to the elimination of neonatal tetanus.

In pursuit of resolution WHA41.28 of the World Health Assembly a draft plan for the eradication of poliomyelitis in the region has been prepared. The Regional Director has also established a Technical Advisory Group on this matter. Plans have been made to recruit a full-time medical officer at the Regional Office for poliomyelitis eradication. The Regional Committee at its most recent meeting in Geneva in October 1988 passed a resolution endorsing the regional plan for poliomyelitis eradication.

Western Pacific Region

In the Western Pacific Region, progress has been achieved in all countries during the past year. This is due at least in part to accelerated activities, particularly in China, Democratic Kampuchea, the Lao People's Democratic Republic, Papua New Guinea, the Philippines, and Viet Nam.

China has set a target of 85% coverage at provincial level by the end of 1988 and 85% coverage at district level by 1990. Immunization coverage surveys conducted in the first half of 1988 showed that 12 of 20 provinces surveyed had reached the target ahead of schedule.

In the Lao People's Democratic Republic the Government is strongly committed to achieving universal childhood immunization by 1990. While immunization coverage for the country as a whole remains low, it has improved in areas with access to immunization services as a result of social mobilization and health education. Following an intensive acceleration in the first half of 1988, coverage in the Vientiane Municipality rose to 77% for BCG, 70% for measles, 71% for a third dose of oral polio vaccine, and 62% for a second dose of tetanus toxoid.

Significant improvements have occurred in the Philippines, where the proportion of children fully immunized increased from 21% in 1985 to 62% in 1987. The Philippines EPI disease surveillance system also improved after its computerization and the adoption of standardized formats and schedules for reporting.

Most developing countries in the region receive the bulk of their vaccines from UNICEF. However, several countries are involved in vaccine production. China produces all the EPI vaccines, and UNICEF has provided substantial support to upgrade their quality. World Bank funds for the construction of new vaccine-manufacturing facilities are still under negotiation. Viet Nam is producing oral poliovirus vaccine, although it does not yet meet WHO standards. It also produces BCG and DPT vaccine, although not in adequate quantities. The Philippines is self-sufficient in the production of BCG and tetanus toxoid, both of which meet national quality-control standards that are similar to WHO standards.

The technology and equipment for large-scale production of hepatitis B vaccine have been successfully transferred through WHO collaboration from Japan to China. China produced more than 9 million doses of hepatitis B vaccine in 1986 and 17 million doses in 1987. Hepatitis B vaccine has been added to the EPI schedule for infants in highly endemic rural areas and big cities of China. WHO also collaborated with Fiji, Samoa, and Tonga to establish laboratory facilities to collect and concentrate plasma from high-titer carriers of hepatitis B antigen. The concentrated plasma has been processed into vaccine in Japan and returned to these countries for the immunization of infants in 1988-1989.

At its session in September 1988 the Regional Committee passed a resolution to eradicate poliomyelitis from the 35 countries or areas of the region, where incidence has been declining steadily over the past eight years. Seventeen have reported no cases of poliomyelitis for at least 13 years; an additional eight have reported no cases for at least four years; four have reported occasional imported or vaccine-associated cases. Notable decreases have been seen in China, Malaysia, the Philippines, and the Republic of Korea. With further acceleration of EPI activities the prospect remains high for dramatic decreases in poliomyelitis incidence and its eradication from the region by 1995.

REACHING 1990: THE REMAINING BARRIERS

The figures for coverage in 1987 at first seem daunting. How, by the end of this decade, can immunization levels which took almost 15 years to raise to the 50% mark be boosted to 80% or more? And the issue is not only 1990 and not only immunization. For immunization services must be sustained for the foreseeable future and they must be established in ways that strengthen other elements of primary health care.

The prospects are, in fact, encouraging. The coverage now being achieved rests on a health infrastructure that has been developed since the beginning of EPI. It was never envisaged that coverage would increase by equal stages each year. Rather, it was expected to remain at low levels for several years to be followed by rapid growth. This is in fact what has happened.

The program started by emphasizing training. This had two major objectives: (1) to permit the development of sound national plans which external donors could support; and (2) to provide a "critical mass" of competent immunization managers in each country. Those responsible for national programs were encouraged to begin operations in relatively limited geographic areas and to extend them in a phased manner, so that problems of logistics and training and supervision of peripheral staff could be recognized and solved in the initial areas and systems established or reinforced for effective expansion.

Only since the mid-1980s had the majority of developing countries a core immunization infrastructure in place that would permit national immunization coverage to be rapidly increased in a sustained manner. Now global emphasis is on acceleration of national programs.

The low levels of immunization coverage in Africa have been noted. But most unimmunized or partially immunized infants in the developing world are found not in Africa but in the largest countries: half are in India, China, Nigeria, Bangladesh, and Indonesia, and a third are in India alone (FIG. 3). This is good news because all of these five countries have a high commitment to universal childhood immunization and three of the five have strong existing health infrastructures which permit high coverage levels to be reached and sustained (Nigeria and Bangladesh less so). Despite continued efforts for acceleration they may not attain coverage levels of 80% or above until sometime in the next decade (although experience has shown that surprising progress is possible where political will is strong).

There are a limited number of countries in which immunization programs are still in their initial stages. Bangladesh and Ethiopia have coverage of less than 10% for a third dose of oral polio and DPT vaccines. Despite being considered large, they only have about 6.0% of the newborn infants in developing countries as a whole. Eight of the smaller countries which are included in section C of FIGURE 3 have similarly low coverage rates (Angola, Chad, Democratic Kampuchea, Democratic Yemen, Equatorial Guinea, Guinea, Mali and Niger). They account for 2.5% of all newborn infants in developing countries. While efforts to accelerate programs in these countries are urgently needed, they will not be major determinants of coverage rates in the developing world as a whole.

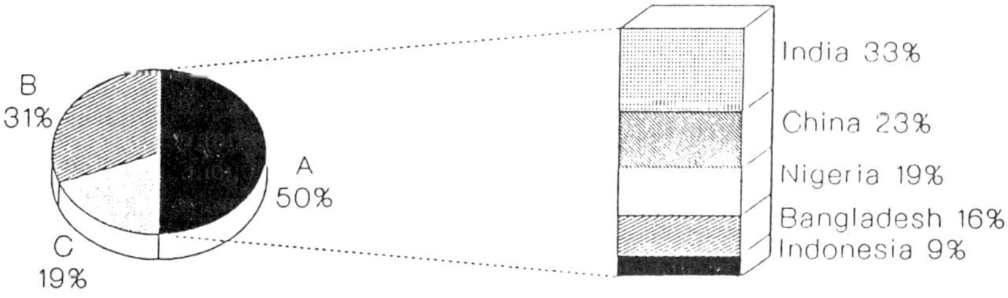

FIGURE 3. Proportion of infants not immunized or partially immunized (polio or DPT vaccines) in developing countries as reported in 1987. A = India, China, Nigeria, Bangladesh, Indonesia; B = 21 largest remaining developing countries (see TABLE 1); C = other developing countries.

FIGURE 4 provides estimates of what might be expected in developing countries by the end of 1990. It is based on the highest coverage for either a third dose of oral poliovirus or DPT vaccines reported as of December 1988, and projected (by subjective judgment) to the end of 1990, including coverage with measles vaccine and BCG in addition to poliovirus and DPT vaccines.

The projections are:

—an average *increase of some 20% in coverage in the five largest developing countries;*

—an *increase of some 15% in the twenty-one remaining largest countries* (listed in TABLE 1); and

—an *increase of 15% in the other developing countries.*

Thus, with vigorous efforts, a coverage of some 75% may be obtained by the end of 1990. Projections are always a risk. There are those who will consider them too optimistic, while others will expect even greater performance. In any case 80% coverage targets should be attempted since it sets the stage for the reduction, elimination and eradication proposed for the next decade. In almost all countries far more can be done to increase coverage immediately, using the health staff facilities that are already in place; many children who receive a first dose of vaccine are at present failing to return for subsequent doses. Coverage levels which reach 60% for a third dose of oral poliovirus or DPT vaccines indicate that some 80% of children have already had contacts with health workers for a first dose; with better health education and follow-up, supported by social mobilization, the majority of these children can be fully immunized.

Many opportunities for immunization are being missed. A particular problem is the failure to immunize eligible children who are brought to health facilities because of sickness. The Gambia demonstrates the importance of providing immunization as a part of curative care; most maternal and child health clinics there provide integrated curative and preventive care; 75% coverage for measles immunization is reported (one of the seven highest in Africa); of the children immunized against measles, 76% had been vaccinated during a visit for other treatment (not for well-child care), the most

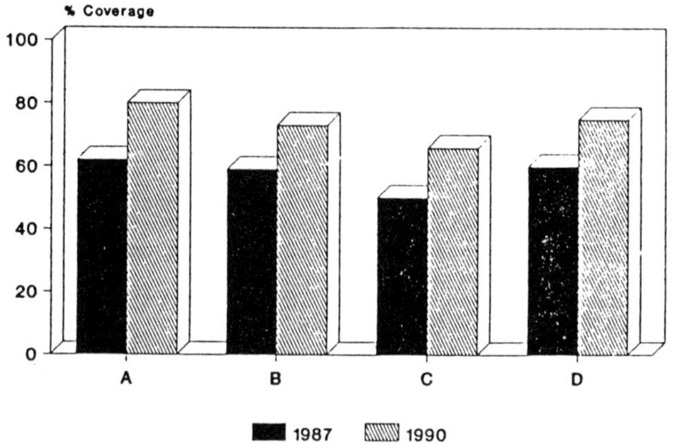

FIGURE 4. Highest coverage for third dose of polio or DPT vaccines in developing countries reported for 1987 and projected for 1990. A = India, China, Nigeria, Bangladesh, Indonesia; B = 21 largest remaining developing countries; C = other developing countries; D = total.

common reason (38%) for nonimmunization of those eligible being that the clinic attended did not immunize those attending for other treatment.

Measles immunization coverage in developing countries has in past years been substantially lower than that for a third dose of poliovirus or DPT vaccines, mainly because several of the large countries in Southeast Asia have only now begun to introduce the vaccine in routine programs (India, for example, while reporting 64% coverage for a third dose of oral polio vaccine, reported only 44% measles coverage in 1987). There should not be major difficulties in quickly raising measles coverage to levels comparable to those of the third dose of polio or DPT vaccines, although the fact that the vaccine should not generally be given before the age of nine months (to avoid interference from maternal antibodies) may place some extra demands on the health services to ensure that eligible children are not lost to follow-up.

Tetanus toxoid coverage for pregnant women is still lower: a mere 23%. The data are not as accurate as for the other EPI antigens, and actual rates of protection of pregnant women and their newborn infants from tetanus may be somewhat higher, as doses of toxoid received prior to the current or most recent pregnancy are often not counted in routine reporting systems or in immunization coverage surveys. Nevertheless, the coverage is almost certainly much lower than that for the other vaccines.

Although the use of every contact women have with the health services to administer tetanus toxoid to those of childbearing age will help to improve coverage, additional strategies, including special immunization campaigns in certain high-risk areas, will be needed before immunization rates become satisfactory. As noted earlier, several regions are now intensifying their activities to prevent neonatal tetanus.

While better immunization strategies are sought, however, the priority in most national programs is simply to improve the performance of existing staff and facilities. Within the health services this calls for intensified training with particular emphasis on assigning particular responsibility for each task essential for the program and providing supervision to ensure that it is carried out.

Community action is also needed. Members of the community can identify eligible children and direct them to immunization services. Members of the community can also exert the pressure required to make immunization services available at times and places convenient to the community and not only to the health worker. And an aroused community can exert the political pressure to ensure a comprehensive array of primary health care services, including immunization.

More spectacular forms of community mobilization may also be appropriate, as demonstrated by the striking success of national immunization days in a number of countries; for example, Colombia (see above). But care must be taken that acceleration efforts do not preclude sustainability, for unless they can strengthen the permanent health care delivery mechanisms they may actually hamper health services development.

Augmenting and sustaining immunization coverage implies for many developing countries augmenting and sustaining outside financial support. It would be a tragedy if the international community misunderstood the long-term investment needs of the immunization initiative. For immunization is a permanent service of the health care delivery infrastructure, and many developing countries will require continuing support well into the twenty-first century.

The outside support required is little enough; the costing studies done in the early 1980s still provide a reasonable guide, particularly if approximate estimates suffice. For the purposes of this report, the cost estimates have been further simplified (United States dollar at 1988 rates):

(1) At 10.00 US$ per fully immunized child, and assuming that 50 million children are immunized yearly with a third dose of oral polio or DPT vaccines, *the total cost will be 500 million US$ per year.*

(2) If external support covers 30% of total costs, *the external cost will be 150 million US$ a year.*

(3) If costs are doubled to account for full coverage, *the total cost will be 1,000 million US$ a year; the share to be borne by external support will be 300 million US$ a year.*

(4) If costs are doubled again to include new vaccines and population growth, *the total cost will be 2,000 million US$ a year; the share to be borne by external support will be 600 million US$ a year.*

Even taking 600 million US$ per year as a rather generous estimate of what might be required in outside support during the next decade, it remains tiny in the context of international development support (the estimate includes funds required for the poliomyelitis eradication initiative, currently estimated to cost some 155 million US$ for the period 1989-2000).

Optimism can be expressed about the continuing availability of outside support for EPI. At the first Bellagio meeting, in 1984, the international development agencies gave the assurance that if developing countries placed immunization high on their own national agendas, outside funds would not be lacking.

External funding for EPI has up to now largely kept pace with the needs. The poliomyelitis eradication initiative, however, has placed immediate demands on extrabudgetary resources, which need to be increased from their present level of some 5 million US$ to a level of some 15 million to 20 million US$ per year. In anticipation that these additional funds will be forthcoming, EPI has already begun to provide support for poliomyelitis eradication, taking the risk that should they not, WHO headquarter's support to regions and countries for routine EPI activities will be compromised.

TOWARDS THE YEAR 2000: ACTION NEEDED

Full Use of Existing Vaccines

The EPI is already preparing for the challenges of the 1990s: to raise immunization coverage rates where these are not yet satisfactory, and to sustain high coverage in countries where this has been achieved, in continuation of present Programme activities.

Disease Control

The primary objective of EPI is not immunization for its own sake, but rather the use of immunization for the control of the target diseases. EPI is already putting increased emphasis on disease control, and will make this an even higher priority during the 1990s; it is concentrating on poliomyelitis, measles and neonatal tetanus.

In May 1988 the Forty-first World Health Assembly committed the Organization to the *global eradication of poliomyelitis by the year 2000* (resolution WHA41.28). The Health Assembly noted that this initiative represented a fitting challenge on the Organization's fortieth anniversary, and an appropriate gift, together with the eradication of smallpox, from the twentieth to the twenty-first century. The Americas and the European and Western Pacific Regions helped to pave the way for this initiative by having already established regional eradication targets to be achieved by or before the year 2000.

A plan of action for the global eradication of poliomyelitis by the year 2000 was drafted in May 1988 (see the subsequent paper in this volume), based on the work and experiences in the Region of the Americas, and on discussions with national program managers in Europe during a meeting in Budapest in April 1988 (attended by the EPI Regional Adviser for the Americas). The initial plan has been revised and extended after a series of further discussions and consultations with national program managers, WHO staff, and outside experts. These have included:

☐ Discussions during meetings of national program managers and regional staff held in the African, Southeast Asian, Eastern Mediterranean, and Western Pacific Regions between May and August 1988;

☐ Discussions during a meeting of experts convened by the Regional Office for the Eastern Mediterranean on 18 and 19 July 1988, on poliomyelitis eradication in the region;

☐ Discussions among several divisions and units at WHO headquarters, including the Divisions of Communicable Diseases (and the Diarrheal Diseases Control Programme), Family Health, Health Manpower Development, Public Information and Education for Health, and Strengthening of Health Services, and the Biologicals and Rehabilitation units of the Division of Diagnostic, Therapeutic and Rehabilitative Technology, held in July and August 1988;

☐ Detailed review and discussion during an informal consultation of global poliomyelitis experts held in Geneva on 5 and 6 September 1988; and

☐ A further review by the EPI Global Advisory Group (attended by EPI advisers from all regions) during its meeting of 17-21 October 1988.

The Plan of Action is given as the subsequent paper in this volume. While the broad strategies outlined in the plan remained largely the same during the consultation process, many of the specific details have changed, and further change is seen as a natural consequence of further program evolution. This plan has already been used as a framework for developing eradication plans in the African, Southeast Asian, European, Eastern Mediterranean, and Western Pacific Regions.

The Plan of Action emphasizes the following strategies:

☐ Raising immunization coverage as quickly as possible with a protective course of administration of poliovirus vaccine and all other antigens included within national immunization programs to include at least 80% of infants by their first birthday, and throughout the age-group of 1-4 years, in each "district" (a geopolitical subdivision within a country whose population might range from a few hundred thousand to a few million), and to sustain those levels;

☐ Improving disease surveillance, including reporting by district, reporting of "zero cases," investigating outbreaks, and applying control measures;

☐ Strengthening laboratory capabilities for isolating and characterizing polioviruses, for vaccine quality control and for viral and serologic surveillance;

☐ Creating and maintaining public awareness in order to sustain political and financial commitment to poliomyelitis eradication;

☐ Providing information and education for parents and other community members in order to increase immunization coverage and to improve the detection of cases;

☐ Improving poliomyelitis rehabilitation services; and

☐ Promoting research so as to develop better eradication strategies, including improved poliovirus vaccines or combinations of vaccines.

As recommended in resolution WHA41.28, these strategies will be carried out in ways that strengthen EPI as a whole, fostering its contribution, in turn, to the development of primary health care.

The Health Assembly noted that poliomyelitis eradication will depend on the political will of countries and the investment of adequate human and financial resources in the program. The external resources called for in the Plan of Action amount to some 155 million US$ for the period 1989-2000, and some 17 million US$ for the period 1989-1990, over and above the resources required for full implementation of EPI. (The estimate for the overall cost of eradication may well be on the low side; between 155 and 500 million US$ is probably more realistic. For comparison, the cost of the smallpox eradication program is estimated to have been 300 million US$.)

As noted earlier, external resources for EPI are currently 150 million US$ per year and will need to rise to 300 million to 600 million US$ during the 1990s. Contributions to the Special Account for the Expanded Programme on Immunization forming part of the Voluntary Fund for Health Promotion will need to increase from their present level of some 5 million US$ per year to 15 million to 20 million US$ to support the poliomyelitis eradication initiative.

The difficulty of poliomyelitis eradication is not being underestimated. But poliomyelitis is only one of the EPI target diseases, and intensified action is also needed to control two other EPI target diseases which continue to threaten health: measles and neonatal tetanus.

Despite the success of EPI, *measles* continues to kill almost 1.6 million children each year (TABLE 3). Even with better coverage, measles cases that occur before the currently recommended age of immunization of 9 months, may continue to pose problems. Research is already under way to evaluate a strain of measles vaccine (the Edmonston-Zagreb strain) that may possibly be administered at 6 months. At the same time, immunization strategies are being examined with a view to bringing this highly infectious and highly lethal disease under better control with the vaccine strains now in widespread use. A target has been set for 1995 to reduce reported measles incidence in all countries to below 40 cases per 100,000 population, a reduction of over 90% from pre-program levels.

The drive to control *neonatal tetanus* provides a direct link between those concerned with immunization and those concerned with safe motherhood, for tetanus immunization and clean-delivery practices are both effective in preventing this disease. Neonatal tetanus still causes some 750,000 deaths per year, second only to measles among the EPI target diseases (TABLE 3). A target date of 1995 has been set for its elimination.

Introducing New or Improved Vaccines

One of the original goals of EPI was to put in place a delivery system in developing countries capable of using the new vaccines promised by current investments in research and development. Already, individual developing countries are adding, or are considering adding, vaccines such as yellow fever, hepatitis B and Japanese encephalitis B vaccines to their national programs. There are hopes that rotavirus vaccines and improved vaccines against typhoid, *Shigella* and cholera will become available during the coming decade. Leprosy vaccine is currently undergoing field trials, and research continues on vaccines against many other diseases.

The vaccines already being used in EPI are being improved. New manufacturing techniques have permitted the introduction of an improved inactivated poliovirus vaccine, and oral poliovirus vaccines which diminish the threat of paralysis and improve efficacy in tropical environments seem a possibility. A less reactogenic vaccine against pertussis is being evaluated. The work on the Edmonston-Zagreb strain of measles vaccine has already been mentioned. During the 1990s the EPI will continue to advocate the widespread application of vaccines of public health significance, and, through research and development, will collaborate with others to bring new or improved vaccines from the laboratory to broad application.

Promoting Other Primary Health Care Interventions

The EPI will increasingly promote other primary health care practices which are compatible with the EPI delivery system and target populations. The coverage being achieved by the Programme in infants in their first year of life and their mothers makes it imperative that EPI should promote the application of other practices (including those relating to improved maternal and child nutrition, diarrheal diseases control, appropriate birth spacing and, in selected populations, vitamin A and iodine supplementation) which can also contribute to their health.

Research and Development

Research and development will constitute a major priority for EPI in the 1990s. When the Programme was established, it was with the notion that the vaccines, supplies and equipment and knowledge about immunization were all already sufficient to make the Programme a success. The main emphasis was placed on the application of existing knowledge. Even so, research and development have been a part of EPI from the beginning. For it quickly became apparent that the material and methods that had served industrialized countries so well needed adaptation for application in developing countries. So equipment for the cold chain was improved, time/temperature monitors were introduced for vaccines, more efficient immunization schedules were proposed, and a more appropriate policy regarding contraindications to immunization was adopted.

The questions for research and development are multiplying, however, owing partly to the advent of new vaccines and new technologies, but partly to the advanced state of immunization programs in developing countries, which has revealed many limits to current knowledge about immunization. In particular, questions are being raised concerning approaches needed to assure optimal control of EPI target diseases (and in the case of poliomyelitis, eradication).

EPI took the first steps to strengthen its research and development capacity in 1987. At that time, funds for the purpose were solicited and received from the Rockefeller Foundation and from UNDP, and an EPI Research and Development Group was established to advise on priorities and monitor progress. The Netherlands added its support to these activities in 1988. EPI will focus on applied research (encompassing the broad areas of biotechnology and epidemiology), in contrast to and to complement more basic research under other WHO programs (including vaccine development, vaccinology, and the work of the Special Programme for Research and Training in Tropical Diseases, the Special Programme of Research, Development and Research Training in Human Reproduction and the Diarrheal Diseases Control Programme).

The research and development activities of EPI are expected to play an essential role in guiding program activities in the areas mentioned in the preceding paragraphs.

CONCLUSION

The promise of the Expanded Programme on Immunization is being fulfilled. The public health revolution that has quietly been taking place for less than 15 years is continuing. More important than the prevention of some 1.9 million deaths per year from measles, pertussis and neonatal tetanus, EPI has contributed to changing social value systems so that immunization is now recognized as a high priority by both national and international leaders. This support must be sustained to ensure continued program progress and to set the stage for disease control and eradication, the introduction of new vaccines and the reinforcement of other primary health care interventions which are planned for the decade of the 1990s and which represent steppingstones to the goal of health for all by the year 2000.

The World Health Organization's Plan of Action for Global Eradication of Poliomyelitis by the Year 2000[a]

R. H. HENDERSON

Director, Expanded Programme on Immunization
World Health Organization
1211 Geneva 27, Switzerland

INTRODUCTION

In May 1988, the Forty-first World Health Assembly committed WHO to the global eradication of poliomyelitis by the year 2000 (resolution WHA41.28). The Health Assembly emphasized that eradication efforts should be pursued in ways which strengthen the development of the Expanded Programme on Immunization (EPI), fostering its contribution, in turn, to the development of primary health care.

The Health Assembly had as a background document the "Declaration of Talloires,"[b] which also cited this poliomyelitis eradication goal. The Declaration was issued by the Task Force for Child Survival (comprising WHO, UNICEF, the World Bank, UNDP and the Rockefeller Foundation) after a meeting in March 1988 in Talloires, France, attended by world leaders in the area of health and development.

This Plan of Action draws on experience gained in the Region of the Americas, which began its drive for poliomyelitis eradication in 1985, and the resulting optimism about the feasibility of using the specialized efforts required for eradication to boost broader aspects of immunization and strengthen other health services.

The progress of EPI has resulted in optimism about the eradication of poliomyelitis during the next decade. In 1988, coverage rates for a third dose of polio or DPT vaccines in developing countries were more than 60%. In response to the EPI goal of providing immunization for all children of the world by 1990 (universal child immunization by 1990, or "UCI-1990"), national and international efforts are being intensified to increase coverage to 80% or more for all antigens included in the Programme by this date. Achieving and sustaining this level is a prerequisite for the global eradication of poliomyelitis.

Improved surveillance of poliomyelitis is essential so that useful information about cases and outbreaks can be used to guide and refine eradication strategies. For example, experience to date suggests that the circulation of wild polioviruses in communities

[a] This paper was originally published as Annex 2 of the preceding paper, and is reproduced in slightly modified form by permission of the World Health Organization.

[b] Document WHA41/1988/REC/1, Annex 6.

is heavily dependent on intimate person-to-person contact. Large urban areas seem to be foci for particularly intense transmission of polioviruses, and this may play an important role in the transfer of virus to less densely settled populations.

Once freed of endemic transmission, areas within individual countries, and groups of countries, may be less likely to return to an endemic state than had been thought previously, suggesting that global eradication may be approached by eliminating endemic transmission from groups of countries, and underlining the importance of achieving high immunization coverage in urban areas, particularly among socially disadvantaged groups.

In 1987, only some 10% of the 250,000 cases of poliomyelitis estimated to occur in that year were officially reported. Trends in reported cases may be difficult to interpret in coming years since the real decline in incidence may be masked by improvements in disease surveillance, making it appear that the incidence of poliomyelitis is increasing—a phenomenon experienced in the course of the smallpox eradication program.

The strategies outlined in this plan need to remain flexible and evolve on the basis of experience gained in national programs. Thus the budget estimates which have been provided at this stage (particularly for the later years of the initiative) are mainly intended to indicate orders of magnitude. Both the Plan of Action and the budget estimates will need continuing review and updating in coming years.

OBJECTIVES

Goals for the Year 2000

1. There should be no case of clinical poliomyelitis associated with wild poliovirus.
2. There should be no wild poliovirus identified anywhere in the world after sampling of communities and environments.
3. The process of independent certification of global poliomyelitis eradication should begin so that consideration can be given to stopping poliomyelitis immunization (a three-year period during which active surveillance reveals neither cases nor the circulation of wild polioviruses is currently envisaged).

Goals for the Year 1995

1. Poliomyelitis eradication, defined as the cessation of indigenous transmission of wild poliovirus, should be achieved in the European and Western Pacific Regions, with formal certification in the Region of the Americas.
2. Indigenous transmission of wild poliovirus should cease in five or more countries each in the African, Eastern Mediterranean and South-East Asia Regions, preferably in epidemiologically defined zones, and the evidence of "polio-free zones" should be documented in the majority of the remaining countries.
3. There should be expansion and strengthening of the network of laboratories which: (*a*) reliably measure serum antibodies to poliovirus by type; (*b*) isolate, identify

and, if necessary, carry out intratypic differentiation of polioviruses from clinical and sewage samples; and (*c*) refer samples as needed for further characterization.

4. Systems should be established that permit all countries to refer specimens for laboratory diagnosis as required.

5. There should be intratypic characterization of poliovirus isolates from all poliomyelitis-like cases/outbreaks through appropriate methods in areas previously considered to be polio-free so that a probable source or sources can be identified.

6. There should be annual review/revision of national poliomyelitis eradication plans in countries not yet free from wild poliovirus and development of special action programs in countries whose infrastructure appears insufficient to permit achievement of the goal by the year 2000. In countries where external resources are required to supplement national resources, national plans are to be developed in collaboration with donors who will be co-signatories to the plan.

Goals for the Year 1990

1. Poliomyelitis incidence and immunization coverage should be monitored in all countries by "district" (a geopolitical subdivision with a population that could range from a few hundred thousand to a few million).

2. Poliomyelitis incidence should be reported at least monthly by district to regional and global levels.

3. Poliomyelitis status of all countries should be reviewed, and poliomyelitis eradication plans developed in endemic countries.

4. Confirmation should be made that all countries use vaccines that meet WHO requirements.

5. A standard case definition for cases of poliomyelitis and standard laboratory diagnostic methods should be adopted.

6. Poliomyelitis eradication training materials should be introduced for field staff (relating particularly to surveillance and outbreak control) and for laboratory personnel (relating particularly to poliovirus isolation and identification, to vaccine potency testing and to serological tests for poliomyelitis immunity). Inter-regional, inter country, and national training programs should be initiated.

7. A network of poliomyelitis reference laboratories should be established that are able to isolate and type poliovirus and differentiate vaccine-like from wild poliovirus and that are willing to test specimens from one or more countries for diagnostic purposes.

8. Simple, rapid tests should be validated to confirm the presence of poliovirus in samples taken from individuals and from the environment.

9. Epidemiologic research should be done to better characterize the patterns of spread of wild viruses and to define rapid, effective outbreak control procedures.

10. Current oral polio vaccine formulations should be reviewed to decide whether changes in WHO requirements are warranted. The combined use of inactivated and oral vaccines should be evaluated, and the further development and testing of new oral poliovirus vaccines should be promoted with a view to being able to introduce them by 1995.

11. Advisory bodies should be established in each region that will: (*a*) review at least annually the progress being achieved to eradicate poliomyelitis in the context of EPI; (*b*) offer advice concerning the improvement of programs in the region; and (*c*) promote coordination and collaboration among the supporters of national programs,

including organizations of the United Nations system, multi- and bilateral development agencies, and private/nongovernmental organizations.

STRATEGIES

Seven major areas in which action is required have been identified:
1. Immunization coverage
2. Surveillance
3. Laboratory services/vaccine quality control
4. Training
5. Social mobilization
6. Rehabilitation services
7. Research and development

1989-1990

Immunization Coverage

All countries should attain coverage of at least 80% with a protective course of polio vaccine among infants by their first birthday and among children in each one-year cohort between the ages of 1 and 4 years. This coverage level should be regarded as a management goal for all districts. Interruption of transmission of wild poliovirus may require coverage in excess of 80%, however, especially in areas of high population density, such as periurban slums. By the year 2000, immunization coverage should exceed 90% in all countries. To achieve this, emphasis will be placed on general strengthening of the EPI infrastructure through (*a*) training, (*b*) improved supervision, (*c*) reduction of missed immunization opportunities, (*d*) adoption of appropriate immunization schedules and strategies, and (*e*) improved social communication activities.

Surveillance

National managers should obtain reports of cases, including reports of "zero cases," from each district (or other major geopolitical subdivision) on at least a monthly basis. Monthly reporting, by district, will be introduced progressively, so that by 1995 it will involve all countries. Weekly reporting will become necessary as endemic transmission is stopped. It is expected that in most countries this information will contribute to the national management information system for primary health care.

Countries should report cases, by district, to the regional and global level on a monthly basis. This should be achieved as rapidly as possible. Countries and regions close to achieving poliomyelitis eradication will need to establish weekly reporting. Feedback should be provided from the global and regional levels beginning at six-monthly intervals, but becoming monthly or weekly as soon as possible.

A clear poliomyelitis *case definition* is essential for surveillance. All countries should be encouraged to adopt a standard case definition by 1990. For reporting purposes the following is proposed: *A case of poliomyelitis is defined as that occurring in any patient with acute flaccid paralysis (including any child less than 15 years of age diagnosed to have Guillain-Barré syndrome) for whom no other cause can be identified.* Countries with fewer than 50 cases per year should establish an expert review committee responsible for the final diagnosis of cases reported as poliomyelitis and for their classification as: (*a*) vaccine-associated, (*b*) wild virus/imported, (*c*) wild virus/indigenous, or (*d*) unknown/other.

Laboratory Services/Vaccine Quality Control

Laboratory capabilities for isolating and characterizing polioviruses will be strengthened. A network of international poliomyelitis reference laboratories already exists, and a regional network is being established in the Americas. This reference network will be extended by 1990. Systems for the exchange of samples among reference laboratories and between these laboratories and national programs will be developed. Prototype kits for the collection and transport of laboratory specimens will be introduced.

The World Health Organization will work with countries and vaccine producers to assure that all immunization programs use vaccines that meet WHO requirements. Continued emphasis on cold-chain management is a complementary strategy for ensuring that vaccine potency is maintained up to the time of administration.

Training

The EPI is at present revising its training materials to reflect the advanced state of most national programs in developing countries and their increasing similarity to programs in industrialized countries. One or more EPI modules will be devoted exclusively to poliomyelitis eradication activities for health workers at different levels. Training materials will also be developed for laboratory personnel, relating particularly to poliovirus isolation, identification and strain differentiation, vaccine potency testing, and serologic tests for poliomyelitis immunity. Inter-regional, inter-country, and national training programs will be initiated. EPI will also continue its efforts, in conjunction with other WHO programs, to integrate its training materials into the curricula of institutions training health staff.

Social Mobilization

Creating and maintaining public awareness of the poliomyelitis eradication initiative will be important for sustaining political and financial commitment to the goal of poliomyelitis eradication. WHO should collaborate with other agencies and voluntary organizations to develop appropriate messages for the media and material for lay education. Development of national communication plans including regular media coverage of national, regional, and global progress in immunization coverage and disease control should be encouraged. Progress reports should also be regularly issued to agencies providing support to the EPI.

In recent years political, religious, and community leaders have successfully and enthusiastically participated in social mobilization for acceleration of immunization. Their continued support will be necessary to increase and sustain immunization coverage and may be useful in the development of community surveillance.

Rehabilitation Services

The poliomyelitis eradication initiative is expected to provide an excellent opportunity for strengthening rehabilitation services in developing countries. Eradication efforts will focus public attention on the tragic consequences of poliomyelitis, and will create an environment in which rehabilitation efforts can be expected to receive additional support, particularly from local resources. As the number of cases diminishes, these efforts can become more comprehensive, covering an ever larger proportion of all cases which occur and providing a more extensive array of services to each case.

Rehabilitation efforts undertaken in conjunction with poliomyelitis eradication will support the eradication effort itself, helping to ensure among other things that all cases of poliomyelitis come to the attention of health authorities. The efforts should also contribute to the development of more comprehensive national rehabilitation services by strengthening the health infrastructure and by building community support which can focus on other causes of disability as poliomyelitis disappears from the scene.

Some polio rehabilitation initiatives are already being undertaken internationally, most notably by IMPACT (an organization devoted to the prevention of avoidable disability co-sponsored by WHO, UNICEF and UNDP) and by Rotary International, which is providing some 10 million US$ to support poliomyelitis rehabilitation work. However, the major contributions to these efforts are expected to come from endemic countries, and national rehabilitation services should become increasingly evident during the 1990s.

Research and Development

The development of simple, rapid diagnostic tests for poliomyelitis is an immediate priority. Special studies will be initiated to improve surveillance for poliomyelitis, including: (*a*) the use of simplified tests for confirming infection, (*b*) techniques for detecting wild poliovirus in the environment, and (*c*) methods for stimulating active case reporting.

Operational research will be conducted to define cost-effective methods of interrupting transmission of wild poliovirus. These include strategies for reaching people in periurban slums, who are a major challenge to immunization and other primary health care programs.

Current studies on the optimal formulation of oral polio vaccine for developing countries will be pursued with the objective of making definitive recommendations by

1990 concerning any changes that might be warranted. The combined use of oral and inactivated polio vaccines will be examined. Basic research to develop improved oral vaccines will be promoted.

1991-1995

This period will see increasing application of the strategies developed during the previous period. By 1995 health workers in all countries not considered free of poliomyelitis will have received specific training in eradication techniques. By 1995 reliable surveillance information will be available from every country, by district, on at least a monthly basis. In countries reporting fewer than 10 cases per year, all cases of flaccid paralysis with no other immediately obvious cause will be investigated (including the appropriate application of laboratory confirmation and characterization of the virus[es] concerned), and reported as vaccine-associated, wild virus/imported, wild virus/indigenous, or unknown/other.

1996-2000

This will be the period during which the global drive to eradicate poliomyelitis will be intensified. By 1996, endemic transmission of wild poliovirus should be confined to well-defined areas in 10 to 20 countries. While continuation of routine operations may suffice for some of the countries that are not yet free of poliomyelitis, it is likely that exceptional eradication measures, such as immunization campaigns conducted on a national or smaller scale, will be required in other countries. Some countries will require additional support from outside collaborators for supplies, equipment, and operating costs. In some circumstances the services of international consultants may be called upon to support national managers in the planning, implementation, and analysis of the effectiveness of eradication strategies.

Application of Strategies at the National Level

In the development of national plans for the eradication of poliomyelitis, consideration should be given to immunization coverage rates and the number of cases reported. In the absence of an alternative regional or sub-regional strategy, countries (or areas within countries) can be placed according to these variables in four groups:

Group A: Countries Considered to be Free of Poliomyelitis

These are countries with reliable reporting systems, which have reported no indigenous case of poliomyelitis for at least three years and have achieved a coverage of 80% or more among infants by their first birthday and among children in each one-year cohort between the ages of 1 and 4 years. These countries should maintain their immunization program. "Zero case" reporting from all districts should be continued. Any reported case should be investigated promptly with full laboratory support to confirm the diagnosis. An expert review committee should be established that would be responsible for final diagnosis of cases and their classification as vaccine-associated, wild virus/indigenous, wild virus/imported, or unknown/other. Outbreak-control measures should be rapidly instituted if transmission of wild poliovirus appears likely.

Group B: Countries with Fewer than 10 Cases per Year and Coverage Rates of More Than 50%

Many of these countries may already be free of indigenous transmission of wild poliovirus, cases being imported or vaccine-associated. These countries should review their surveillance systems to assure that all cases are being reported and investigated. Clinical diagnoses should be confirmed through full laboratory testing. Consideration should be given to establishing an expert review committee responsible for final diagnosis of cases and their classification as vaccine-associated, wild virus/indigenous, wild virus/imported, or unknown/other. Countries with indigenous cases should identify common risk factors and undertake special immunization to interrupt transmission. Countries in this group should continue their efforts to achieve high immunization coverage levels.

Group C: Countries with 10 or More Cases per Year and Coverage Rates of More Than 50%

In these countries primary emphasis should be placed on improving immunization coverage and strengthening surveillance systems. National or local immunization days or other special strategies may be considered as a means for increasing coverage. Surveillance systems should define areas of continued transmission. Outbreak control and case investigation should be increasingly emphasized in countries or areas within countries in which endemic transmission is almost eliminated. Countries that report fewer than 50 cases per year should provide specimens from each case for laboratory confirmation. They should consider establishing an expert review committee responsible for the final diagnosis of cases reported as poliomyelitis and for their classification as vaccine-associated, wild virus/indigenous, wild virus/imported, or unknown/other.

Group D: Countries with 10 or More Cases per Year of Unknown Incidence and/or Coverage Rates of 50% or Below or Unknown

In these countries primary emphasis should be placed on increasing routine immunization coverage. National immunization days or other special strategies may be considered as a means for increasing coverage. These strategies represent a complement to routine services and should include all EPI antigens. Group D countries should also develop surveillance systems, initially focusing on sentinel surveillance. Outbreak control and investigation of cases or outbreaks will be particularly encouraged in areas of the country where coverage exceeds 50%. Laboratory confirmation of clinical diagnoses is not a priority, except in countries or areas within countries where endemic transmission has stopped.

Variations in these strategies may be appropriate. For example, efforts will be made to establish epidemiologically defined zones consisting of groups of contiguous countries that would benefit from inter-country coordination of eradication strategies. In such circumstances, it may be advisable to emphasize surveillance and outbreak control measures in a Group D country if it is thought to be a major focus for export of wild poliovirus to neighboring countries.

A provisional classification of countries, based on data available to the Programme at headquarters in Geneva as of 1 August 1988, is provided in FIGURE 1. Of the total global population, 17% lives in Group A countries, 7% in Group B countries, 60% in Group C countries, and 16% in Group D countries (TABLE 1).

WHO RESPONSIBILITIES AT NATIONAL, REGIONAL AND GLOBAL LEVELS

The World Health Organization will provide technical leadership in the management and coordination of global poliomyelitis eradication until its completion. Success will depend on the recognition of this as a universal challenge, and WHO will actively solicit the collaboration of as wide a spectrum of institutions and individuals as possible. Commitment from governments and individual political/community leaders will be essential. Financial and technical support will be required from multi- and bilateral development agencies, other international agencies, nongovernmental organizations, technical institutions, universities, private and voluntary groups, and concerned individuals.

While additional coordinating groups may need to be established at global level, emphasis in the beginning stages will be placed on coordination through the existing activities of the EPI Global Advisory Group and on coordinating groups established within countries and within regions.

WHO activities associated with the poliomyelitis eradication initiative will be conducted as part of the Expanded Programme on Immunization (EPI) in collaboration with other WHO programs as appropriate. Responsibilities for this initiative will be distributed at national, regional and global levels in the same manner as responsibilities for EPI are distributed.

The most important activities will be those of *national* health authorities in strengthening their immunization programs and in stopping the transmission of wild poliovirus within national boundaries. The main responsibilities for planning, resource mobilization, donor coordination, training, implementation, monitoring, evaluation and research are national. WHO will collaborate in these activities through the office of the WHO representative, where such an office has been established, and through support from WHO/EPI staff and consultants assigned at country, inter-country, regional and interregional levels.

WHO *regional* offices will:

(1) provide technical support and coordination within the region;

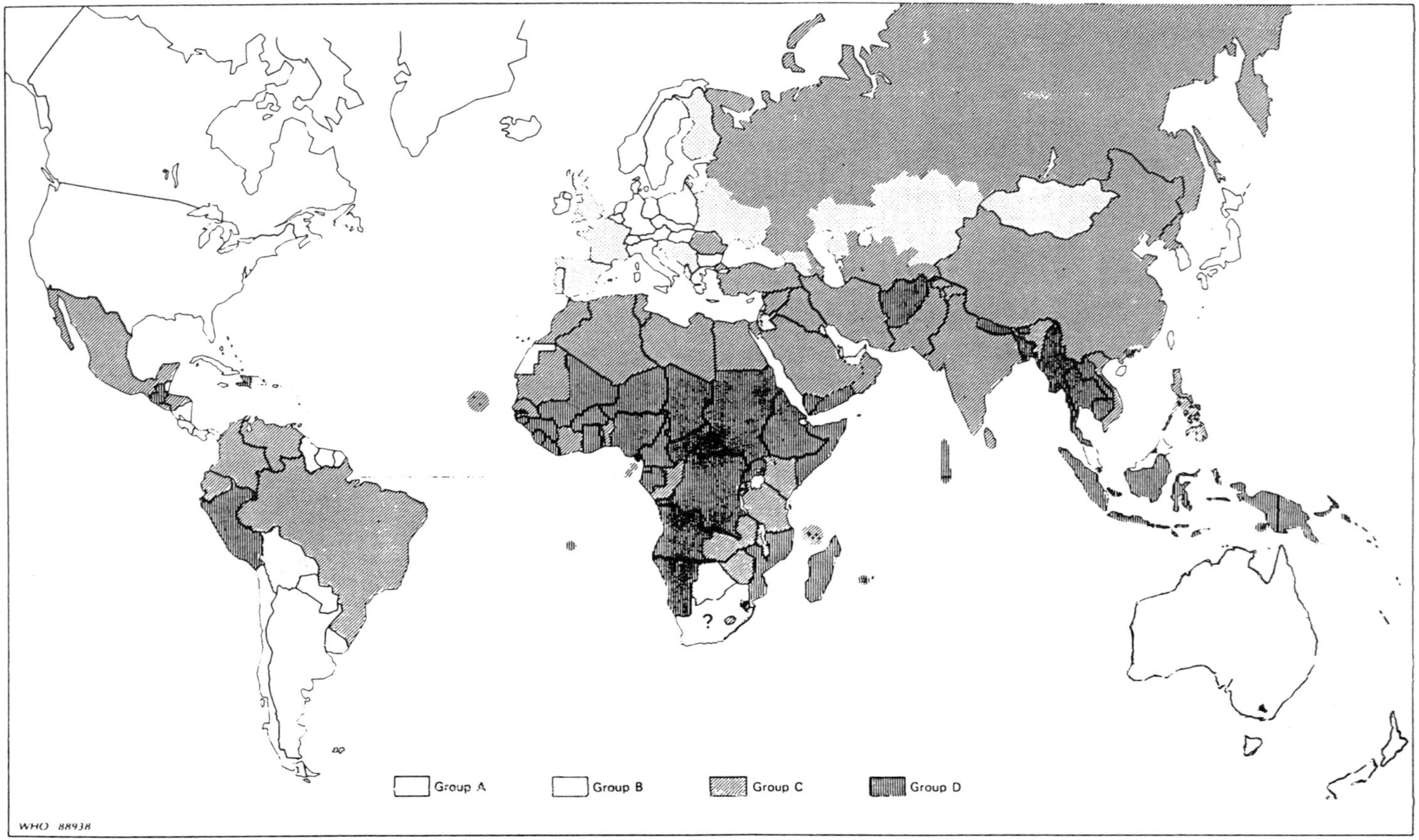

FIGURE 1. Countries/areas according to category of polio incidence/coverage (1 August 1988).

(2) prepare regional plans of action based on the results of assessments of national programs;

(3) support national managers in planning, donor coordination, training, monitoring, evaluation and research;

(4) place special emphasis on poliomyelitis surveillance, making available as required reference laboratory services for the diagnosis of poliomyelitis and/or the characterization of the poliovirus isolates;

(5) provide technical support to national programs to adapt and develop computer software for management information systems (including disease surveillance); and

(6) provide training to national laboratory staff.

TABLE 1. Population (in Millions) by Category of Poliomyelitis Incidence/Coverage, by Region (1 August 1988)

	Population			
Region	A	B	C	D
Africa[a]	1	1	132	307
Americas	350	13	291	35
Eastern Mediterranean	3	10	282	56
Europe[b]	287	292	254	0
Southeast Asia	0	2	819	387
Western Pacific	186	25	1 205	16
Total	827	344	2 983	801
%	17	7	60	16

NOTE: Group A: No indigenous cases due to wild virus for the last 3 years and immunization coverage > 80%. Group B: Fewer than 10 cases per year for the last 3 years and immunization coverage > 50%. Group C: More than 10 cases per year and immunization coverage > 50%. Group D: More than 10 cases per year or unknown incidence and/or immunization coverage < 50% or unknown.

[a] South Africa excluded.

[b] The 15 republics of the Soviet Union have each been counted as a separate country/area.

The regional plans of action will address research needs of regional scope, for which purpose regional offices will support national programs. Regions will engage in regional resource mobilization to the extent possible. Progress within regions will be reviewed and discussed annually by regional EPI advisory bodies and by annual regional or subregional meetings of national program managers. It will be reviewed periodically by the WHO regional committees.

At the *global* level EPI will provide overall technical direction for this initiative. It will:

(1) provide leadership in resource mobilization and donor coordination;

(2) develop prototype training materials and technical support documents as required;

(3) promote the development and application of improved disease surveillance and program monitoring and evaluation techniques;

(4) support regional offices and national programs by providing expertise, by assigning short- and long-term staff and by providing funds, particularly to strengthen donor coordination, planning, training, supervision, monitoring and evaluation (including surveillance) and research;

(5) update and share with regional offices and countries, at least twice a year, global information on immunization coverage, disease incidence and other selected variables obtained from national managers through the regional offices;

(6) promote vaccine quality-control activities so as to assure that all countries have the benefit of using polio vaccines that meet WHO requirements;

(7) promote the development and introduction of improved polio vaccines;

(8) develop a system of poliomyelitis reference laboratories to which specimens can be sent from national level for poliovirus isolation, serologic testing, and/or poliovirus characterization;

(9) strengthen the capacities of national laboratories through training, provision of standard reagents, and proficiency testing;

(10) promote operational research at a national level, in collaboration with the regional offices, addressing program priorities;

(11) ensure annual review of the global poliomyelitis eradication initiative by the EPI Global Advisory Group, and periodic review by the WHO Executive Board and World Health Assembly; and

(12) certify the global eradication of poliomyelitis.

RESOURCE REQUIREMENTS

Resource requirements for the 1990s over and above current support for the EPI are estimated as follows: more than 100 million children in developing countries are being immunized each year, and so the total cost of the program (estimated as 10.00 1988 US$ per fully immunized child) will come to more than 1000 million US$ per year—and maybe double that if one considers the new vaccines that can be expected to be added to the program, and the growth in world population. For the most part, external contributions will cover the costs of vaccines, cold-chain equipment, syringes and needles and sterilization equipment. In the least-developed countries, it is probable that a portion of operational costs will also need to be covered from external resources.

Most of the costs are being met by developing countries themselves, but external support will continue to be needed, probably in the range of 20%-30% of the total costs. The 150 million US$ per year being invested from external sources in EPI according to an approximate estimate in 1988 will need to be increased to some 300 million US$ in the early 1990s. The partners already engaged in the EPI, particularly UNICEF, multi- and bilateral development agencies and private and voluntary groups, would have to increase and sustain their current contributions to meet this need.

The projections below are also for funds over and above those that are currently being provided to EPI for its global operations. EPI at headquarters in Geneva now receives some 3.7 million US$ in extrabudgetary support per year. The poliomyelitis initiative requires an additional 10-15 million US$ per year. Except for a small contribution from headquarters, the poliomyelitis eradication activities of the Americas are being supported by funds raised within the region; its requirements, which have already been met through the early 1990s, are not included in the estimates provided below.

Estimated resource requirements are summarized in TABLE 2. No line items have been provided for social mobilization or rehabilitation; it is expected that they will for the most part be supported from community resources.

1989-1990

Staff Requirements

The primary need during this period is for additional international staff who can help assess the status of national programs and contribute to program planning (including donor coordination), monitoring and evaluation. Aided by the findings, they will help in further developing eradication strategies, in developing prototype training materials, and in the further development and application of simplified computer-based management information systems at global, regional, and national levels (see below).

Initial help will be sought largely through the use of short-term consultants; full-time (core) staff will, however, be recruited as soon as suitable persons can be identified. The full-time staff who are recruited will be expected to constitute a majority of the core staff who will be required at least up to 1995.

A total additional "core" staff of some 20 professionals will be needed, in addition to secretarial staff. Efforts will generally be made, when selecting staffs for inter-regional posts, to provide flexibility of transfer between regions according to the needs of the Programme. Five professionals will be based at headquarters, five in regional offices, and ten in countries within regions, who will have inter-country responsibilities.

National professional staff will be recruited to supplement the work of the international staff. Efforts will be made to recruit young national staff who can profit from the experience for career development.

Short-term consultant services will also be required, and an initial projection of a total 10 person/years per year has been made. Funds for administrative support and travel have also been budgeted.

Total "core" and consultant staff costs will be some 9,000,000 US$.

In addition to the "core" staff and consultants, resources will be needed to support activities in the following areas:

1. Coordination Meetings of Regional and Global Advisory Bodies and National Program Managers

Advisory bodies have already been established in the Region of the Americas and the European Region. They will be established in the remaining regions during 1989. At present, an annual meeting of each regional advisory body is foreseen. Annual regional meetings of national program managers will be convened, where possible, in conjunction with the meeting of the regional advisory body. Two meetings will be required in the African Region, one in French and one in English. The combined cost is estimated at 75,000 US$ per meeting. Excluding the Region of the Americas, six annual meetings, at a total cost of 450,000 US$ per year will be needed, beginning in 1989, together with meetings of experts at global level to advise on specific aspects of the poliomyelitis eradication initiative. Their recommendations will be considered by the EPI Global Advisory Group, which will remain the central advisory body for

TABLE 2. Estimate of Additional EPI Resource Requirements[a] for Eradication of Poliomyelitis, 1989-2000 (United States Dollars at 1988 Rate)

Component	1989-1990 (2 years)	1991-1995 (5 years)	1996-2000 (5 years)
Personnel			
Staff/consultants	6,000,000	15,000,000	20,000,000
National professional staff	1,500,000	7,500,000	20,000,000
Administrative support	500,000	2,500,000	3,000,000
Travel	1,000,000	3,000,000	4,000,000
Subtotal	9,000,000	28,000,000	47,000,000
Coordination			
Meetings	1,000,000	3,000,000	3,000,000
Subtotal	1,000,000	3,000,000	3,000,000
Monitoring and surveillance			
Transport	1,000,000	10,000,000	10,000,000
Software installation	300,000	750,000	750,000
Software development	100,000	250,000	250,000
Subtotal	1,400,000	11,000,000	11,000,000
Training			
Development of educational materials	400,000	400,000	400,000
Courses for:			
program staff	700,000	2,000,000	2,000,000
laboratory staff	200,000	600,000	600,000
Subtotal	1,300,000	3,000,000	3,000,000
Laboratory Support			
Meetings	100,000	500,000	500,000
Supplies	500,000	2,000,000	1,000,000
Fellowships	—	500,000	500,00
Subtotal	600,000	3,000,000	2,000,000
Research and Development			
Development of laboratory diagnostic methods	500,000	500,000	—
Operational studies	600,000	2,500,000	2,000,000
Vaccine development	600,000	2,000,000	1,000,000
Subtotal	1,700,000	5,000,000	3,000,000
Total			
without program support costs	15,000,000	53,000,000	69,000,000
with program support costs	17,000,000	60,000,000	78,000,000

[a] External resource requirements for routine EPI operations, estimated to range from 300 million US$ to 600 million US$ per year during the 1990s, are *excluded* from this table.

EPI. A total of 50,000 US$ per year is budgeted for global meetings conducted in addition to the annual meeting of the EPI Global Advisory Group.

The total cost of coordination meetings will be 1,000,000 US$.

2. Monitoring and Surveillance

Two major changes need to be introduced:

First, national managers must begin analyzing their data district by district. General data for the country as a whole, whether they relate to immunization coverage or to disease incidence, will no longer suffice. In a number of countries, building an effective surveillance system will require regular visits to district facilities. The proposal therefore includes the provision of 1 million US$ to ensure the availability of vehicles and fuel for this purpose.

Secondly, in order to analyze and respond to district data promptly, simplified computerized management information systems are required at the national level, and should be linked as rapidly as possible to more peripheral systems as these are progressively introduced. Regional and global systems should be compatible with the data being obtained and analyzed at the national level.

A considerable amount of software for EPI is already being developed. This work will need to be continuous, however, since these systems will evolve as improved software and hardware become available, and as the needs of national managers evolve. The major need during this period, however, will be for installation of software for national systems and training of national staff in its use. It is hoped that this can be accomplished in approximately 15 countries per year, at a cost of 10,000 US$ per country. An additional 50,000 US$ per year will be needed to continue software development, particularly linking national with district and peripheral systems and making EPI a component of the national management information system for primary health care.

The total monitoring and surveillance cost will be 1,400,000 US$.

3. Development of Training Materials and Support for Training Courses

The development and field-testing of training materials is expected to proceed rapidly, given the work already done in the Pan American Health Organization.

After the course materials for immunization program staff have been developed and field-tested, they will be introduced in the current routine EPI training activities within national programs. As was done to introduce the original EPI materials, intercountry courses of national program managers will be held in each region (with the exceptions of the region of the Americas and the European region), courses in both English and French being held in the African region. The cost per course is estimated to be 80,000 US$. Special practical courses to permit surveillance supervisors to recognize clinical cases of poliomyelitis and to teach these skills to health workers in communities will also be needed. Five such courses are planned for 1989-1990, at 60,000 US$ per course.

The training for laboratory support will focus on poliovirus isolation and strain differentiation, vaccine potency testing, and serologic tests for poliomyelitis antibodies. Only a limited number of laboratories will be engaged in poliomyelitis diagnostic work during this period, and only two courses, both inter-regional, are envisaged (at 60,000 US$ per course).

The total training costs will be 1,300,000 US$.

4. Establishment of Poliomyelitis Reference Laboratories

Meetings will have to be convened to obtain a consensus on various standardized test procedures which will form the basis for training (1 meeting per year at 50,000 US$ per meeting). Extra staff, supplies and equipment will be needed to permit the reference laboratories to perform the diagnostic tests required; 500,000 US$ have been budgeted for these purposes.

The total poliomyelitis reference laboratory costs will be 600,000 US$.

5. Research and Development

500,000 US$ will be used to support the development of improved laboratory diagnostic tests for poliomyelitis that can be reliably used in laboratories with relatively limited capabilities, including the purchase of specialized equipment and the hiring of extra laboratory staff. 600,000 US$ are provided for operational research on cost-effective methods of interrupting the transmission of wild poliovirus.

The optimal formulation of oral poliomyelitis vaccine will require expensive and time-consuming field studies and will only be possible in a limited number of sites. Support for two studies, at a cost of approximately 200,000 US$ each, and for the further development of improved vaccines (another 200,000 US$) is requested. Support is also required to accelerate the testing and introduction of new oral polio vaccines, but probably will not be needed for field trials until after 1990.

The total research and development costs will be 1,700,000 US$. The total resource requirements for 1989-1990 will thus be 17,000,000 US$ (including program support cost).

1991-1995

While the activities will be modified to meet the changing needs of the program, the total annual resources required will remain approximately the same in terms of international staff and training, monitoring, and surveillance. Increased resources will be needed for country assessment activities. Recruitment of national professional staff will increase and the cost of staff participation in coordination meetings will increase. Projected travel costs will increase from 500,000 US$ per year during 1989-1990 to 600,000 US$ per year. Laboratory costs will also increase as more national laboratories are developed. While fellowships for laboratory staff have not been projected for the period 1989-1990, they will be used as a training method in 1991-1995. In addition, proficiency testing programs will be increasingly developed during this period. Laboratory support costs will double, from approximately 300,000 US$ per year to approximately 600,000 US$ per year during 1991-1995. Support for research and development will increase from 850,000 US$ per year to 1,000,000 US$ per year during the period 1991-1995.

Increased resources will be needed to support specific poliomyelitis eradication strategies forming part of national programs during this period. These will mainly be covered by bilateral or multilateral support from organizations other than WHO, and are not included in these estimates. The total costs for 1991-1995 will thus be 60,000,000 US$ (including program support cost).

1996-2000

This is the period during which an increased need for WHO-managed resources can be envisaged, as specific intensive eradication strategies are implemented in countries which might otherwise not achieve the goal, relying in part on the help of short- and long-term international consultants. Realistic estimates of these needs will be developed during the period 1991-1995. It can be anticipated, however, that personnel costs will be at least two-thirds more than what has been projected for the period 1991-1995. The total costs for 1996-2000 are estimated at 78,000,000 US$, (including program support cost).

Vaccinia Virus Expression Vectors[a]

BERNARD MOSS AND CHARLES FLEXNER

Laboratory of Viral Diseases
National Institute of Allergy and Infectious Diseases
National Institutes of Health
Bethesda, Maryland 20892

INTRODUCTION

We depend on a variety of specific and nonspecific mechanisms for defense against microbial invaders. Although the value of vaccination for protection against infectious disease is well established, neither the significant target antigens nor the relative roles of humoral and cell-mediated immunity have been adequately defined in most cases. Nevertheless, a thorough understanding of these parameters is critical for the engineering of new vaccines. Recent advances in recombinant DNA technology, peptide synthesis, and hybridoma production are providing important tools for analyzing the protective immune response. In this review we focus on one new approach, namely, the use of vaccinia virus as a general expression vector for stimulation of humoral and cell-mediated immunity to specified proteins and for determination of target antigens of cytotoxic T lymphocytes (CTL). The protective effect of vaccination with live recombinant vaccinia viruses and their potential as vaccines for veterinary and medical purposes are discussed.

TYPES OF EXPRESSION VECTORS

Recombinant DNA technology has made it possible to synthesize proteins in cells from diverse sources including bacteria, yeast, and mammals. Generally speaking, homologous systems are best for producing proteins that are properly folded and processed. Continuous high-level expression of mammalian proteins can be obtained by gene amplification in stably transformed cell lines. The use of viruses as expression vectors, however, provides advantages of rapid construction and portability to different cell types and even whole animals. For technical reasons, DNA viruses and retroviruses have been developed as vectors. The small- and intermediate-sized viruses, including SV40, bovine papilloma virus, retroviruses, and adenoviruses offer simplicity of vector construction and relatively high-level expression. As a trade-off, however, these viruses have a limited host range and/or can accommodate little extra genetic information

[a] This article is reproduced in slightly modified form from the *Annual Review of Immunology* (1987 **5:** 305-324) by permission of Annual Reviews, Inc. Additionally, the U.S. Government has the right to retain a nonexclusive, royalty-free license in and to any copyright covering this paper.

before becoming defective in replication. The large DNA viruses, such as vaccinia virus and herpes simplex virus, are intrinsically more difficult to engineer genetically than are the viruses listed above, but they have a wider host range and can accommodate substantial amounts of foreign DNA while retaining infectivity. Since vaccinia virus has been used extensively for gene expression, identification of targets for humoral and cell-mediated immunity, and protection of experimental animals against viral diseases, further discussion is limited to this vector. Although vaccinia virus has some unique characteristics, many of the approaches described here could be readily adapted to other poxviruses as well as to members of the herpesvirus and adenovirus families.

HISTORICAL PERSPECTIVES

The distinctive scars left by smallpox and the severity of the disease led to the early recognition that recurrences were rare. This observation was put to practical use, perhaps first in China, by inoculating susceptible individuals with infectious material from mild cases of smallpox. Although this process, known as variolation, had a mortality as high as 1%, it otherwise effectively prevented even more severe natural infections.

The recognition, in England, that milkmaids who had contracted cowpox also were protected against smallpox led to the next advance. Edward Jenner, a country physician and noted naturalist, tested the validity of this folklore by inoculating several children with cowpox and then challenging them by variolation.[1] The absence of smallpox lesions in these children convinced Jenner that vaccination would protect against naturally transmitted smallpox, and he correctly predicted that this means of prophylaxis would eventually eradicate the disease. The value of vaccination was quickly and generally accepted and fostered a burgeoning interest in immunization by Pasteur and others in the 1800s. In this sense, smallpox vaccination played a major role in the inception of the science of immunology.

In Jenner's time, poxvirus infections occurred naturally in cattle and horses, and more than one virus type may have been prevalent. Jenner's vaccine was passaged initially in humans and subsequently in cattle and sheep. In some places it was even mixed with smallpox virus. For these reasons the pedigree of vaccinia virus, as it came to be known, is somewhat clouded. Comparisons of the restriction endonuclease maps of the genomes of vaccinia virus isolates from all over the world, however, revealed a remarkable uniformity indicating a common origin. It is interesting that vaccinia virus DNA maps are similar to but distinct from those of modern cowpox and variola (smallpox) viruses, confirming their classification as three separate species within the orthopoxvirus genus.[2]

The success of the vaccination program in eradicating smallpox was due both to the properties of the vaccine and the characteristics of the disease.[3] With regard to the latter, the simplicity of diagnosis, antigenic stability of variola virus, and absence of animal reservoirs are of special note. Important properties of the live vaccinia virus vaccine include its close antigenic relationship to variola virus, its high immunogenicity, economy of manufacture in animal skin or tissue culture, stability in freeze-dried form (making continuous refrigeration unnecessary), and simplicity of administration—by skin scratch with a bifurcated needle or jet gun. It is important that many of these advantages could also apply to a recombinant vaccinia virus designed to protect against other diseases.

BIOLOGY OF VACCINIA VIRUS

Poxviruses comprise a large family with members that infect both vertebrate and invertebrate hosts.[4] Unlike other DNA viruses, they replicate in the cytoplasm of infected cells. The best known members of this family, vaccinia virus and variola virus, are in the orthopoxvirus genus. All orthopoxviruses, including cowpox and ectromelia (mousepox), are very closely related, as judged by electron micrographic appearance, DNA analysis, and immunologic cross-reactivity.

The genome of vaccinia virus consists of a long linear double-stranded DNA molecule of about 185,000 base pairs. Hairpin structures at the two ends of the molecule link the DNA strands together. The DNA is packaged within the virus core, which also contains a complete transcription system. The presence of a virus-specific RNA polymerase, as well as modifying enzymes for capping, methylation, and polyadenylation of mRNA, are unique features of poxviruses that are intimately tied to their cytoplasmic life-style. The outer portion of the poxvirus particle is composed of lipoprotein membranes.

After entry into a cell, the viral transcription system is activated and approximately 100 early genes are expressed. The viral proteins synthesized include a DNA polymerase and other factors needed for replication of the vaccinia genome. Replication then signals the onset of expression of the late class of genes, which also number about 100, as well as the decline of early gene expression. The sequences that regulate early and late RNA formation are located just upstream of the coding regions and differ significantly from eukaryotic promoters.[5]

The products of the late genes include the majority of structural proteins assembled into virus particles within the cytoplasm. Some virions remain intracellular, while others become wrapped in golgi membrane and are extruded through the plasma membrane with an additional envelope. Both the intracellular and extracellular forms of vaccinia virus are infectious.

FORMATION OF RECOMBINANT VIRUSES

Insertion of foreign DNA into nonessential regions of the vaccinia virus genome has been carried out by homologous recombination.[6,7] Expression of foreign genes within the DNA may occur because of transcriptional regulatory elements at or near the site of insertion or by more precise genetic engineering. Plasmid vectors that greatly facilitate insertion and expression of foreign genes have been constructed.[8,9] These vectors contain an expression site, composed of a vaccinia transcriptional promotor and one or more unique restriction endonuclease sites for insertion of the foreign coding sequence, flanked by DNA from a nonessential region of the vaccinia genome. The choice of promoter determines both the time (e.g., early or late) and level of expression, whereas the flanking DNA sequence determines the site of homologous recombination.

Only about one in a thousand virus particles produced by this procedure is a recombinant. Although recombinant virus plaques can be identified by DNA hybridization, efficient selection procedures have been developed. By using segments of the nonessential vaccinia virus thymidine kinase (TK) gene as flanking sequences, the foreign gene recombines into the TK locus and by insertion inactivates the TK gene.

Selection of TK^- virus is achieved by carrying out the virus plaque assay in TK^- cells in the presence of 5-bromodeoxyuridine. Phosphorylation of this nucleoside analogue and consequent lethal incorporation into viral DNA occurs only in cells infected with TK^+ parental virus. Depending on the efficiency of the transfection and recombination, up to 80% of the plaques are desired recombinants, and the rest are spontaneous TK^- mutants.

Plasmid vectors that contain the *E. coli* β-galactosidase gene, as well as an expression site for a second gene, permit an alternative method of distinguishing recombinant from parental virus.[10] Plaques formed by such recombinants can be positively identified by the blue color that forms upon addition of an appropriate indicator. By combining both TK^- selection and β-galactosidase expression, recombinant virus is readily and quickly isolated. The recombinants are then amplified by propagation in suitable cell lines and expression of the inserted gene is checked by appropriate enzymologic, immunologic, or physical procedures.

An upper limit to the amount of genetic information that can be added to the vaccinia virus genome is not yet known. However, the addition of nearly 25,000 base pairs of foreign DNA had no apparent deleterious effect on virus yield.[11] Were it necessary, large segments of the vaccinia virus genome could be deleted to provide additional capacity.[12,13]

SYNTHESIS, PROCESSING, AND TRANSPORT OF PROTEINS

Apparently any continuous open reading frame, whether derived from prokaryotic or eukaryotic sources, can be expressed by vaccinia virus vectors. The kinetics of protein synthesis depends on the vaccinia promoter chosen. When early transcriptional signals are used, expression occurs within the first 6 hours; when late signals are used, expression occurs from 6 hours on.[8,14] The most widely used promoter, referred to as P7.5, contains both early and late signals and leads to continuous expression for 1-2 days, depending on the conditions.[8,15] Significantly longer periods of protein synthesis are not possible since vaccinia virus infection leads to cell death. Nevertheless, there is little lysis, and the majority of cells remain intact. Production of 1-2 mg of foreign protein per liter of cell culture has been achieved, although the levels of gene expression have not yet been optimized. Synthesis of multiple foreign proteins by a single recombinant virus is also possible.[10,16]

When the proteins expressed by vaccinia virus vectors are of mammalian or mammalian virus origin, posttranslational modifications appear to occur faithfully. TABLE 1 lists examples of proteins that have been shown to be proteolytically processed, glycosylated, secreted, and inserted into the plasma membrane. Perhaps most dramatic was the demonstration of correct polarity of transport: The influenza hemagglutinin was directed to the apical surface of infected cells, whereas murine leukemia and vesicular stomatitis virus envelope glycoproteins were directed to the basolateral surface.[17] Because of the extraordinarily wide host range of vaccinia virus, the cell-type specificity of processing can be analyzed. Variation in the efficiency of proteolytic cleavage of the envelope protein of human immunodeficiency virus type 1, the causative agent of AIDS,[18] and preproenkephalin[19] was noted in different cell lines.

TABLE 1. Proteins Expressed by Recombinant Vaccinia Viruses

Origin	Protein	Glycosylation	Cleavage	Cell Location or Biological Activity	Reference
DNA Viruses					
Epstein-Barr	Membrane antigen (gp 340)	+	Signal[a]	Cell surface	22
Hepatitis B	Surface antigen (S, MS, LS)	+		Secreted particle	15, 24-27
Herpes simplex I	Glycoprotein D	+	Signal	Cell surface	24,28
	Thymidine kinase			Active enzyme	6,7
RNA Viruses					
Friend murine leukemia	Envelope protein	+	Signal, subunit	Basolateral cell surface	17,43
Human immunodeficiency (HIV-1)	Envelope protein	+	Signal, subunit	Cell surface	18, 44
Influenza A	Hemagglutinin	+	Signal	Apical cell surface	17, 20, 30, 31
	Nucleoprotein			Internal	33, 34
Rabies	Glycoprotein	+	Signal	Cell surface	39, 41
Respiratory syncytial	Glycoprotein	+		Cell surface	36, 37
	Fusion protein	+	Signal, subunit	Cell surface	38
Sindbis	Structural proteins (C, E1, E2)	+	Signal, polyprotein	Cell surface, virion	46
Transmissible gastroenteritis	Spike protein (gp 195)	+	Signal		45
Vesicular stomatitis	Glycoprotein	+	Signal	Basolateral cell surface	17, 21
	Nucleoprotein			Internal	21
Protozoa					
P. knowlesi	Circumsporozoite			Internal	48
P. falciparum	Circumsporozoite			Internal	49
	S antigen		Signal	Secreted	50

TABLE 1.—*Continued*

Bacteria					
E. coli	β-galactosidase			Active enzyme	10
	Chloramphenicol acetyltransferase			Active enzyme	8
Mammalian					
Human	Factor IX[b]	+	Signal, precursor	Secreted, coagulant	57
	Interleukin 2	+	Signal	Secreted, lymphokine	53
	Preproenkephalin		Signal, precursor	Secreted	19
Bovine	γ-interferon		Signal	Secreted, antiviral	51

[a] Cleavage of signal peptide assumed because of translocation.
[b] Evidence for γ-carboxylation.

STIMULATION OF NEUTRALIZING ANTIBODY

A broad spectrum of antibodies directed against multiple protein components of a virus frequently appears after natural infection. Determination of which antibodies are responsible for neutralizing virus infectivity, however, is an important task. Immunization of animals with vaccinia virus vectors that express only one gene of an infectious agent provides a direct approach to the resolution of this problem. When possible, sera from such vaccinated animals can be analyzed for neutralizing ability *in vitro* and *in vivo.* Although similar experiments can be carried out with subunit proteins, requirements for extensive purification of the native form of the antigen may be technically difficult. Vaccinia virus vectors have particular advantages when the neutralizing antigens are membrane proteins, since they will be presented in a manner that closely mimics the natural infection.

Antibody production has been elicited with live recombinant vaccinia viruses in a variety of animals including rabbits, mice, hamsters, cotton rats, and cattle (TABLE 2). Usually intradermal inoculations have been used, but in some cases the route was intravenous, intraperitoneal, or intranasal. In the latter case secretory IgA as well as circulating IgG was demonstrated.[20]

In most instances, intradermal inoculation leads to the production of a pox lesion that lasts one to two weeks; there is no evidence for persistent infection of animals. Antibody is frequently detected by the end of the second week after vaccination and remains elevated for extended periods. Since the experimental animal also is immunized against the vaccinia virus vector, subsequent vaccinations may produce a mild or no discernible skin lesion, depending in part on the dose and interval of time between inoculations. Nevertheless, significant boosting of antibody production to a recombinant protein has been reported in several cases and should be tried if higher levels of immunity are required.[16,21,22]

STIMULATION OF CELL-MEDIATED IMMUNITY AND IDENTIFICATION OF TARGET ANTIGENS

Natural virus infections stimulate specific cell-mediated as well as humoral immune mechanisms. Cytotoxic T cells (CTL) are effectors in cell-mediated immune reactions that specifically recognize a foreign antigen in conjunction with a syngeneic MHC protein on the surface of target cells and cause their lysis. The identification of viral antigens that prime T lymphocytes *in vivo* and serve as CTL targets, however, may be quite difficult. Although the most direct approach involves the use of isolated proteins, proper protein presentation is an important consideration. Virus vectors consequently appear to be most suitable for such purposes.

Virus-specific and MHC-restricted CTL effectors have been demonstrated after *in vitro* stimulation of spleen cells from mice that had been vaccinated with recombinant vaccinia virus.[23] In this paradigm, the recombinant vaccinia virus used to immunize the animal expressed only a single candidate immunogen of the test virus (e.g., the hemagglutinin of influenza virus). Spleen cells were then isolated, and effectors were stimulated *in vitro* with cells infected with the recombinant vaccinia or the test virus itself. Target cells infected *in vitro* with the test virus and loaded with ^{51}Cr were incubated with the effector cells, and lysis was measured by ^{51}Cr release. Several

TABLE 2. Immune Response to Vaccinia Vectors and Disease Protection

Infectious Agent	Protein Expressed	Antibody Response	T-Cell Response	Protection	Reference
DNA Viruses					
Epstein-Barr	Membrane antigen (gp 340)	Neutralizing (rabbit)			22
Hepatitis B	Surface antigens (pre-S and S)	Anti-S and pre-S (rabbit), priming (chimpanzee)		Hepatitis (chimpanzee)	15, 24-27
Herpes simplex I	Glycoprotein D	Neutralizing (mouse, rabbit, cow)	Proliferative (mouse), CTL target (human)	Lethal and latent infections (mouse)	24, 28, 29
RNA Viruses					
Friend murine leukemia	Envelope	Priming, neutralizing (mouse)	Proliferative, CTL priming (mouse)	Leukemia (mouse)	43
Influenza A	Hemagglutinin (HA)	Anti-HA, neutralizing (hamster, mouse)	Type-specific: CTL priming, target (mouse)	Lower respiratory infection (hamster, mouse)	17, 20, 30, 31, 34
	Nucleoprotein		Cross-reactive: priming, target (mouse, man)	Lethal infection (mouse)	33, 34
Rabies	Glycoprotein	Neutralizing (mouse, rabbit, fox)	CTL priming (mouse)	Encephalitis (mouse, rabbit, fox)	40-42
Respiratory syncytial	Glycoprotein	Neutralizing (cotton rat)		Lower respiratory infection (cotton rat)	37
	Fusion	Neutralizing (cotton rat)		Lower respiratory infection (cotton rat)	38
Sindbis	Structural (C, E1, E2)	Neutralizing (cow)			47
Transmissible gastroenteritis	Spike (gp 195)	Neutralizing (mouse)			45
Vesicular stomatitis	Glycoprotein	Neutralizing (mouse, cow)	Type-specific: CTL priming, target (mouse)	Lingual infection (cow)	21, 39

TABLE 2.—*Continued*

Infectious Agent	Protein Expressed	Antibody Response	T-Cell Response	Protection	Reference
	Nucleoprotein	Anti-N (mouse, man)	Cross-reactive; CTL priming, target (mouse)		39, 58
Protozoan					
P. knowlesi	Circumsporozoite antigen	Anti-sporozoite (rabbit, mouse)			48
P. falciparum	Circumsporozoite antigen	Anti-sporozoite (rabbit, mouse)			49
	Blood stage secretory (S) antigen	Anti-S (rabbit)			50

examples in which recombinant vaccinia viruses have been successfully used to demonstrate CTL priming are shown in TABLE 2.

A complementary approach is to obtain effector cells from animals naturally infected with the test virus and to prepare target cells *in vitro* with a recombinant vaccinia virus that expresses a single test virus protein.[23] Although target cells can also be prepared by other recombinant DNA techniques, vaccinia virus vectors have several advantages. It is most important that the same recombinant vaccinia virus can be used to prime animals and prepare targets (in different experiments), to determine the influence of MHC by infecting several inbred mouse strains or cell lines, and to prepare target cells from individuals of outbred animals such as humans.

PROTECTIVE IMMUNIZATION

Protection of animals against infection may rely on humoral and cell-mediated immune mechanisms, depending to a large extent on the nature of the microbial agent. Although many different approaches are requires to understand fully the complex host reactions and their protective roles, recombinant vaccinia viruses can be used as one facet in such investigations. In several cases, immunization with live recombinant vaccinia expressing a single protein of a pathogenic virus has protected experimental animals against subsequent challenge with that virus. Examples include both RNA and DNA viruses, viruses that cause local or systemic infections, and viruses that produce acute or latent infections (TABLE 2). A synopsis of information obtained in this manner is presented below.

HEPATITIS B VIRUS

Hepatitis B virus (HBV) is an important cause of acute and chronic liver disease and a factor in the development of hepatocellular carcinoma. Worldwide, the number of cases of chronic hepatitis B is believed to be about 200 million. The development of effective plasma-derived and recombinant yeast subunit vaccines has considerably brightened the prospect for reducing the incidence of hepatitis B and perhaps eliminating the disease entirely. Studies with recombinant vaccinia viruses have been undertaken to learn more about the expression and immunogenicity of HBV proteins and to provide an economical mass delivery system for a hepatitis B virus eradication campaign similar to that successfully used for smallpox.

Recombinant vaccinia viruses that express the major HBsAg gene have been described.[15,24] The hepatitis protein is glycosylated and secreted as particles that are indistinguishable by sedimentation or electron microscopy from human plasma-derived material. Moreover, vaccinated rabbits mounted a high and sustained antibody response. Although two chimpanzees that were inoculated intradermally with recombinant vaccinia virus had little or no detectable circulating anti-HBsAg, they were protected against any signs of hepatitis after intravenous challenge with HBV.[25] Since the HBV challenge was promptly followed by a vigorous anti-HBsAg response, which was not seen for several months in control animals, it was evident that the vaccination had a priming effect. Most likely the challenge HBV caused a mild inapparent infection which produced a protective anamnestic neutralizing antibody response. A role for cell-mediated immunity in prevention of HBV infections has not been determined. Despite the qualified success of this experiment, monitoring the efficacy of vaccination would be difficult without antibody to HBsAg. Use of recombinants that express higher amounts of HBsAg or improvement in the vaccination protocol may be necessary.

Another alternative is the use of recombinant vaccinia viruses that express the larger forms of HBsAg containing the highly immunogenic pre-S region that has been implicated in binding of HBV to hepatocytes. Vaccinia recombinants that selectively express the large and middle forms of HBsAg have both been constructed. It is interesting that the middle protein is secreted from infected tissue culture cells in a form similar to particles made of the major small HBsAg.[26] By contrast, the large form of the protein (not yet selectively made by other recombinant DNA methods) is not secreted as a particle and even interferes with secretion of the major HBsAg when cells are infected simultaneously with two recombinants.[27] Rabbits vaccinated with recombinants that express the middle or large forms of HbsAg produce antibodies to both pre-S and S epitopes. The immunogenicity of these pre-S recombinant vaccinia viruses in chimpanzees, however, has not yet been tested.

HERPES SIMPLEX VIRUS (HSV)

Like other members of the herpesvirus family, HSV is a large complex DNA virus. The two serotypes of HSV cause acute infections at the portal of entry and latent infections in nerve ganglia. Recurrent infections can occur despite the presence of antibody. Nevertheless, experimental animals immunized with purified glycoprotein D (gD), one of several glycoproteins in the HSV envelope, display considerable protection against subsequent challenge.

Recombinant vaccinia viruses that express HSV-1 gD protect mice against lethal and latent infections with HSV-1.[24,28] The high degree of immunity was indicated by cross-protection against HSV-2,[28] and the presence of neutralizing antibody in mice after vaccination suggested that this was an important component of protection.[28] It is surprising that no evidence of MHC class-1 restricted CTL priming was obtained, although spleen cells did exhibit a proliferative response (J. Bennink, personal communication). This was consistent with the failure of cells infected with the gD recombinant virus to serve as targets for CTL from HSV-infected mice. Thus, the target antigens of mouse CTL remain to be determined. On the other hand, human CTL clones that lyse autologous cells infected with HSV-1 or HSV-2 were generated by stimulating lymphocytes with the recombinant vaccinia virus that expresses HSV-1 gD.[29] Furthermore, CTL clones generated with HSV-1 or cloned HSV-1 gD lysed autologous cells infected with the vaccinia recombinant.

INFLUENZA VIRUS

Influenza viruses contribute significantly to respiratory diseases in man and domesticated animals. Protection against influenza virus is type-specific and is mediated primarily by antibody to the hemagglutinin (HA), one of the two surface proteins.

Changes in the antigenicity of the HA, and to a lesser extent the neuraminidase, allow influenza virus to elude host defenses and make long-term immunization difficult. In contrast to the type specificity of neutralizing antibody, cytotoxic T cells are cross-reactive. Until recently, it was not known whether the cross-reactivity was due to conserved regions of the HA or to other more highly conserved internal proteins of influenza virus. Direct evidence for the latter has been obtained by using recombinant DNA-transformed and recombinant vaccinia virus-infected cells as targets.

Recombinant vaccinia viruses that express the influenza HA have been constructed.[30,31] The protein is properly glycosylated, is transported to the plasma membrane where it is cleavable into two subunits, and is reactive with a panel of monoclonal antibodies.[31,32] Antibody production has been demonstrated in experimental animals that have been vaccinated.[30,31] Moreover, intradermal vaccinations of hamsters and mice were shown to prevent lower respiratory infections in a type-specific manner.[31] Intranasal vaccination of mice, however, led to production of secretory IgA antibodies to HA and prevented both upper and lower respiratory infections.[20]

Vaccination of mice with the influenza HA recombinant vaccinia virus also produced a CTL priming effect that was predominantly type-specific.[23,32] An even greater CTL priming effect occurred after vaccination with an influenza nucleoprotein (NP) recombinant vaccinia virus, and CTLs from these animals had cross-type specificity.[33,34] Vaccination with the NP recombinant, however, did not prevent lower respiratory infection, although partial protection against lethality has been reported.[34] This result confirms the primary defensive role of neutralizing antibody against influenza virus. Nevertheless, efforts to enhance the immunogenicity of NP are being pursued because of the anticipated cross-type specificity.

HA and NP are not the only targets of influenza virus CTL. In mice, CTL directed against the nonstructural and polymerase proteins also have been demonstrated (J. R. Bennink, J. W. Yewdell, personal communication). The latter studies also revealed that CTL recognition of individual viral antigens occurs in conjunction with only a limited number of available class-I MHC restriction elements.

Determination of the target specificity of human CTL is difficult for several reasons. The HLA specificity of the CTL response poses a particular problem. By using recombinant vaccinia virus to prepare target cells *in vitro,* however, both target and effector cells can be derived from the same individual. With this type of protocol, evidence has been obtained that NP[35] and other internal proteins (F. Gotch, A. McMichael, personal communications) are human CTL targets.

RESPIRATORY SYNCYTIAL VIRUS

Respiratory syncytial virus (RSV) is the most important pediatric lower respiratory pathogen. At present an effective vaccine against this disease has not been developed, although there are data from animal models that neutralizing antibody can be protective. The two surface glycoproteins, G and F, are considered to be the most likely targets of a successful vaccine.

Recombinant vaccinia viruses that express either G[36,37] or F[38] have been constructed. The proteins produced by the recombinant viruses are glycosylated, processed, and transported to the plasma membrane of infected tissue culture cells. Intradermal vaccination of cotton rats, an experimental model for RSV, with either G or F recombinant, produced neutralizing antibodies and protected against lower respiratory infection.[37,38] In the case of the F recombinant, the level of neutralizing antibody was even higher than that which occurred after intranasal RSV infection, and protection against lower respiratory infection was as good. The intradermal route of inoculation with the F recombinant vaccinia virus diminished but did not prevent upper respiratory infection. The studies with influenza virus, summarized in the previous section, suggest the likelihood that intranasal inoculation would prevent both upper and lower respiratory infections. Continued studies with these and other RSV/vaccinia recombinants should provide valuable information regarding the targets and role of cell-mediated immunity.

VESICULAR STOMATITIS VIRUS AND RABIES VIRUS

Vesicular stomatitis virus (VSV) and rabies virus are both members of the rhabdovirus family. VSV causes significant infection of horses, cattle, and pigs, whereas rabies virus infects a variety of wild and domesticated animals as well as man. Both viruses contain a surface glycoprotein (G) that can induce neutralizing antibody, and inactivated and attenuated rabies virus vaccines have been developed.

The VSV G protein produced by recombinant vaccinia virus is glycosylated and expressed on the surface of infected cells.[21] When polarized cells were used, transport to the basolateral surface of the plasma membrane was demonstrated as in natural VSV infection.[17] Cattle that were vaccinated intradermally with the recombinant virus produced neutralizing antibody, and the majority were protected against direct lingual injection of VSV.[21]

CTL studies similar to those carried out with influenza virus were extended to VSV. The results were entirely consistent: CTL recognition of G was type-specific, whereas recognition of the internal nucleoprotein was cross-reactive.[39]

Recombinant vaccinia viruses that express the rabies virus G protein induce high levels of neutralizing antibody and protect a variety of animals against direct intracerebral inoculation with lethal doses of rabies virus.[40,41] Of potential practical importance, foxes inoculated orally were also protected against rabies.[42] This result raises the possibility of using bait vaccines to immunize wildlife.

FRIEND MURINE LEUKEMIA VIRUS (FMuLV)

The recent finding that certain human leukemias and the acquired immune deficiency syndrome (AIDS) are caused by retroviruses has greatly increased the interest in immune defenses against this class of viruses. While murine retrovirus infection should not be considered as a model for AIDS, considerable useful information may be derived. Friend virus complex, which consists of replication-competent FMuLV and replication-defective spleen-focus-forming virus, causes erythroleukemia and splenomegaly in newborn and adult mice. As with other retroviruses, FMuLV contains two envelope glycoproteins that are generated by cleavage of a precursor. Evidence has been obtained that repeated immunization with the envelope proteins can protect against murine leukemia.

The FMuLV envelope protein made by a recombinant vaccinia virus was glycosylated, transported to the plasma membrane, and correctly processed into large and small subunits.[43] In polarized cells, the protein appeared on the basolateral cell surface.[17] Mice that were vaccinated intradermally with the recombinant virus were protected against splenomegaly and leukemia when challenged with Friend virus complex several weeks later.[43] In order to understand the nature of the protection, several immune parameters were measured both before and after challenge. Before challenge, neutralizing antibody and CTL were difficult to detect, but spleen cells exhibited a specific proliferative response. After challenge, both neutralizing antibody and CTLs rapidly appeared, indicating that the animals had been primed. By contrast, control animals had a more delayed neutralizing antibody response and never developed a measurable CTL response. A second interesting finding was that seeding of the spleen with FMuLV was not entirely prevented by vaccination, but the vaccinated animals were able largely to clear their spleens of virus. Whether protection and recovery are due to CTL or antibody or both may be determined by further investigations.

EXPRESSION OF GENES OF OTHER VIRUSES AND PARASITES

We have not described in detail reports of expression of genes from certain other viruses because of the absence thus far of protection data. Nevertheless, it is worth mentioning the expression and processing of the envelope protein of the virus causing AIDS,[18,44] a surface glycoprotein of Epstein-Barr virus,[22] the spike glycoprotein of transmissible gastroenteritis virus of swine,[45] and Sindbis virus structural proteins.[46,47] The approaches described here may also find use in studies of other classes of infectious agents as demonstrated by expression of malarial circumsporozoite[48,49] and blood-stage secretory[50] antigens.

FUTURE PROSPECTS

It seems likely that vaccinia virus expression vectors will continue to be improved both with regard to efficiency of expression and convenience of construction. Increased expression may be achieved by using stronger natural or synthetic promoters, altering the site of gene insertion, and introducing multiple gene copies. One novel approach being explored involves the integration of a bacteriophage RNA polymerase gene into the genome of vaccinia virus. This allows the efficient and selective expression of coding segments containing bacteriophage promoters in transfected plasmids[51] or in a second recombinant vaccinia virus (T. Fuerst, B. Moss, personal communication).

Enhancement of the immunologic response either through antigen presentation or immune modulation also has been considered. An increased antibody response which resulted from the placing of a membrane anchor sequence on the end of a plasmodial secretory protein is an example of the former.[50] The placement of genes for interferon gamma[52] and interleukin-2[53] into the vaccinia virus genome represent attempts at the latter approach.

A third active area of research is directed toward altering the biological properties of the vaccinia virus vector. By inactivating the TK gene or deleting other gene segments, the pathogenicity of vaccinia virus can be sharply reduced.[54] Even the host range of vaccinia virus can be restricted by mutation.[55]

The value of recombinant vaccinia viruses for experimental immunology has been established, and new uses will undoubtedly be found. Serious consideration is also being given to the development of recombinant vaccinia viruses as vaccines for veterinary and medical purposes. It is a fact that the most widely used viral vaccines (e.g., for smallpox, poliomyelitis, measles, rubella, mumps, and yellow fever) are live attenuated viruses. Recombinant vaccinia viruses maintain many of the advantages of live virus vaccines, particularly with regard to stimulation of cell-mediated immunity, economical production, and simple delivery for mass immunization, while eliminating certain hazards such as reversion to virulence. The impressive degree of protection obtained in immunizing foxes with a rabies G protein recombinant opens up the possibility of wildlife vaccination.[42] Similarly, the resistance of cotton rats to RSV induced by recombinant vaccinia viruses that express the RSV G or F proteins suggests possible human application.[37–39] Development of effective and safe recombinant vaccinia virus vaccines for hepatitis B, Epstein-Barr, and malaria would surely benefit underdeveloped areas of the world. Individual and environmental safety is, of course, a major concern with all live vaccines, whether developed by attenuation or by recombinant DNA methods.[56] Experience with smallpox vaccination indicates that serious complications varied with the vaccine strain and were relatively rare with some. Even more attenuated strains were developed, but were not used on a large scale because of the overriding necessity of eradicating smallpox. Either these attenuated strains or new ones developed by genetic engineering may provide vectors with low risk relative to potential benefits.

REFERENCES

1. JENNER, E. 1778. An Inquiry into the Causes and Effects of the Variolae Vaccinae, a Disease Discovered in Some of the Western Counties of England, Particularly Gloucestershire, and Known by the Name of the Cow Pox. Sampson Low. London.
2. MACKETT, M. & L. C. ARCHARD. 1979. Conservation and variation in orthopoxvirus genome structure. J. Gen. Virol. **47:** 683-701.
3. FENNER, F. 1985. Poxviruses. *In* Virology. B. N. Fields, D . M. Knipe, R. M. Chanock, J. L. Melnick, B. Roizman & R. E. Shope, Eds.: 661-84. Raven. New York.
4. MOSS, B. 1985. Replication of poxviruses. See Ref. 3: 685-704.
5. COCHRAN, M. A., C. PUCKETT & B. MOSS. 1985. In vitro mutagenesis of the promoter region for a vaccinia virus gene: Evidence for tandem early and late regulatory signals. J. Virol. **54:** 30-37.
6. PANICALI, D. & E. PAOLETTI. 1982. Construction of poxviruses as cloning vectors: Insertion of the thymidine kinase gene from herpes simplex virus into the DNA of infectious vaccinia virus. Proc. Natl. Acad. Sci. USA **79:** 4927-4931.
7. MACKETT, M., G. L. SMITH & B. MOSS. 1982. Vaccinia virus: A selectable eukaryotic cloning and expression vector. Proc. Natl. Acad. Sci. USA **79:** 7415-7419.
8. MACKETT, M., G. L. SMITH & B. MOSS. 1982. A general method for the production and selection of infectious vaccinia virus recombinants expressing foreign genes. J. Virol. **49:** 857-864.
9. MACKETT, M., G. L. SMITH & B. MOSS. 1985. The construction and characterization of vaccinia virus recombinants expressing foreign genes. *In* DNA Cloning, Vol. II. D. M. Glover, Ed.:191-212. IRL Press. Oxford.
10. CHAKRABARTI, S., K. BRECHLING & B. MOSS. 1985. Vaccinia virus expression vector: Coexpression of β-galactosidase provides visual screening of recombinant virus plaques. Mol. Cell. Biol. **5:** 3403-3409.
11. SMITH, G. L. & B. MOSS. 1983. Infectious poxvirus vectors have capacity for at least 25,000 base pairs of foreign DNA. Gene **25:** 21-28.

12. PANICALI, D., S. W. DAVIS, S. R. MERCER & E. PAOLETTI. 1981. Two major DNA variants present in serially propagated stocks of the WR strain of vaccinia virus. J. Virol. **40:** 1000-1010.
13. MOSS, B., E. WINTERS & J. A. COOPER. 1981. Deletion of a 9,000 base pair segment of the vaccinia virus genome that encodes non-essential polypeptides. J. Virol. **40:** 387-395.
14. WEIR, J. P. & B. MOSS. 1984. Regulation of expression and nucleotide sequence of a late vaccinia virus gene. J. Virol. **51:** 662-669.
15. SMITH, G. L., M. MACKETT & B. MOSS. 1983. Infectious vaccinia virus recombinants that express hepatitis B virus surface antigen. Nature **302:** 490-495.
16. PERKUS, M. E., A. PICCINI, B. R. LIPINSKAS & E. PAOLETTI. 1985. Recombinant vaccinia virus: Immunization against multiple pathogens. Science **229:** 981-984.
17. STEPHENS, E. B., R. W. COMPANS, P. EARL & B. MOSS. 1986. Surface expression of viral glycoproteins is polarized in epithelial cells infected with recombinant vaccinia viral vectors. EMBO J. **5:** 237-245.
18. CHAKRABARTI, S., M. ROBERT-GUROFF, F. WONG-STALL, R. C. GALLO & B. MOSS. 1986. Expression of the HTVL-III envelope gene by a recombinant vaccinia virus. Nature **320:** 535-537.
19. THOMAS, G., E. HERBERT & D. E. HRUBY. 1986. Expression and cell-type-specific processing of human preproenkephalin with a vaccinia recombinant. Science **232:** 1641-1646.
20. SMALL, P. A., G. L. SMITH & B. MOSS. 1985. Intranasal vaccination with a recombinant vaccinia virus containing influenza hemagglutinin prevents both influenza virus pneumonia and nasal infection: Intradermal vaccination prevents only viral pneumonia. *In* Vaccines 85. Molecular and Chemical Basis of Resistance to Parasitic, Bacterial and Viral Diseases. R. A. Lerner, R. M. Chanock, F. Brown. Eds.: 175-176. Cold Spring Harbor, NY. Cold Spring Harbor Laboratory.
21. MACKETT, M., T. YILMA, J. K. ROSE & B. MOSS. 1985. Vaccinia virus recombinants: Expression of VSV genes and protective immunization of mice and cattle. Science **227:** 433-435.
22. MACKETT, M. & J. R. ARRAND. 1985. Recombinant vaccinia virus induces neutralizing antibodies in rabbits against Epstein-Barr virus membrane antigen gp 340. EMBO J. **4:** 3229-3234.
23. BENNINK, J. R., J. W. YEWDELL, G. L. SMITH, C. MOLLER & B. MOSS. 1984. Recombinant vaccinia virus primes and stimulates influenza virus HA-specific CTL. Nature **311:** 578-579.
24. PAOLETTI, E., B. R. LIPINSKAS, C. SAMSONOFF, S. R. MERCER & D. PANICALI. 1984. Construction of live vaccines using genetically engineered poxviruses: Biological activity of vaccinia virus recombinants expressing the hepatitis B virus surface antigen and the herpes simplex virus glycoprotein D. Proc. Natl. Acad. Sci. USA **81:** 193-197.
25. MOSS, B., G. L. SMITH, J. L. GERIN & R. H. PURCELL. 1984. Live recombinant vaccinia virus protects chimpanzees against hepatitis B. Nature **311:** 67-69.
26. CHENG, K.-C & B. MOSS. 1987. Selective synthesis and secretion of particles composed of the hepatitis B virus middle surface protein directed by a recombinant vaccinia virus; induction of antibodies to pre-S and S epitopes. J. Virol. **61:** 1286-1290.
27. CHENG, K.-C, G. L. SMITH & B. MOSS. 1986. Hepatitis B virus large surface protein is not secreted but is immunogenic when selectively expressed by recombinant vaccinia virus. J. Virol. **60:** 337-344.
28. CREMER, K. J., M. MACKETT, C. WOHLENBERG, A. L. NOTKINS & B. MOSS. 1985. Vaccinia virus recombinant expressing herpes simplex virus type 1 glycoprotein D prevents latent herpes in mice. Science **228:** 737-740.
29. ZARLING, J. M., P. A. MORAN, L. A. LASKY & B. MOSS. 1986. Herpes simplex virus (HSV)-specific human T-cell clones recognize HSV glycoprotein D expressed by a recombinant vaccinia virus. J. Virol. **59:** 506-509.
30. PANICALI, D., S. W. DAVIS, R. L. WEINBERG & E. PAOLETTI. 1983. Construction of live vaccines by using genetically engineered poxviruses: Biological activity of recombinant vaccinia virus expressing influenza virus hemagglutinin. Proc. Natl. Acad. Sci. USA **80:** 5364-5368.
31. SMITH, G. L., B. R. MURPHY & B. MOSS. Construction and characterization of an infectious vaccinia virus recombinant that expresses the influenza hemagglutinin gene and induces

resistance to influenza virus infection in hamsters. Proc. Natl. Acad. Sci. USA **80:** 7155-7159.
32. BENNINK, J. R., J. W. YEWDELL, G. L. SMITH & B. MOSS. 1986. Recognition of cloned influenza virus hemagglutinin gene products by cytotoxic T lymphocytes. J. Virol. **57:** 786-791.
33. YEWDELL, J. W., J. R. BENNINK, G. L. SMITH & B. MOSS. 1985. Influenza A virus nucleoprotein is a major target antigen for cross-reactive anti-influenza A virus cytotoxic T lymphocytes. Proc. Natl. Acad. Sci. USA **82:** 1785-1789.
34. ANDREW, M. E., B. E. H., COUPAR, G. L. ADA & D. B. BOYLE. 1986. Cell-mediated immune response to influenza virus antigens expressed by vaccinia virus recombinants. Microb. Path. **1:** 443-452.
35. MCMICHAEL, A. J., C. A. MICHIE, F. M. GOTCH, G. L. SMITH & B. MOSS. 1986. Recognition of influenza A virus nucleoprotein by human cytotoxic T lymphocytes. J. Gen. Virol. **67:** 719-726.
36. BALL, L. A., K. K. Y. YOUNG, K. ANDERSON, P. L. COLLINS & G. W. WERTZ. 1986. Expression of the major glycoprotein G of human respiratory syncytial virus from recombinant vaccinia virus vectors. Proc. Natl. Acad. Sci. USA **83:** 246-250.
37. ELANGO, N., G. A. PRINCE, B. R. MURPHY, S. VENKATESAN, R. M. CHANOCK & B. MOSS. 1986. Resistance to human respiratory syncytial virus (RSV) infection induced by immunization of cotton rats with a recombinant vaccinia virus expressing the RSV G glycoprotein. Proc. Natl. Acad. Sci. USA **83:** 1906-1910.
38. OLMSTED, R. A., N. ELANGO, G. H. PRINCE, B. R. MURPHY, P. R. JOHNSON, B. MOSS, R. M. CHANOCK & P. L. COLLINS. 1986. Expression of the F glycoprotein of respiratory syncytial virus by a recombinant vaccinia virus: Comparison of the individual contributions of the F and G glycoproteins to host immunity. Proc. Natl. Acad. Sci. USA **83:** 7462-7466.
39. YEWDELL, J. W., J. R. BENNINK, M. MACKETT, L. LEFRANCOIS, D. S. LYLES & B. MOSS. 1986. Recognition of cloned vesicular stomatitis virus internal and external gene products by cytotoxic T lymphocytes. J. Exp. Med. **163:** 1529-1539.
40. KIENY, M. P., R. LATHE, R. DRILLIEN, D. SPEHNER, S. SKORY, D. SCHMITT, T. WIKTOR, H. KOPROWSKI & J. P. LECOCQ. 1984. Expression of rabies virus glycoprotein from a recombinant vaccinia virus. Nature **312:** 163-166.
41. WIKTOR, T. J., R. I. MACFARLAN, K. J. REAGAN, B. DIETZSCHOLD, P. J. CURTIS, W. H. WUNNER, M.-P. KIENY, R. LATHE, J.-P. LECOCQ, M HOCKETT, B. MOSS & H. KOPROWSKI. 1984. Protection from rabies by a vccinia virus recombinant containing the rabies virus glycoprotein gene. Proc. Natl. Acad. Sci. USA **81:** 7194-7198.
42. BLANCOU, J., M. P. KIENY, R. LATHE, J. P. LECOCQ, P. P. PASTORET, J. P. SOULEBOT & P. DESMETTRE. 1986. Oral vaccination of the fox against rabies using a live recombinant vaccinia virus. Nature **322:** 373-375.
43. EARL, P. L., B. MOSS, K. WEHRLY, J. NISHIO & B. CHESEBRO. 1986. T cell priming and protection against Friend murine leukemia by a recombinant vaccinia virus expressing env gene. Science. **234:** 728-731.
44. HU, S., S. G. KOSOWSKI & J. M. DALRYMPLE. 1986. Expression of AIDS virus envelope gene in recombinant vaccinia viruses. Nature **320:** 537-540.
45. HU, S., J. BRUSZEWSKI, R. SMALLING & J. K. BROWNE. 1985. Studies of TGEV spike protein gp 195 expressed in *E. coli* and by a TGE-vaccinia virus recombinant. Adv. Exp. Med. Biol. **185:** 63-82.
46. RICE, C. M., C. A. FRANKE, J. H. STRAUSS & D. R. HRUBY. 1985. Expression of sindbis virus structural proteins via recombinant vaccinia virus: Synthesis, processing, and incorporation into mature sindbis virions. J. Virol. **56:** 227-239.
47. FRANKE, C. A., E. S. BERRY, A. W. SMITH & D. E. HRUBY. 1985. Immunization of cattle with a recombinant togavirus-vaccinia virus strain. Res. Vet. Sci. **39:** 113-115.
48. SMITH, G. L., G. N. GODSON, V. NUSSENZWEIG, R. S. NUSSENZWEIG, J. BARNWELL & B. MOSS. 1984. Plasmodium knowlesi sporozoite antigen: Expression by infectious recombinant vaccinia virus. Science **224:** 397-399.
49. CHENG, K. C., G. L. SMITH B. MOSS, F. ZAVALA, R. NUSSENZWEIG & V. NUSSENZWEIG. 1986. Expression of malaria circumsporozoite protein and hepatitis-B virus surface an-

tigen by infectious vaccinia virus. *In* Vaccines 86. F. Brown, R. M. Chanock & R. A. Lerner, Eds.: 165-168. Cold Spring Harbor Laboratory. Cold Spring Harbor, NY.

50. LANGFORD, C. J., S. J. EDWARDS, G. L. SMITH, B. MOSS, D. J. KEMP, R. F. ANDERS & G. F. MITCHELL. 1986. Anchoring a secreted plasmodium antigen on the surface of recombinant vaccinia virus-infected cells increases its immunogenicity. Mol. Cell. Biol. **6:** 3191-3199.
51. FUERST, T. R., E. G. NILES, F. W. STUDIER & B. MOSS. 1986. Eukaryotic transient expression system based on recombinant vaccinia virus that synthesizes bacteriophage T7 RNA polymerase. Proc. Natl. Acad. Sci. USA **83:** 8122-8126.
52. YILMA, T., K. ANDERSON, K. BRECHLING, & B. MOSS. 1987. Expression of an adjuvant gene (interferon-γ) in infectious vaccinia virus recombinants. *In* Vaccines 87. R. M. Chanock, R. A. Lerner and H. Ginsberg, Eds.: 393-396. Cold Spring Harbor Laboratory. Cold Spring Harbor, NY.
53. FLEXNER, C., A. HÜGIN & B. MOSS. 1986. Expression of human interleukin-2 by live recombinant vaccinia virus. *In* Ref. 52: 380-383.
54. BULLER, R. M. L., G. L. SMITH, K. CREMER, A. L. NOTKINS & B. MOSS. 1985. Decreased virulence of recombinant vaccinia virus expression vectors is associated with a thymidine kinase-negative phenotype. Nature **317:** 813-815.
55. GILLARD, S. D., SPEHNER, R. DRILLIEN & A. KIRN. 1986. Localization and sequence of a vaccinia virus gene required for multiplication in human cells. Proc. Natl. Acad. Sci. USA **83:** 5573-5577.
56. BROWN, F., G. C. SCHILD & G. L. ADA. 1986. Recombinant vaccinia viruses as vaccines. Nature **319:** 549-550.
57. DE LASALLE, W. ALTENBURGER, R. ELKAIM, K. DOTT, A. DIETERLÉ, R. DRILLIEN, J.-P. CAZENAV, P. TOLSTOSHEV & J.-P. LECOCQ. 1985. Active γ-carboxylated human factor IX expressed using recombinant DNA techniques. Nature **316:** 268-270.
58. JONES, L, S. RISTOW, T. YILMA & B. MOSS. 1986. Accidental human vaccination with vaccinia virus expressing nucleoprotein gene. Nature **316:** 543.

Strategies for Genetic Modification of Parasites

RONALD W. DAVIS

Department of Biochemistry
Stanford University School of Medicine
Palo Alto, California 94305

To define the genetics of a new organism is usually very expensive and time-consuming, as exemplified by the few organisms for which extensive genetic analysis has been carried out. However, modern genetics is an extraordinarily powerful tool that ought to be applied to a large number of organisms, particularly those that cause disease.

This is an exciting time for genetics. We are in the midst of developing new technologies that can profoundly simplify genetic approaches to new organisms. One example is the development of restriction fragment length polymorphism (RFLP) mapping,[1] which is being applied to the human genome. That mapping strategy has proceeded a great deal faster than had been expected, and, in fact, we presently have a 3-centimorgan map of chromosome 7, and overall, about a 10-centimorgan map of the human genome.[2] (A centimorgan is approximately a million base pairs). Because of the increased emphasis on mapping the human genome and the search for human disease associations, it is clear that we will probably have a 1-centimorgan map of the human genome in a matter of a few years.

To effectively analyze the genetics of an organism has in the past required a well-defined sexual cycle. That is indeed true for humans, but there are a great number of organisms of interest and importance that do not exhibit a sexual cycle, or, if they do, it is extremely difficult to manipulate. However, we would like to apply the power of genetics to identify and characterize genes for important functions. Indeed, the basic reason one carries out genetic mapping is to identify single, or even multiple genes involved in particular functions or susceptibilities. But, for those organisms without a well-defined sexual cycle, a new approach is needed for carrying out genetics, essentially in mitotic cells. Because I believe that progress is being made towards achieving this goal, I would like to discuss some general approaches to what I hope will become a generic approach for genetics of important organisms. It would allow the same kinds of mutational analysis that are classically done in other organisms that have a defined sexual cycle, as well as permitting the mapping and localization of genes and functions.

Let me begin by outlining a few very simple principles, many of which were first learned and developed in a simple eukaryotic organism, baker's yeast. The approach was a rational general strategy, which has been extremely successful in developing yeast genetics, many aspects of which should be applicable to a whole variety of organisms, including protozoa as well as humans and higher plants. In carrying out this kind of manipulative genetics, including the application of recombinant DNA technology, it is obvious that one needs a dominant drug-resistance marker, or its equivalent and one similar to the classical selectable marker traditionally used in bacteria (FIG. 1). A dominant drug-resistance marker enables one to select for acquisition of a new segment of DNA by covalently coupling it to the marker and selecting for drug resistance after DNA-mediated transformation.

What is less widely appreciated and equally important is the need for another marker that does just the opposite, that is, provides the ability to eliminate DNA. One means of achieving this type of negative selection is to develop a dominant drug-sensitive marker. There are currently about eight such dominant drug-sensitive markers in use for yeast. An example is a gene coding for a permease that promotes the import of a toxic drug. If the organism already contains such a permease gene, then a mutant organism can often be directly selected that will not take up the particular drug because of a lesion in the permease gene. The gene for the permease becomes a dominant drug-sensitive marker. If the permease gene is now introduced, for example in a plasmid, the organism now becomes sensitive to the drug and can be selected against. Other examples of dominant drug-sensitive markers are genes encoding enzymes that carry out reactions that become toxic to cells. Dominant drug-sensitive markers allow one to select against organisms containing these DNA molecules, and the power of how they can be used will be illustrated through several examples.

In general, then, what is needed to carry out genetic analysis and manipulation are DNA molecules containing two markers—a dominant drug-resistance and a dominant drug-sensitivity marker. The strategy described below has been effective in *Saccharomyces cerevisiae* or baker's yeast, *Candida albicans,* and *Schizosaccharomyces pombe,* and appears to be equally effective for the *Mycobacteria.* For example, in organisms that synthesize their own uracil, a drug is used which, if metabolized and taken up in the uracil pathway, produces toxic products. Cells that are resistant to this drug are no longer able to make uracil. In the case of yeast, the gene that is generally targeted is the URA 3 gene. For example, if we have a segment of DNA, as illustrated in FIGURE 1, connected to this uracil gene, we can select for its presence by withdrawing uracil from the medium. If this gene is present, the cells will grow; in the absence of the gene, they will not. However, in the presence of uracil and in the presence of a chemical analogue, 5-FOA (5-fluoroorotic acid), the same enzyme makes a toxic product for the cell, presumably because of incorporation of 5-FOA

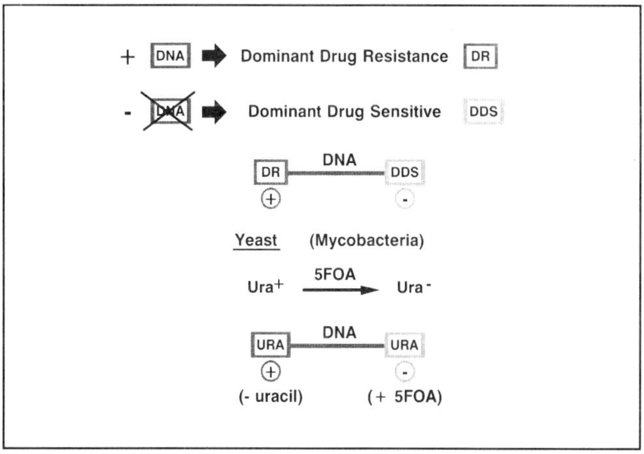

FIGURE 1.

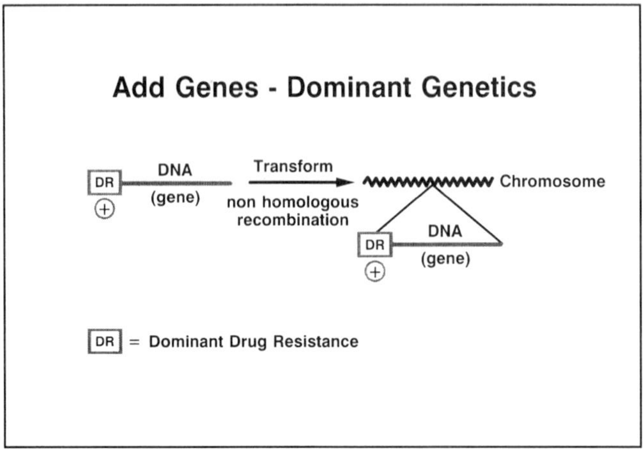

FIGURE 2.

into RNA.[3] Thus, by depriving cells of uracil, we can select for genes in DNA fragments linked to URA 3, which provide uracil. In the presence of 5-FOA and uracil, we can kill cells that have the same gene. Here a single gene provides both dominant drug-resistance and a dominant drug-sensitive function.

Dominant drug-resistance markers can be used in precisely the same way that classical drug-resistance markers have been used in bacteria: to be able to add a gene to a cell (FIG. 2). In the simplest case, one connects the gene of interest to a resistance marker and then transforms the cell. This allows new genes to be introduced into the cell and to be integrated into some chromosome by selecting for the resistance marker. While this strategy is widely used in plants and mammalian cells, it is not so widely used for doing genetic experiments in yeast because it only allows one to do dominant genetics. Adding genes can be useful, but usually the study of dominant genes is not

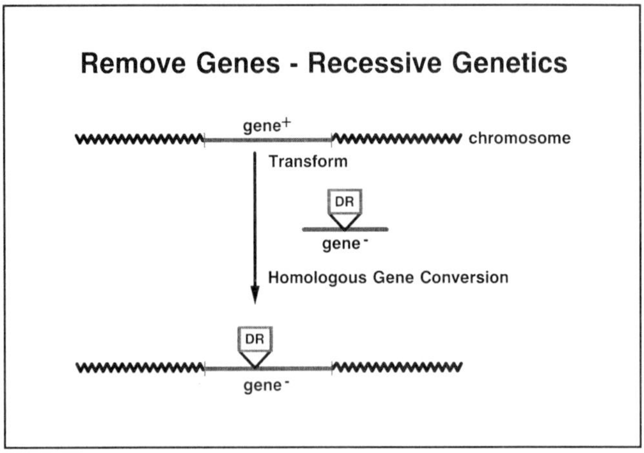

FIGURE 3.

sufficient to allow understanding of how the organism works. What is sought is the ability to understand and manipulate genes that already exist within the organism. Adding extra copies does not give us much of a clue as to how the gene functions. Making mutations in such genes that become dominant in some way or become dominant nonfunctional (such as anti-sense RNA) is often complex, may not always be possible, and can be misleading. This is an intrinsic limitation to dominant genetics.

Selective gene disruption or deletion is a much more powerful tool for genetic analysis. Removing a gene, often called transplacement,[4] gives one the ability to analyze recessive genes, which represent the bulk of all genetics in all organisms. In yeast, in the generic approach, there are several ways of accomplishing this task. One can introduce the drug-resistance markers into the middle of the gene such that the insertion disrupts the function of the gene, and, by homologous gene conversion, one can replace or transplace (transformation followed by gene replacement) the wild-type gene with the insertionally inactivated gene containing the resistance marker (FIG. 3). The key here is homologous recombination. All organisms are likely to have

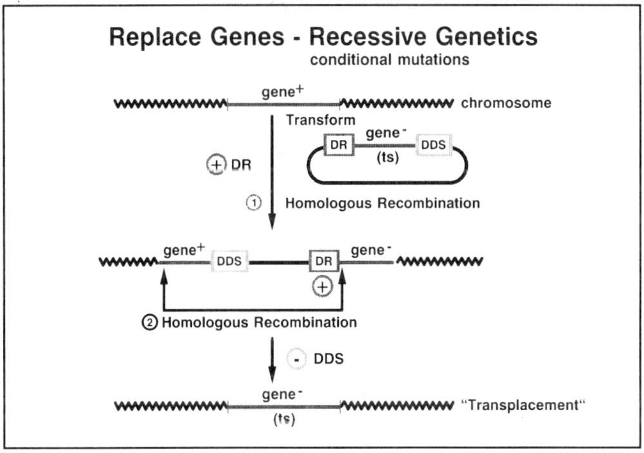

FIGURE 4.

homologous recombination and the major limitation geneticists have experienced is that many organisms also have nonhomologous recombination, which limits the application of this powerful approach. The other limitation of this approach is the fact that the introduction of the resistance marker in the middle of the gene of interest generally totally destroys the function of that gene. Although this is the original intent and is wonderful for analyzing the function of the gene, it is not so useful if the gene is essential for viability of the organism. It is not very helpful to learn that the gene's function is essential to life and that mutation or gene disruption simply leads to death of the organism. It is obviously difficult to do genetic experiments on an organism and gain an understanding of precisely what the gene does, when the mutation in the gene of interest is lethal.

Consequently, another approach is needed, such as conditional mutations, rather than gene disruption. This approach works very well in yeast and bacteria, and phage lambda, which has extraordinarily well-studied genetic systems. This approach is a bit more complicated, and is illustrated in FIGURE 4. The task is to transplace a functional gene with a new version that is, for example, temperature-sensitive. The most straightforward way to accomplish this is to insert the gene of interest between the two markers, the dominant drug-resistance marker and the dominant drug-sensitive marker. One then transforms and identifies the homologous recombinants. In yeast, this is very easy because that is all one gets and the recombinants are identified by selecting for the resistance marker. Thus, there are two copies of the gene: one will be the wild-type gene and the other the conditional functioning gene. The two markers will be located between the two gene copies. The wild-type gene is then eliminated. This is accomplished by a second homologous recombination, on the other side of the gene. That can occur spontaneously either by mitotic loopout or, most commonly, by sister chromatid exchange or gene conversion. Such recombination eliminates all the DNA between the two gene copies and can be readily found by selecting for organisms that lost the dominant drug-sensitive marker. Some of the recombinants have replaced the wild-type gene with the conditional lethal gene. This genetic strategy is extraordinarily efficient in yeast, and could probably be effectively applied to many

Problems

1. DR & DDS Markers
2. Gene Structure
   Functional Unit
3. Homologous Recombination
   Autonomous Replication & Segregation
4. Transformation

FIGURE 5.

other organisms. Transplacing genes is a powerful tool that is necessary to analyze the genetics of any organism.

It would appear that scientists contemplating genetic approaches to protozoa have been concerned about a long list of problems in trying to attack the genetics of these new organisms (FIG. 5). What is not appreciated perhaps is that these are the same problems that all new organisms have faced. Most researchers would list transformation as the first problem, but, in fact, that is probably a mistake. It is very easy to get preoccupied with the difficulties and technical problems in efficient transformation of a new organism. Transformation is not yet a science, it is an art; so one does not rationally know what one is doing. The approach remains essentially empirical in varying a not very clearly defined set of variables. The best approach is to first make a real effort at getting selectable markers that one can be certain will function when placed in an organism, and then to provide a method for maintenance of that sequence either autonomously or by chromosomal integration. As it has turned out, in all organisms where these conditions (i.e., the development of appropriate selectable markers) are met, transformation has not been the limiting problem. For example, several groups had been attempting to transform yeast for about 20 years with a total lack of success. They incorrectly concluded that yeast could not be transformed. But they were unsuccessful because they did not develop markers that they knew would function and could be selected and that they knew would not give cell growth without transformation. Once those markers were developed, the transformation took approximately one week to solve! You can spend an endless amount of time wondering how in the world you could possibly get a DNA molecule that will occupy a space larger than the cell into a cell, and you would not find solid answers. The best strategy is to construct molecules with appropriate selectable markers that can be found and selected even as rare events. Once those rare events are found, transformation becomes more of a science and one can readily optimize conditions for those events.

Another approach that we have been developing for a variety of organisms may overcome some of the empirical difficulties associated with transformation. It will also have significant implications for analyzing gene structure and homologous recombination. The strategy is to try to create artificial chromosomes. This has been done in yeast and we are currently trying to do this with human chromosomes, and those of higher plants and protozoa.

On the basis of what we know, it should be possible to construct artificial chromosomes, which, when incorporated back into the organisms, are fully capable of functioning and replicating (FIG. 6). This approach not only will allow us to overcome the need to achieve homologous recombination, but will also permit us to modify these chromosomes *in vitro* or in various hosts such as yeast, and then return them to the organism of interest. The components that are necessary for chromosomal stability in yeast are: (i) a centromere, which is required for maintaining a chromosome in a cell; (ii) autonomous replicating sequences, which are origins of replication that initiate replication appropriately in the cell cycle; (iii) telomeres, which are required for chromosomal replication; and, of course, (iv) appropriate selectable markers (FIG. 7). Autonomous replicating sequences (ARS) are origins of replication that are found frequently in chromosomes, on the order of 100 kilobases apart. The centromere is the most complex of the structures, although it has turned out to be relatively simple for yeast. We have just successfully identified and purified to homogeneity one of the proteins that interacts with a yeast centromere and we have now cloned the gene.[5] We hope that it will lead to a better understanding of the kinetochore structure that is involved in maintaining and segregating chromosomes. These elements can then be used to make vectors for eukaryotic cells, very similar to phage lambda cloning vectors in bacteria. The principal difference is capacity. For example, a yeast artificial chromosome[6] can be made by introducing high molecular weight DNA fragments, between 0.1 and several megabases in size, between two fragments, one containing a selectable marker and a telomere, and the other containing a centromere and a telomere. In the case of yeast, we use auxotrophic complementation and not drug selection, because they are generally nonreverting. By appropriate molecular ligation events, it is possible to drive these reactions almost to completion to produce effective vectors.

We have made libraries starting with total human genomic DNA and a yeast artificial chromosome vector (YAC)[7] (FIG. 8). In addition, we[8] have made human chromosome-7-specific libraries, and have begun to physically map human chromosome 7. Physical mapping is not actually as difficult as it may seem, because the hybrid molecules are linear and the vector ends are very short with unique sequences. One has only to partially digest the hybrid molecules, separate the resulting fragments by pulse field gel electrophoresis (FIG. 9), and probe for unique vector sequences on

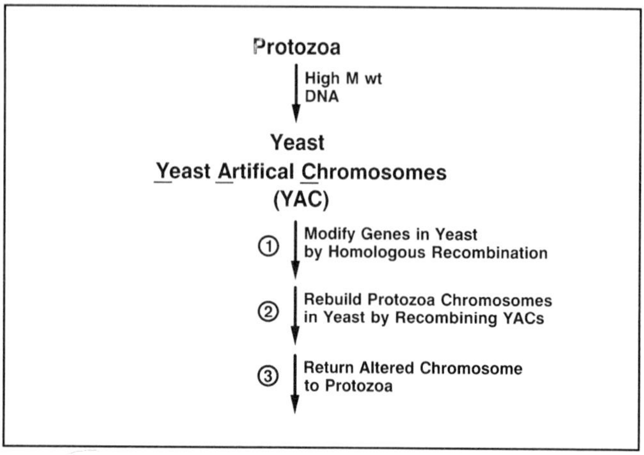

FIGURE 6.

either side of the cloned DNA. The pulse field electrophoresis apparatus that we have developed in our laboratory is called contour clamped homogeneous field (CHEF) electrophoresis; it switches the electric field 120 degrees using a hexagonal array of electrodes, where all the electrode potentials are uniquely defined electronically such that a homogeneous electrical field is generated[8] (FIG. 10). The electric field is switched with a given frequency usually ranging from a few seconds to a few hours. When the field angle is switched at 120 degrees, the molecules realign, ultimately leading to different mobilities on the basis of molecular weight. FIGURE 11 illustrates an example of chromosomal separations from *Saccharomyces cerevisiae* by CHEF gels, the smallest chromosomes being 230 kilobases, and the largest in the range of 2.5 megabases. Molecules as large as 15 megabases have been separated.[9] What is perhaps most

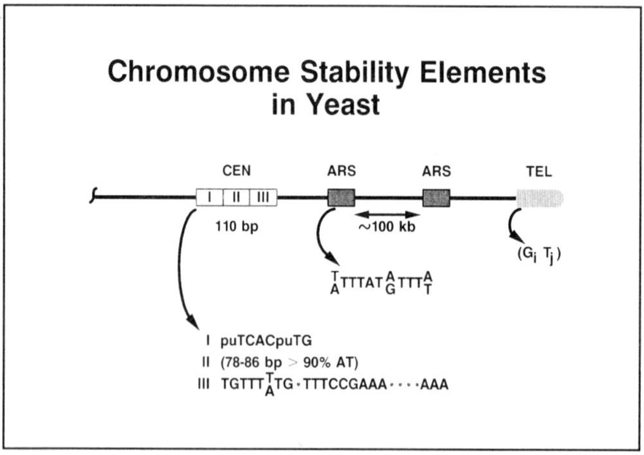

FIGURE 7.

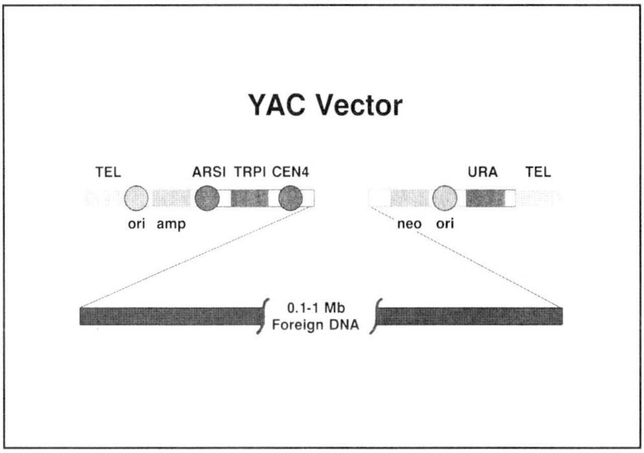

FIGURE 8.

extraordinary, since we are using DNA molecules that in extended linear form would be approximately 1 centimeter long, is that there is so little DNA degradation. As the DNA increases in size, the bands broaden.

In the case of yeast cloning, because of shearing during DNA transfers, our practical current cloning limits appear to be in the range of about 3 megabases. Further, since higher efficiencies of transformation seem to be obtained with smaller molecules, libraries of smaller molecules may be more efficient. We can now "replica plate" directly from the transformation plates, minimizing multiple manipulations with total genomic libraries. An entire genomic library from an organism can be stored on a few petri dishes and replicated onto nitrocellulose and frozen with glycerol at −80°C.[7] Thus, individual chromosomes or recombinants can be isolated, arrayed, and re-replicated readily and distributed to a number of laboratories.

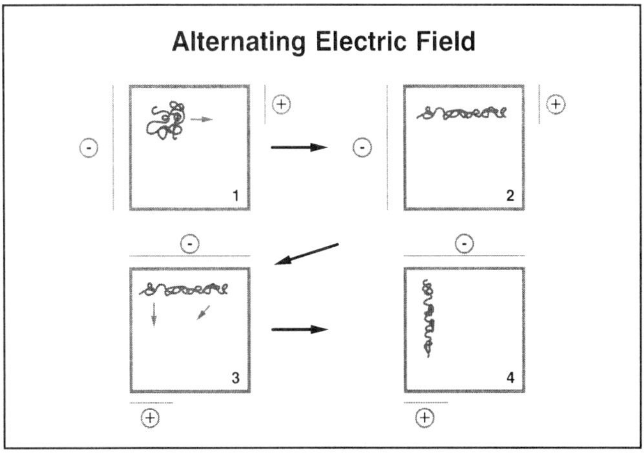

FIGURE 9.

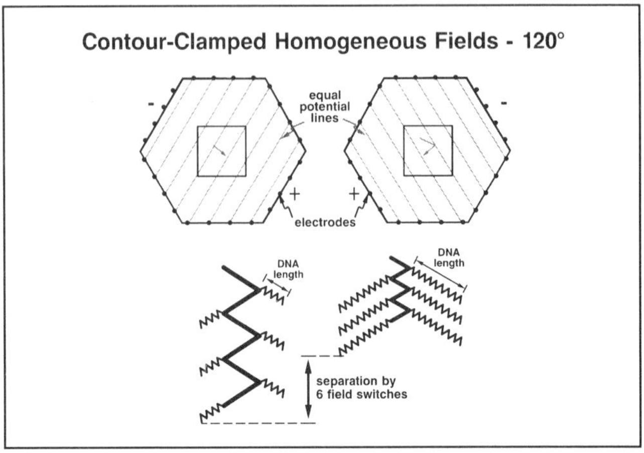

FIGURE 10.

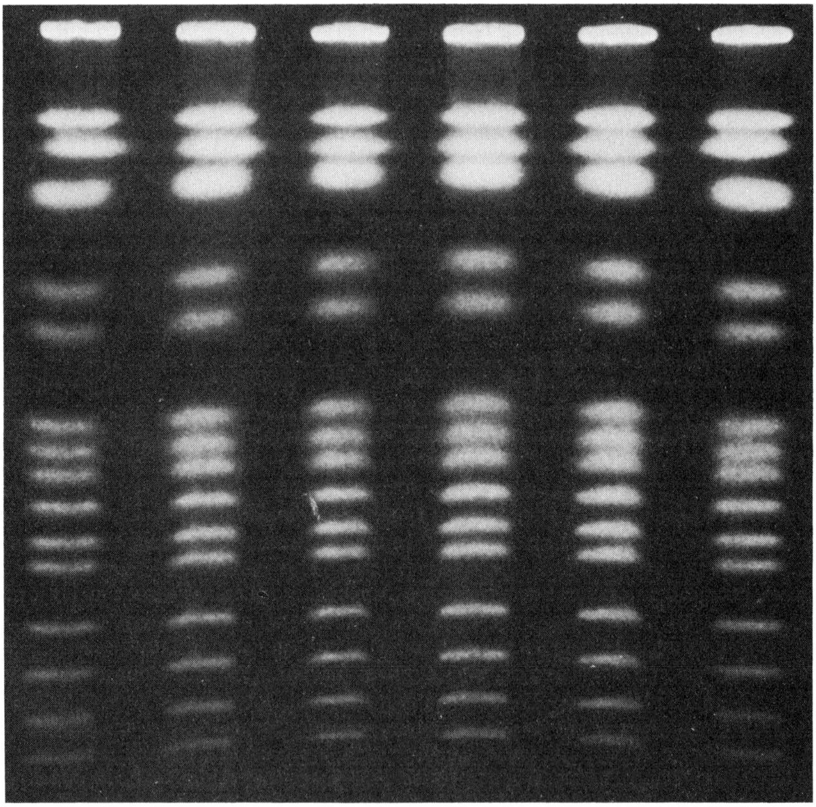

FIGURE 11.

These methods should be very applicable and effective with smaller genomes, including the protozoal and possible metazoal parasites. One should be able to readily physically map an organism with a genome size of about 50 million base pairs. This is a reasonable project for a single scientist to accomplish in one year. The technology is advancing so rapidly that things that five years ago were considered impossible to do are now highly feasible.

A great deal can be done with such clones, largely because of the way these new vectors are constructed. For example, if it is important to have adjacent or contiguous clones ("contigs"), this can be accomplished using a "walking" strategy. In principle, the number of manipulations involved in walking can be minimized by using vectors built with dominant resistance markers (in this case auxotropic complementation markers) on one end and dominant sensitive markers on other.[10] This is illustrated in FIGURE 12. A library is made in a yeast cell line having one mating type (*a* mating type). One can then find all clones in that library that have homologous DNA

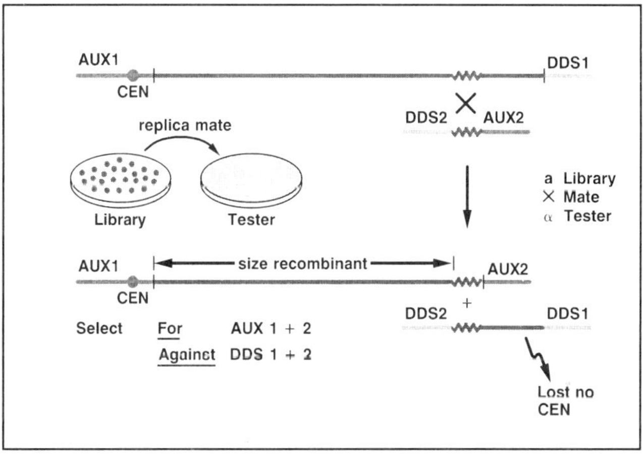

Yeast Chromosome Walking

FIGURE 12.

sequences by making a "tester" sequence in the opposite mating type (α mating type) which is placed in a small linear vector that lacks a centromere. To find the clones with homologous DNA sequences, all one has to do is to replica plate the library onto a "lawn" of the tester strain. Recombination can occur if there are homologous sequences. When such a recombination occurs, both dominant drug-sensitive markers will end up on the same linear molecule, which is then lost very easily because it has no centromere. At the same time, both of the auxotrophic markers will end up on the same chromosome, and one can readily select for both markers. The recombinants are identified as having lost both drug-sensitive markers while retaining both auxotrophic markers. The advantage of this strategy is that one can size both the original and the homologous recombinant with the tester sequence clones directly on CHEF gels. This will directly determine the position and orientation of the particular sequence relative to the whole clone, so that a restriction map does not have to be made for this determination. This is a general strategy that should work for identifying homologous sequences and mapping clones. It has the virtue of not even requiring

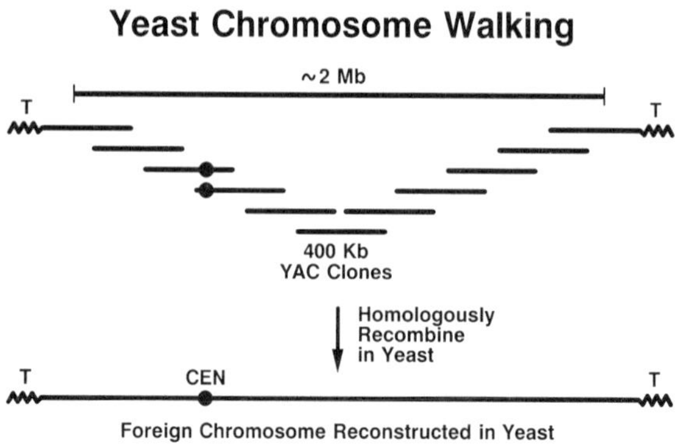

FIGURE 13.

radioactive labeling, merely simple replica plating. Using this strategy to find overlapping clones, one can "walk," as shown in FIGURE 13. With 400-kilobase clones it would take very few "steps" to walk about 2-megabase pairs, which is in the range of entire chromosomes of many parasites.

In the case of organisms containing chromosomes of about 2 megabases, even if the entire chromosome cannot be cloned directly, one could reconstruct and maintain it in yeast. Presumably the chromosome reconstructed in yeast would be maintained, and could function when transformed back into the organism from which it is derived. This type of reconstruction would allow understanding of how chromosomes are maintained in the species of interest, for example, whether there is a centromere, where it is, and so forth. We are currently engaged in applying this approach to parasites and simpler plants that have small chromosomes. We hope to isolate all the chromosomal components by these walks and actually rebuild the chromosomes in yeast and then transfer them back into their organism of origin.

Yeast also allows one to conduct other kinds of whole-chromosome manipulations. FIGURE 14 illustrates a strategy for producing large terminal chromosome deletions and constructing a physical map, without the necessity of first restriction mapping.[11] Assume that there is a gene that you want to map, labeled G, that you introduce into two simple yeast vectors that each have selectable markers, but are not competent

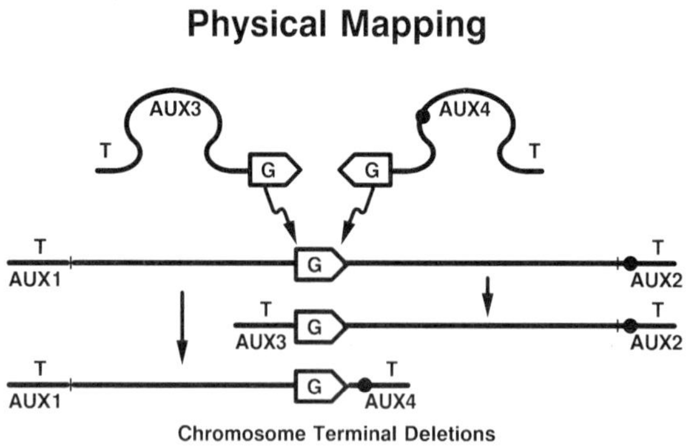

FIGURE 14.

for yeast transformation because they have only one telomere and no origin of replication. These two vectors are transformed into yeast that contains the artificial chromosome. In order for them to be maintained and provide the selectable marker in a stable inheritable form they must integrate by homologous recombination. A break is created in the artificial chromosome at the point of the gene G by the introduction of a telomere. These broken molecules then allow one to physically map the DNA for any gene and, in addition, to make terminal deletions. This kind of a strategy, in fact, has enormous capacity to generate many types of genetic rearrangements on large molecules that can be done normally on only small molecules of a few kilobases. One can generate duplicate sequences, internal deletions, and reciprocal translocations.

An intrinsic problem in genetic manipulation in screening for a conditional phenotype by transformation with mutagenizing DNA is that, while one hopes that the phenotype will be caused by the mutation in the gene of interest, it is not uncommon to learn that the altered phenotype results from a mutation gene at another unlinked location. One of the reasons why this arises, and which most scientists fail to appreciate, is because transformation itself is mutagenic; when one transforms an organism, one is invariably mutagenizing it. Consequently, simple methods must be developed for ascertaining that a mutation one hopes to have introduced and identified by screening is actually in the gene of interest. This has been a major problem in yeast, but recently has been solved by several different laboratories in essentially the same way.[12,13] The method is called a "plasmid shuffle," and I believe that it is likely to be useful in studying genetics in a wide variety of organisms.

The plasmid shuffle was originally worked out for generating conditional mutations. Once again, it uses dominant drug-resistance and -sensitive markers. The first step is to transplace the gene of interest with a selectable marker (dominant drug or auxotropic marker). The result is that one copy of the gene in a diploid eukaryotic cell like yeast is inactivated. That cannot always be directly accomplished, because one encounters problems involving gene dosage effects that directly or indirectly lead to chromosomal segregation mistakes. Cells that have duplicated the chromosome containing the one remaining functional copy of the gene of interest are selected. This results in three copies of the chromosome; two containing the functional gene and one containing the disrupted gene. This type of problem is easily prevented by making an artificial chromosome that carries another functional copy of the gene. Thus the genetic manipulations can be carried out in organisms that are diploid for the gene of interest, even though one chromosomal copy has been inactivated. In the case of yeast, we can carry the organism through meiosis to ascertain whether or not the gene inactivated is actually essential. When diploid yeast undergoes meiosis haploid products are obtained. Obviously, this would have to be done in some other way for organisms that do not have a sexual cycle. In many cases this test indicates that the gene is essential and that mutant haploid cells are dead. However, failure to obtain the haploid cell with the disruption does not establish that the gene is essential. The following approach used to establish the function of the gene can be used in other organisms as well: A gene to be tested is placed on an autonomous vector that is easily identified by the phenotype of the resulting cell. In the case of yeast we use a tyrosine-inserting tRNA suppressor. The cell contains a suppressible defect in the adenine pathway that causes the accumulation of an intermediate, which is converted to a dark red pigment. Cells containing the defect are red, while cells containing the suppressor are white. Thus, if cells do not have the plasmid, they are red; if they do have the plasmid containing the suppressor, the cells are white. For example, if the gene is essential when one obtains colonies of red progeny, they do not have the plasmid, and examination of their genome structure invariably shows them to be wild-type for the chromosomal gene. On the other hand, the cell line that has a wild-type gene and the plasmid will lose the plasmid occasionally during growth and the colony will "sector," that is, white colonies will be formed amidst the red sectors. When the colony sectors, you know that the plasmid is not essential. However, if the chromosomal gene copy is disrupted, then ability to lose the plasmid is indicative of the essential nature of the gene. If the plasmid can be lost (sector), then the gene is not essential. If the plasmid cannot be lost, as evidenced by total lack of sectors, then the gene is essential. This test can also be performed by killing cells with the plasmid through use of a dominant drug-sensitive marker on the plasmid.

Using this same approach, one is now in the position to construct and screen for conditional mutations in the gene. This is the circumstance in which one carries out a "plasmid shuffle." One mutagenizes a gene of interest in a vector (plasmid) with a different selectable marker and transforms a cell line containing a disrupted gene in the chromosome and a plasmid copy providing the essential gene. One can easily determine whether an additional copy of the gene is wild-type and will continue to

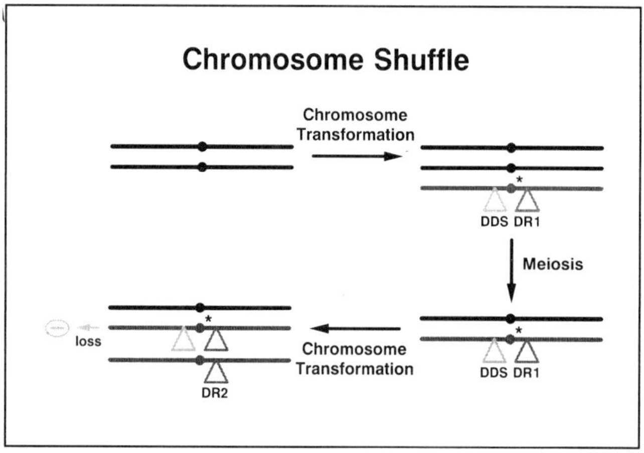

FIGURE 15.

provide red sectors, or whether it is defective and nonsectoring. This allows one to look for mutations that are conditional, such as temperature-sensitive sectors. This provides nonsectoring progeny at high temperature, but allows sectoring to occur at low temperatures. Thus, one can identify mutations or defects in essential genes carried on the plasmid or genetically linked to the plasmid and now somewhere else in the genome. This whole process can also be conducted using a dominant drug-sensitive marker instead of sectored colonies.

Because this strategy has been so useful for conducting genetic manipulations and studying essential genes using small artificial chromosomes in yeast, it should be able to be applied to very large chromosomes in what I would call a "chromosomal shuffle" (FIG. 15). First one builds a chromosome, say in yeast, marked by dominant resistance and dominant sensitive markers on both sides of the centromere. Then one transforms the marked chromosome into the organism of origin. Obviously in order to use this approach, a centromere has first to be defined. To provide the shuffle one can make a defect in the centromere. In yeast, a conditional centromere can be constructed by placing a strong promoter that is regulatable directed into the centromere.[14] If the promoter is off, the centromere is fully functional. If the promoter is on, it causes total dysfunction of the centromere and the chromosome is lost. This then provides a means by which we can very simply induce a whole chromosome loss for a specific chromosome. If the organism can undergo meiosis, one can generate an organism that can lose a particular chromosome upon induction of the promoter. That enables one to bring in copies of the chromosome that have been manipulated or are otherwise of interest to study by transformation. Such a host organism is then set-up to do the genetic study, since one can easily get rid of the unaltered chromosome. In studying a diploid organism, this has to be repeated twice to eliminate and replace two copies of the same chromosome. This kind of genetics provides the capacity to conduct most of the genetic manipulations classically carried out on small pieces of DNA in bacteria and now in yeast as yeast artificial chromosomes. It offers the possibility of rigorous genetic testing of very complex functions. I believe that these approaches for manipulating organisms will greatly facilitate developing genetics of higher organisms, including protozoan and metazoan parasites. By means of these kinds of strategies, it is possible for workers in a single laboratory to establish, in a reasonable time, the genetics for a completely new organism.

REFERENCES

1. Botstein, D., R. L. White, M. Skolnick & R. W. Davis. 1980. Am. J. Hum. Genet. **32:** 314-331.
2. Donnis-Keller, H. *et.al.* Cell **51:** 319-337.
3. Boeke, J. D., F. LaCroute & G. R. Fink. 1984. Mol. & Gen. Genet. **197:** 345-346.
4. Scherer, S. & R. W. Davis. 1979. Proc. Natl. Acad. Sci. USA **76:** 4951-4955.
5. Cai, M. & R. W. Davis. 1989. Unpublished results.
6. Burke, D. T., G. F. Carle & M. V. Olson. 1987. Science **236:** 806-812.
7. Traver, C., S. Klapholz, R. Hyman & R. W. Davis. 1989. Proc. Natl. Acad. Sci. USA. In press.
8. Traver, C. & R. W. Davis. 1989. Unpublished results.
9. Chu, G., D. Vollrath & R. W. Davis. 1986. **234:** 1582-1585.
10. Orbach, M. J., D. Vollrath, R. W. Davis & C. Yanofsky. 1988. Mol. & Cell. Biol. **8:** 1469-1473.
11. Klapholz, S. & R. W. Davis. 1989. Unpublished results.
12. Vollrath, D., R. W. Davis, C. Connelly & P. Hieter. 1988. Proc. Natl. Acad. Sci. USA **85:** 6027-6031.
13. Elledge, S. J. & R. W. Davis. 1988. Gene **70:** 303-312.
14. Boeke, J. D., J. Truehart, G. Natsoulis & G. R. Fink. 1988. Meth. Enzymol. **154:** 164-175.
15. Snyder, M., R. J. Sapolsky & R. W. Davis. 1988. Mol. Cell. Biol. **8:** 2184-2194.

Strategies for Malaria Control: Realities, Magic, and Science

LOUIS H. MILLER

Laboratory of Parasitic Diseases
National Institute of Allergy and Infectious Diseases
National Institutes of Health
Bethesda, Maryland 20892

I am commenting on methods for malaria eradication and control, while realizing my limitations in first-hand experience with malaria-control programs. I will not deal, therefore, with the potential impact of improvement of primary health care or the relative advantages and disadvantages of a vertical program organized centrally, as was the malaria eradication program of the 1950s and the 1960s. I will also not discuss economic considerations, although these are important. We are critical of economists for not considering the impact of health on development. Improvement of the standard of living of families in the developing world combined with health education is likely to have a marked effect on health. Who are more committed to the health of children than their parents? Because of my limited knowledge and experience in the above issues, I will draw strongly from the interaction of discoveries in the laboratory and their impact in the field and from my own experiences in the laboratory today.

THE SITUATION TODAY

To set the stage, malaria and its impact vary with the area of the world. In village Africa, malaria has a heavy impact on children and primigravid women who suffer and die from the disease. Multiple studies have consistently found a major effect of malaria control on mortality in children aged 1 to 4 years.[1,2] In contrast, the disease in Madang, Papua New Guinea appears quite different, causing little mortality in children.[3] Why this difference? Both places are hyperendemic for *Plasmodium falciparum.* Is the parasite more virulent in Africa? I doubt it. Is the host more innately resistant in New Guinea? This is a possibility since 95% of the population in this region have a deletion of one alpha hemoglobin gene[4] and 30% have ovalocytosis, which suppresses parasitemia. Is the epidemiology in the two areas different? First, there may be more ready access to chloroquine in Papua New Guinea.[5] Chloroquine is taken for all illnesses in this area. Second, a greater level of transmission or continuous year-round transmission as occurs in Papua New Guinea may lead to a less severe disease in a population. A possible explanation for this seemingly paradoxical observation is the timing of the first infection. If the first infection comes during the first six months of life, when a baby has partial resistance because of a PABA-deficient milk diet and passive immunity to malaria, the infection will not be severe, but will begin the induction of active immunity. If, on the other hand, the first infection comes later in childhood, when there is no immunity to malaria, such as in an area of seasonal transmission, then the infection may be life-threatening. Unfortunately, different investigators have studied the disease in the two areas, and the reasons for the differences have never been assessed. There is no question that an intervention that would diminish the severity of malaria in children in Africa would greatly affect their survival. That is one of the realities of the disease.

Again in Africa, in part because of the high vector capacity, drug resistance is spreading rapidly across the continent from East to Central to West Africa. If, as occurred in Thailand, drug resistance increases morbidity and mortality, then the situation in Africa may deteriorate in the coming years. The introduction of mefloquine into drug-resistant areas of Thailand led to the almost complete disappearance of cerebral malaria in the Thai province of Chantaburi. What happens in Thailand as mefloquine-resistance becomes widespread? The spread of chloroquine-resistance throughout Africa has increased the severity of disease and will further complicate strategies based on use of drugs to diminish the severity of disease. This will become especially severe as the level of chloroquine-resistance advances from RI to RII and RIII, that is, to where there is little or no response to chloroquine in sick children in village Africa. The dimensions of the potential impact of drug-resistance in Africa can be estimated from the rate of sickle cell trait in some regions of Africa.[1] If one assumes that mortality from *P. falciparum* is the only force selecting for hemoglobin SA and that malaria creates a balanced polymorphism with hemoglobins S and A, then it is possible to estimate the mortality to puberty (including fetal deaths) to maintain a given hemoglobin S gene frequency. As an example, at a hemoglobin S gene frequency of 0.2, the mortality from malaria for hemoglobin AA children would be greater than 20% and would equal mortality from all other diseases combined. One presumes that the lower mortality that is seen today in Africa is the result of chloroquine treatment of sick children. What happens when chloroquine is no longer effective? That may be a sad reality in the near future.

The high level of transmission in Africa is in large measure the result of the mosquitoes of the *Anopheles gambiae* complex. The preference for human blood meals and the longevity of some of these mosquitoes are ideal for high vector efficiency. Furthermore, the peridomestic feeding of these mosquitoes and their failure to land on walls after feeding in some areas make residual insecticides of little value in control.[6] In Asia the continuous cost of vector control is a strain on the health budget in areas where the mosquitoes are still susceptible to insecticides. In cotton-growing areas of Latin America, resistance of mosquitoes to all insecticides is commonplace.

RESEARCH ON THE *ANOPHELES* VECTOR

What do we in the laboratory have to offer for the future? A review of the history of significant advances shows the dissociation between discovery and application. The vector was identified in the 1890s, but the broad applications awaited the discovery of DDT, a "magic" moment in science. There was no way to predict that the addition of chlorine side chains by Müller to a structure in the published literature would lead to the most important insecticide and the one that would spawn the malaria-eradication program.[7] There was no reason to believe in the success of such a molecule from previous observations, other than its similarity to a moth repellent. Müller thought that this first-generation insecticide would lead to others far more effective and safe. None more effective and safe for humans was to come. Was this magic moment predictable? No, but the research in entomology over the previous 50 years set the stage for its application. Bruce-Chwatt evaluated field research and control measures in Africa with this most powerful tool in the hands of public health workers.[8] Bruce-Chwatt spoke from first-hand knowledge of malaria in Africa. Success with insecticides was limited to areas where *Anopheles funestus* was the main vector, such as was the case with the Taveta-Pare Scheme in Kenya. Some mosquitoes do not land on the walls in the house after feeding, but instead fly outside. Others, such as the *Anopheles funestus,* remain in the house and are ideal candidates for control by spraying of residual insecticides on the walls. The *A. gambiae* complex, the major vector in Africa, was not such an easy target, and its capacity to transmit malaria is extremely efficient. That was the reality that forced the acceptance of the impossibility of having any malaria-eradication or -control program based on the residual insecticides in much of Africa.

Entomologists are currently trying to use methods of the 1930s that had minimal effect prior to the introduction of DDT. Will these methods be more successful today? For example, larvivorous fish will have a minimal effect in most areas, although exceptions may exist. Other biological control methods are being considered for introduction into the natural habitat such as fungi and bacteria that either invade mosquito larvae or release a toxin. The addition of toxins to algae and other microorganisms raises exciting possibilities in vector control, but technical and environmental problems must be resolved. It is too early to judge this approach, especially since it is unknown which microorganisms colonize the larvae in the field. At the more immediate level, the use of bednetting impregnated with permethrine is being evaluated.[9] This will clearly require education before it will be possible to evaluate its full effectiveness. It will be crucial to determine the effect of impregnated bednetting on disease as well as the numbers of mosquitoes and attack rate of malaria. The relation of the size and frequency of inoculation of sporozoites to disease during the period of use of bednets is unknown, but may be important. This makes clear the need for careful epidemiology combined with entomologic techniques to evaluate the effect on any population. It is amazing that so little is known about the most important vectors of malaria, the *Anopheles gambiae* complex. This type of research is needed and may lead to a miraculous discovery or, what is more likely, to the more conventional development of novel vector-oriented methods for malaria control. It is of such importance that an institute should be developed in Africa committed to studying the biology of these disease vectors in a manner similar to that used in studying retroviruses throughout the world today. A large effort to study the population biology has been made by Coluzzi and his colleagues, who found that within one species populations have become reproductively separated because of behavior and that this may relate to paracentric inversions.[10] This is a form of incipient speciation. Consequently, the same species may live in different ecological niches and present many biological systems, not one. Each may have to be approached in a different way in terms of control measures.

One approach to this vector would be to introduce a gene that would reduce the viability of the parasite in the mosquito. Such mechanisms occur naturally in mosquito populations and determine the vectors in each area. The parasite may adapt to a local vector but the same species of parasite from other parts of the world may be unable to infect this vector. As an example, encapsulation of malaria parasites by *Anopheles gambiae*[11] involves a primitive host defense mechanism, melanin formation, and may use the same enzymes as for cuticle formation. These enzymes include the diphenol oxidase and other enzymes that control its activation. How does the mosquito recognize the malaria parasite as foreign and where does the initiation of encapsulation occur?

In *Drosophila,* a genetic mutation leads to encapsulation around soft tissue in the hemocoel and the formation of melanotic tumors.[12] The genetic defect has exposed self to the mechanism that is normally reserved for encapsulating invading microorganisms. Interestingly, *P. falciparum* from Africa is largely resistant to encapsulation by lines of *A. gambiae* that encapsulate *P. falciparum* from other parts of the world,[11] an example of evolution of the parasite under pressure from the local mosquito vector. Can an understanding of encapsulation identify a mechanism from which the parasite cannot escape? Some mosquitoes may have absolute blocks so that the malaria parasite cannot undergo full development to the infectious stage in these mosquitoes. For example, mammalian malarias have never been observed in mosquitoes other than *Anopheles.* There must be some step in the life cycle that cannot be completed outside this host, despite the long time and multiple opportunities (e.g., in Culicine mosquitoes). What is the mechanism of the absolute block and could it be introduced into the vector genus *Anopheles*? One fascinating area of insect immunity has been the response to bacterial infection discovered and developed by Bowman and his colleagues.[13] A group of proteins called cecropins and attacins are synthesized in response to bacterial infection. Cecropins are small peptides that have an amphipathic alpha helix at the N-terminus and a hydrophobic stretch at the C-terminus.[14] It is thought that they form channels in the membrane of bacteria that lead to bacterial lysis. Interestingly, these compounds and a related one from frog skin, maiganin, kill malarial parasites within oocysts in the mosquito midgut if injected into the mosquito during infection.[15] Obviously, such a mechanism is nonoperative during natural infection because cecropin synthesis is probably not induced during a malaria infection. Introduction of the genes for cecropins on a promoter responsive to a blood meal could lead to its production at a time when the parasite is susceptible to this killing mechanism. Other secrets await discovery if we just explore this relatively untouched area of host-parasite biology.

CHEMOTHERAPY RESEARCH

Development of synthetic antimalarial drugs was stepwise. It started with methylene blue of Erhlich to the addition of the synthetic side chain that was to be a part of chloroquine and primaquine. Even here the synthesis depended on the discovery in the 1600s of quinine by Peruvian Indians and the analysis of its structure by the French organic chemists of the 1800s. The first synthetic drugs were 8-aminoquinolines instead of 4-aminoquinolines because the 4-aminoquinolines proved difficult to synthesize. It was this accident in organic synthesis, magic if you will, that led to the discovery of a new class of drugs, the 8-aminoquinolines, which are effective against the relapsing form of *P. vivax* and *P. ovale.* These plasmodias can remain dormant in the liver cells of infected persons and, at unpredicted times months to years after infection, lead to an attack of malaria that can be transmitted to others. Such a persistent form of disease can make eradication difficult unless the program can be maintained for years. This is not unlike the case of river blindness caused by onchocerciasis where parasites remain in the skin of infected persons for years. Primaquine, however, has limitations in control and eradication programs, since it must be given daily for 14 days and is toxic. It is curious that despite 60 years of searching for a replacement for primaquine, we have never found another drug against the relapsing malarias.

Today for treatment and prophylaxis, we are largely relying on the blood schizonticidal drugs discovered during the Second World War and modified since, including the drugs developed by the Walter Reed Army Institute of Research. The recent discovery that verapamil, a calcium channel blocker, could reverse chloroquine-resistance may open up a new class of antimalarial drugs.[16] Generally speaking, our drug base is too narrow for such a rapidly changing parasite. One exception is the Chinese herbal medicine, artemisinin, which, like quinine, was discovered by unnamed scientists of an earlier culture. None of the drugs today was developed rationally on the basis of a difference between host and parasite metabolism. Our options could be broadened by a sound biochemical research program; perhaps then we will have the choice of drugs that we so badly need.

RESEARCH TOWARDS MALARIA VACCINES

How could I talk about malaria and the modern approaches in research and not mention vaccine research? For a review of this subject, see Ref. 17. This area is scientifically exciting and full of potential, but it has received more attention than other areas mentioned earlier which are of equal importance. What would the ideal vaccine be for the developing world: a sporozoite vaccine that prevents infection, a vaccine against asexual erythrocytic parasites that prevents severe disease, or a sexual-stage vaccine that prevents transmission of disease? There is not one answer because the solution will depend on the epidemiologic setting in which malaria occurs.

Sporozoite vaccines have a great appeal since they could potentially prevent infection, which would be the ideal. However, if they only prevented infection for a short period, then children, for example, might develop severe infections when the immunity waned. This criticism also holds for the transmission-blocking vaccines; for if transmission were only blocked for one period, the population would be potentially exposed to epidemics of malaria. The centerpiece of a combined vaccine should be a vaccine against parasites at the asexual stage because this is the point at which the parasite causes disease. During the rising parasitemia, at a maximum of 10-fold increase every two days, immunity can be boosted so as to limit the parasite growth and thus decrease or eliminate mortality. If an asexual vaccine is combined with a sporozoite or transmission-blocking vaccine, reintroduction of malaria may not have tragic consequences because the population will carry a level of immunity to the asexual parasite.

The challenge facing development of a subunit vaccine against asexual erythrocytic parasites is formidable but not impossible. One problem is that, unlike some virus infections, malaria can persist at low parasitemia in repeatedly infected adults, indicating sophisticated but poorly understood methods of immune evasion. Second, antigenic diversity among clones in the parasite population has been selected by immune pressure. As an example, all base changes in the coding region of the circumsporozoite (CS) protein in different *P. falciparum* clones lead to a change in the amino acid; none is "silent."[18] One region of mutations was T-cell epitopes in mice[19,20] and humans.[21] Presumably this region was under immune pressure, and mutations were selective. In contrast, a protein on the surface of *P. falciparum* ookinetes, probably not expressed in the human host, has no base changes in the coding region.[22] Third, mutations occur rapidly in the asexual erythrocytic parasite under immune pressure because of the numbers of parasites during a single infection.[23,24] This rate will be slower if the protein is required for survival and single point mutations cannot evade the immune response. Fourth, immunogens against this stage will be difficult to test in humans because of the risk to volunteers and the consequent need for early treatment.[25]

Natural immunity to malaria is slow to develop and, in the extreme situation of *P. malariae,* may persist in the blood for the lifetime of the person, cycling every three days to new uninfected erythrocytes.[26] It appears as if the parasite is invisible to the immune system. Recently, we studied the immune response to malarial proteins in mice. Unlike tetanus toxoid and the hepatitis B surface antigen, where the majority of persons show a good immune response, the response to malarial proteins was highly restricted. The ability of an individual to respond to a given antigen is governed by immune response (*Ir*) genes, which encode the polymorphic major histocompatibility complex (MHC) molecules. The variation in the polymorphic pocket determines the ability to bind a particular antigen and subsequently present it to a T cell. This presentation determines the ability of the host to respond to the antigen. It was expected that most foreign proteins would contain sufficient T epitopes to be recognized by the majority of members of a species. This was not found to be the case for malarial proteins. The response to proteins on the surface of sporozoites[19,27] and gametes[27] was highly restricted in mice. Furthermore, we have evidence that the response to these proteins in humans was also restricted.[21,28] The paucity of T-cell epitopes on proteins that are the target of protective immunity has probably evolved to make these proteins poor immunogens, that is, most humans would not respond to them. Consistent with this interpretation is the observation that an ookinete protein of 25 kDa that is only expressed in the mosquito midgut and not in the human host induces antibodies in all mouse strains tested.[27] Antibodies to this protein are highly effective in blocking transmission, but are not seen in humans because expression of this protein is specific for the stages in the mosquito.

How then do we identify the best immunogen from the asexual erythrocytic parasite? One approach is to identify molecules that may be involved in invasion of erythrocytes or in cytoadhesion of infected erythrocytes to endothelium.[17] Antibodies to these proteins may block a crucial step in the parasite's life cycle. As an example, *P. vivax* cannot infect human erythrocytes that lack the Duffy blood group antigen.[29] The parasite molecule from *P. knowlesi,* a monkey malaria that also uses the Duffy blood group antigen, has been identified.[30] The *P. vivax* analogue, if not variant, would be a vaccine candidate. *P. knowlesi,* however, has alternative pathways for invasion. that bypass the requirement for the Duffy determinant.[30] An analogous protein of *P. falciparum* binds to sialic acid on the erythrocyte glycoproteins.[31] All *P. falciparum* clones have this protein but some can invade erythrocytes that lack sialic acid,[32–34] indicating an alternative pathway of invasion. Thus the strategy for a vaccine that would block invasion might include proteins from multiple or alternative steps in the invasion process. A concern is that the parasite has been under immune pressure and exhibits diversity of sequence surrounding the receptor pocket.

An alternative approach to identify immunogens for human vaccines is the use of rodent malarias. The actual mechanisms of immunity can be defined precisely, and the antigens for inducing these protective mechanisms can be defined. As an example, protection against *P. chabaudi* and *P. vinckei,* two rodent malarias, is cell-mediated and antibody-independent.[35] Cell-mediated immunity, if it works against human malaria, has certain advantages over antibody-dependent mechanisms. A mutant parasite that escapes antibody can overgrow, be transmitted, and replace the wild-type parasites, making the vaccine ineffective. The effector limb of cell-mediated immunity, on the other hand, is nonspecific and would kill mutant and wild-type parasites equally.

CONCLUSION

I have attempted to put together the infection and disease as it occurs in the field, the leads in the laboratory and the field, and some of the hopeful directions for research in years to come. Will there be a magic bullet that will eliminate malaria? I doubt it. Even DDT could not be called such a weapon, at least in retrospect. I do know that the laboratory will bring new tools to public health workers in the countries where malaria is such a serious problem. Ultimately, drugs, vaccines and mosquito control methods will be integrated into a program whose goal will be the eradication of malaria. That is the challenge to all of us in the laboratory.

ACKNOWLEDGMENTS

I thank Drs. L. Molineaux, M. F. Good, J. Cattani, and D. Alling for discussions on the manuscript.

REFERENCES

1. Molineaux, L. 1985. The impact of parasitic diseases and their control, with an emphasis on malaria and Africa. *In* Health Policy, Social Policy and Mortality Prospects. J. Vallin & A. D. Lopez, Eds. International Union for the Scientific Study of Population. Ordina Editions.
2. Greenwood, B. M., A. K. Bradley, A. M. Greenwood, P. Byass, K. Jammeh, K. Marsh, S. Tulloch, F. S. Oldfield, & R. Hayes. 1987. Mortality and morbidity from malaria among children in a rural area of the Gambia, West Africa. Trans. R. Soc. Trop. Med. Hyg. **81:** 478-486.
3. Stace, J., P. Bilton, K. Coates & N. Stace. 1982. Cerebral malaria in children: A retrospective study of admissions to Madang Hospital 1980. Papua New Guinea Med. J. **25:** 230-234.
4. Oppenheimer, S. J., D. R. Higgs, D. J. Weatherall, J. Barker & R. A. Spark. 1984. α-Thalassemia in Papua, New Guinea. Lancet **1:** 424-426.
5. Cattani, J. A., J. L. Tulloch, H. Vrbova, D. Jolley, F. D. Gibson, J. S. Moir, P. F. Heywood, M. P. Alpers, A. Stevenson & R. Claney. 1986. The epidemiology of malaria in a population surrounding Madang, Papua New Guinea. Am. J. Trop. Med. Hyg. **35:** 3-15.
6. Molineaux, L. & S. G. Gramiccia. 1980. The Garki Project. World Health Organization. Geneva.
7. Muller, P. H. 1948. Dichloro-diphenyl-trichloroethane and new insecticides. Nobel Lecture, December 11, 1988.
8. Bruce-Chwatt, L. J. 1984. Lessons learned from applied field research activities in Africa during the malaria eradication era. Bull. World Hlth. Org. **62**(Suppl.): 19-29.
9. Snow, R. W., S. W. Lindsay, R. J. Hayes & B. W. Greenwood. 1988. Permethrin-treated bed nets (mosquito nets) prevent malaria in Gambian children. Trans. Roy. Soc. Trop. Med. Hyg. In press.
10. Coluzzi, M., A. Savatini, V. Petrarca & M. A. DiDeco. 1977. Behavioral divergences between mosquitoes with different inversion karyotypes in polymorphic populations of the *Anopheles gambiae* complex. Nature **266:** 832-833.

11. Collins, F. H., R. K. Sakai, K. D. Vernick, S. Paskewitz, D. C. Seeley, L. H. Miller, W. E. Collins, C. C. Campbell & R. W. Gwadz. 1986. Genetic selection of a *Plasmodium*-refractory strain of the malaria vector *Anopheles gambiae*. Science **234:** 607-610.
12. Riski, T. M. & R. M. Rizki. 1986. Surface changes on hemocytes during encapsulation in *Drosophila melanogaster* Meigen. *In* Hemocytic and Humoral Immunity in Arthropods. A. P. Gupta, Ed. John Wiley. New York.
13. Bowman, H. G., I. Faye, P. V. Hofsten, K. Kockum, J. Y. Lee, K. G. Xanthopoulos, H. Bennick, A. Engstrom, B. R. Merrifield & D. Andren. 1986. Antibacterial immune proteins in insects—A review of some current perspectives. *In* Immunity in Invertebrates. M. Brehelin, Ed. Springer-Verlag. Berlin and Heidelberg.
14. Christensen, B., J. Fink, R. B. Merrifield & D. Mauzerall. 1988. Channel-forming properties of cecropins and related model compounds incorporated into planar lipid membranes. Proc. Natl. Acad. Sci. USA **85:** 5072-5076.
15. Robert Gwadz *et al.* Unpublished data.
16. Martin, S., A. M. J. Oduola & W. K. Milhouse. 1987. Reversal of chloroquine resistance in *Plasmodium falciparum* by verapamil. Science **235:** 899-901.
17. Miller, L. H., R. J. Howard, R. Carter, M. F. Good, V. Nussenzweig & R. S. Nussenzweig. 1986. Research towards malaria vaccines. Science **234:** 1349-1356.
18. De la Cruz, V. F., A. A. Lal & T. F. McCutchan. 1987. Sequence variation in putative functional domains of the circumsporozoite protein of *Plasmodium falciparum:* Implications for vaccine development. J. Biol. Chem. **262: 11935-11939.**
19. Good, M. F., W. L. Maloy, M. N. Lunde, H. Margalit, J. L. Cornette, G. L. Smith, B. Moss, L. H. Miller & J. A. Berzofsky. 1987. Construction of synthetic immunogen: use of new helper epitope on malaria circumsporozoite protein. Science **235:** 1059-1062.
20. Kumar, S., L. H. Miller, I. A. Quakyi, D. B. Keister, R. A. Houghten, W. L. Maloy, B. Moss, J. A. Berzofsky & M. F. Good. 1988. Cytotoxic T cells specific for the circumsporozoite protein of *Plasmodium falciparum.* Nature **334:** 258-260.
21. Good, M. F., D. Pombo, I. A. Quakyi, E. M. Riley, R. A. Houghten, A. Menon, D. W. Alling, J. A. Berzofsky & L. H. Miller. 1988. Human T-cell recognition of the circumsporozoite protein of *Plasmodium falciparum:* Immunodominant T-cell domains map to the polymorphic regions of the molecule. Proc. Natl. Acad. Sci. USA **85:** 1199-1203.
22. Kaslow, D., I. A. Quakyi & D. B. Keister. 1988. Minimal variation in a vaccine candidate from the sexual stage of *Plasmodium falciparum.* Mol. Biochem. Parasitol. In press.
23. Klotz, F. W., D. E. Hudson, H. G. Coon & L. H. Miller. 1987. Vaccination-induced variation in the 140 kD merozoite surface antigen of *Plasmodium knowlesi* malaria. J. Exp. Med. **165:** 359-367.
24. Hudson, D. E., T. E. Wellems & L. H. Miller. 1988. Molecular basis for mutation in a surface protein expressed by malaria parasites. J. Mol. Biol. In press.
25. Miller, L. H. 1988. Malaria. Effective vaccine for humans? Nature **332:** 109-110.
26. Guazzi, M. & S. Grazi. 1963. Description of a case of recrudescing quartan malaria after 53 years of latency. Riv. Malariol. **42:** 55.
27. Good, M. F., L. H. Miller, S. Kumar, I. A. Quakyi, D. Keister, J. Adams, B. Moss, J. A. Berzofsky & R. Carter. 1988. A challenge for malaria vaccine development: limited immunological recognition of critical vaccine candidate antigens. Science. **242:** 574-577.
28. Quakyi, I. A., L. N. Otoo, D. Pombo, L. Y. Sugars, A. Menon, A. S. De Groot, A. Johnson, D. Alling, L. H. Miller & M. F. Good. Differential non-responsiveness in humans to candidate *Plasmodium falciparum* vaccine antigens. Am. J. Trop. Med. Hyg. In press.
29. Miller, L. H., S. J. Mason, D. F. Clyde & M. H. McGinniss. 1976. The resistance factor to *Plasmodium vivax* in blacks. The Duffy-blood-group genotype, *FyFy.* N. Engl. J. Med. **295:** 302-304.
30. Haynes, J. D., J. P. Dalton, F. W. Klotz, M. H. McGinniss, T. J. Hadley, D. E.

HUDSON & L. H. MILLER. 1988. Receptor-like specificity of a *Plasmodium knowlesi* material protein that binds to Duffy antigen ligands on erythrocytes. J. Exp. Med. **167:** 1873-1881.

31. CAMUS, D. & T. J. HADLEY. 1985. A *Plasmodium falciparum* antigen that binds to host erythrocytes and merozoites. Science **230:** 553-557.
32. MITCHELL, G. H., T. J. HADLEY, M. H. MCGINNISS, F. W. KLOTZ & L. H. MILLER. 1986. Invasion of erythrocytes by *Plasmodium falciparum* malaria parasites. Evidence for receptor heterogeneity and two receptors. Blood **67:** 1519-1521.
33. HADLEY, T. J., F. W. KLOTZ, G. PASVOL, J. D. HAYNES, M. H. MCGINNISS, Y. OKUBO & L. H. MILLER. 1987. Falciparum malaria parasites invade erythrocytes that lack glycophorin A and B (M^kM^k). Strain differences indicate receptor heterogeneity and two pathways for invasion. J. Clin. Invest. **80:** 1190-1193.
34. PERKINS, M. E. & E. H. HOLD. 1988. Erythrocyte receptor recognition varies in *Plasmodium falciparum* isolates. Mol. Biochem. Parasitol. **27:** 23-34.
35. GRUN, J. L. & W. O. WEIDANZ. 1981. Immunity to *Plasmodium chabaudi adami* in the T-cell deficient mouse. Nature **290:** 143-145.

Antigenic Variation in Relation to Vaccines[a]

NINA AGABIAN

University of California, Berkeley and San Francisco
Intercampus Program in Molecular Parasitology
Laurel Heights Campus, Suite 150
San Francisco, California 94143-1204

Like those who have preceded me I wish to say that I am delighted to be here on the occasion of the presentation of the Frohlich Award to Dr. Kenneth Warren. For me the venue, as well as the occasion, is special: about nine years ago I came to this auditorium to attend the first meeting of the Rockefeller Great Neglected Diseases (GND) network and with the specific objective of introducing myself to Ken Warren. I was an Assistant Professor and a molecular biologist who wanted to work on parasites; by the end of that year I had been adopted into the GND family and it was really Ken's encouragement and support that sustained my initial commitment to this field during the ensuing years of developing a program in this arena. Through the development of the GND family, Ken drew persons like myself into a community of scientists who together raised each others' expectations and standards. The dramatic progress in the field of parasitology that is reflected in the program of the symposium owes much to Ken and to his untiring effort and spirit. It has been a very exciting part of my life and I am grateful for the opportunity to have been part of that effort.

INTRODUCTION

Parasitism is usually characterized by the establishment of chronic infections which persistently evade the defense mechanisms of the host. Many strategies are employed by parasites to evade immune surveillance, including sequestration in specific cellular and tissue compartments, the entering of periods of hyperbiotic development or latency, the changing of antigens during life-cycle stages in the mammalian host, and immunosuppression of the immune response. One important strategy which has been illuminated through molecular genetic studies is the process of antigenic variation, whereby variability and diversity are genetically introduced amongst a family of molecules that are functional homologues of one another. The rate of antigenic variation and the extent of the antigenic repertoire of a parasite has serious ramifications for the choice and efficacy of antigens selected for vaccine development.

[a] The research underlying the results presented at this meeting was supported in part by funds provided by the John D. and Catherine T. MacArthur, Edna McConnell Clark and Rockefeller Foundations and NIH Grant AI21975 to N.A. N.A. is a Burroughs Wellcome Scholar of Molecular Parasitology.

ANTIGENIC VARIATION BY GENETIC REARRANGEMENT IN AFRICAN TRYPANOSOMES

One of the earliest-documented and best-studied examples of antigenic variation in parasites is displayed by subspecies of *Trypanosoma brucei,* the parasitic protozoan that causes African sleeping sickness.[1,2] The relapsing fevers and recurrent parasitemias of patients with African sleeping sickness were suggested to arise from a changing antigenic phenotype of the infecting trypanosomes. The phenomenon of antigenic variation was described as early as 1910 by Levaditi and McIntosh.[3] Today, we know that the surface of the African trypanosome is covered by a surface glycoprotein molecule—one of as many as several hundred variable surface glycoproteins (VSGs) which may be expressed from the genome of a single infecting parasite. This intrinsic capacity for an amazing repertoire of antigenically diverse, but functionally identical polypeptides allows parasite populations to escape the host immune system by alternative expression of one of these many VSGs. To complicate matters, expression of any one of the hundreds of possible VSGs is sufficiently random as to be unpredictable, thus precluding their use as potential vaccination antigens.

As a result of molecular genetic analysis, it has been possible to learn how this antigenic variability and diversity are regulated. FIGURE 1 schematically presents three potential modes by which surface antigen expression is regulated. A necessary but not sufficient condition for the transcriptional activation of a particular VSG gene is its chromosomal position; only those VSG genes located in a telomeric position can be transcribed and only one of the many telomeric VSG genes is transcriptionally active at any one time. In addition to the many telomeric copies of VSG genes, there are even more that are located internally in the chromosome structure. In order for these VSG genes to achieve expression, they must undergo a rearrangement which changes their relative position within the genome. This occurs either through duplication of an internal chromosomal gene copy and its transposition to a telomeric site, or gene conversion of a telomeric copy, or by a recombinational exchange between telomeric VSG genes within a given expression site. Any of these potential mechanisms may be employed by all members of the bloodstream VSG gene repertoire (reviewed in Ref. 4).

The discovery of the gene conversion, duplication, and transposition events associated with the activation of VSG gene transcription occurred at a time in the study of cell biology when the role of chromosomal rearrangement of genetic sequences was becoming recognized as a generalized regulatory strategy in gene expression. An understanding of the molecular biology of VSG gene expression in trypanosomes contributed significantly to our knowledge of the role of genetic rearrangements and position effects in gene expression and thus it played an important role in characterizing the molecular biology of mobile genetic elements. It also taught us that the genomes of parasites may have the genetic plasticity for producing enormous variability in antigenic repertoire—a property that in the particular case of African trypanosomiasis has significantly thwarted vaccination strategies based on the properties of the immunodominant surface antigens of the bloodstage parasites. In recent years, the molecular analysis of the surface antigens of *Neisseria gonorrheae*[5] and *Borrelia recurrentis*[6] has provided other examples of antigenic diversity generated by the alternative expression of any of a number of possible antigen genes within the parasite genome. To add to these, the phenotypic expression of alternative surface antigenic types in *Giardia lamblia*[7] and of cytoadherence antigens in *P. falciparum*[8] suggests that antigenic variation by a mechanism similar to that found in African trypanosomes

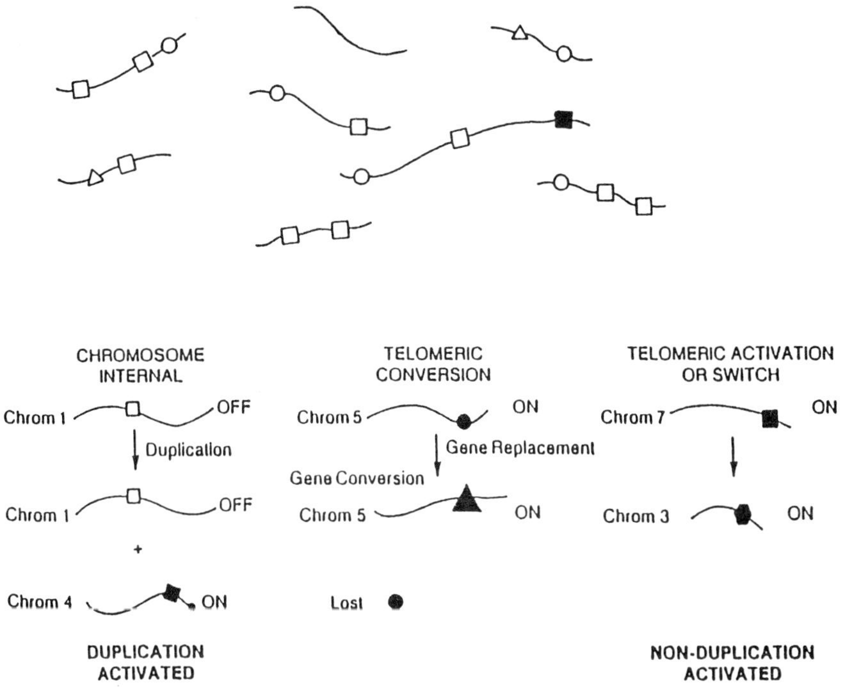

FIGURE 1. Schematic diagram of trypanosome genome illustrating multiplicity of chromosome size classes (*top*). Most chromosomes contain one or more variant antigen genes encoding distinct antigenic types (*square, circle, triangle*) organized in VSG gene families. A filled symbol indicates a transcriptionally active VSG gene. Normally only a single, telomeric VSG gene is expressed at any time; expression is regulated at the level of transcriptional activation; the remaining telomeric and chromosome-internal VSG genes are transcriptionally silent.

will be found in a variety of other infectious organisms. If this is the case, in each of these instances it will become necessary to first discover and then to define alternative targets for the immune system if these parasites are to become subject to immune control.

MAJOR OUTER MEMBRANE PROTEINS (MOMP) AND ALLELIC VARIATION IN *CHLAMYDIA*

The randomized expression of any one gene amongst many of a single genomic repertoire of homologous antigens is only one type of mechanism which provides for antigenic variability and diversity. In other organisms, such as *Chlamydia trachomatis,* the expression of alternative surface antigens occurs in a different way. *Chlamydia trachomatis* is an intracellular microbial parasite which causes not only blinding trachoma, but also sexually transmitted disease and infertility in more than 400 million people in developed and developing countries.[9] Through the work of Richard Stephens and colleagues at the University of California, San Francisco, the molecular biology of antigenic diversity in the MOMP gene family has been elucidated. Distinct from the case of antigenic variation in trypanosomes, each chlamydia genome possesses only a single MOMP antigen gene, which itself is a mosaic of both variable and constant sequence domains.[10] FIGURE 2 shows a Southern blot of chlamydia genomic DNA obtained from three serologically distinct isolates or serovars: L_2, B and C. Genomic DNA restriction digestions of each serovar have been hybridized with a gene probe encoding the L_2 antigen. In each serovar there appears to be only one copy of a MOMP gene.[11] Although each of these isolates is serologically distinct, hybridization is detected using the L_2 probe as a result of the constant domains preserved amongst the MOMP genes.

Comparisons of the DNA sequence between these serovars are shown in FIGURE 3. Each serotype is encoded by an allele for the MOMP gene, which is isolate- or serovar-specific and which encodes conserved as well as variable protein segments. Similar comparisons made amongst the entire spectrum of chlamydia serovars reveal a hierarchical relationship amongst the MOMP proteins, where each of the 15 serotypes can be organized into MOMP families with overlapping antigenic epitopes.[12] These genes thus represent structural mosaics in which there are constant and variable domains that distinguish the serovar and confer antigenic diversity to the population of chlamydia isolates as a whole, rather than conferring on an individual organism the ability to vary its MOMP antigens. On a purely speculative level, it would seem that allelic variation of the type described here is all that is required for a pathogen like chlamydia. As an intracellular parasite it is sequestered from the immune system except for brief periods during each infective cycle. Because chlamydia is a sexually transmitted disease, reinfection rates are likely to be high in endemic populations and

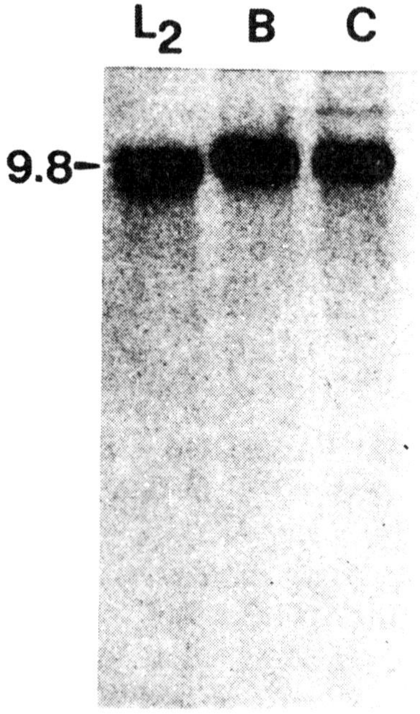

FIGURE 2. Southern analysis of chlamydia serovar L_2, B and C DNA. DNA isolated from each serovar as shown was digested with the restriction endonuclease *Bam*HI and hybridized with ^{32}P-labeled λgt11 containing an insert of the L_2 MOMP gene as described in Ref. 17.

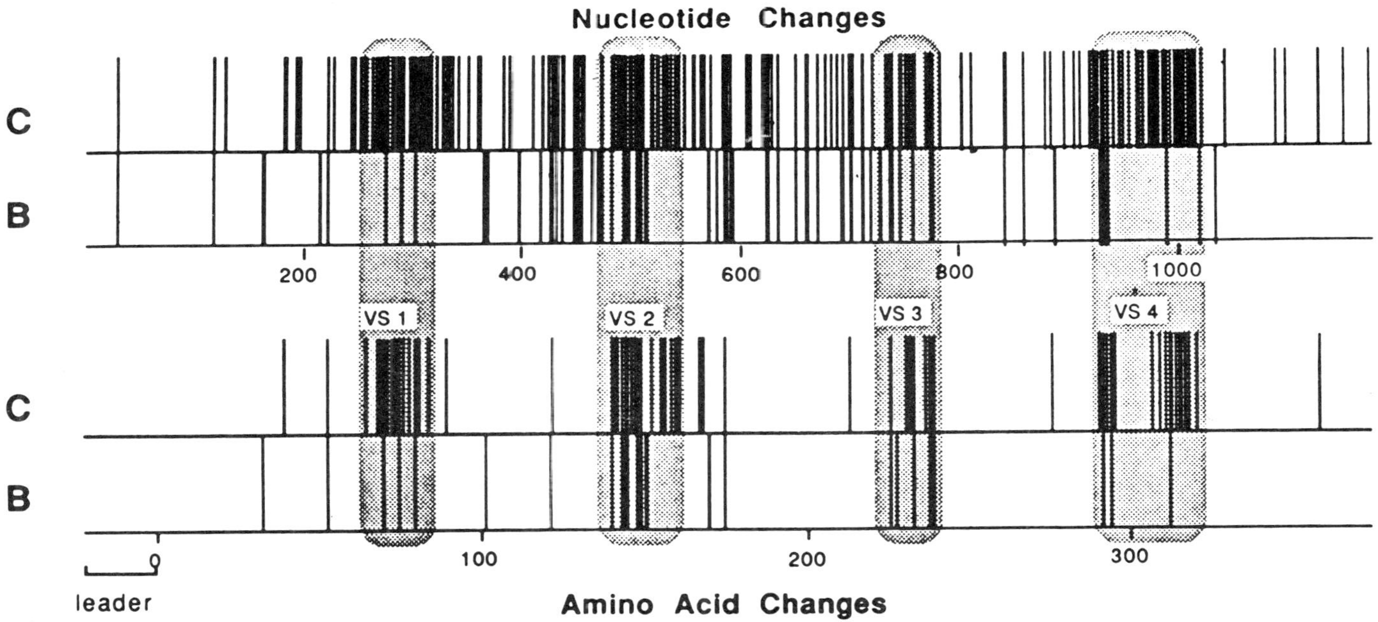

FIGURE 3. Comparison of the frequency and distribution of nucleotide and amino acid differences between the MOMP genes for serovars L_2, B and C. Each *line* represents one nucleotide or amino acid change from that of the L_2 MOMP sequence. **B,** differences for serovar B; **C,** differences for serovar C. *Shaded areas* delineate variable sequence (VS) domains. Details may be found in Ref. 11.

therefore the introduction, over time, of different serotypes might contribute to the chronicity and persistence of infection, thus ensuring the long-term infection of the host (and the survival of the chlamydia reservoir) within a specific population. It is not known whether antigenic diversity between the MOMP alleles can be generated by genetic recombination between serotypes infecting the same host or by other mechanisms. However, as with antigenic variation of the VSG of trypanosomes, the diversity of MOMPs provides an example of antigenic diversity resulting from the alternative expression of functionally homologous molecules; however, in this case each serovar contains only a single species of MOMP antigen. In the case of chlamydia, a major challenge of molecular biology and immunology is to identify and synthesize antigenic mosaics which have overlapping and broad specificity for vaccination against multiple serotypes.

INTERSPECIFIC DIVERSITY AMONGST HEAT-SHOCK PROTEINS

Before the introduction of molecular genetic techniques, the immune system's pattern of reaction against the infecting agent provided the primary access to parasite molecular biology; the antibodies of the host defined the parasite molecules of interest. Because of this long-standing relationship between serologic analysis and infectivity, when molecular technologies allowed access to parasite antigens, many investigations began the screening of recombinant expression libraries of parasite genomes with variously characterized patient sera. Through these studies, novel targets of the immune system have unexpectedly revealed themselves. One of the antigens thus characterized represents a particularly intriguing example. George Newport and colleagues, while screening sera from patients infected with *Schistosoma mansoni,* observed an immunodominant protein antigen of ~70 kD which was uniformly detected by all sera; similarly *S. japonicum*-infected patient sera recognized an *S. japonicum* protein of the same molecular weight. While in both cases these proteins were immunodominant antigens, sera from *S. mansoni* and *S. japonicum* were not reciprocally active in recognizing the protein from the alternative species. The genes encoding the *S. mansoni* and *S. japonicum* sequences, however, were homologous to one another, their genetic sequences hybridizing at high stringency. When the DNA sequence of each of these antigens was evaluated by computerized searches for similar protein sequence, it was discovered that these genes encode the schistosome homologues of the heat-shock protein (HSP) 70. Because the protein sequences deduced from the DNA clones were highly homologous, their lack of immunologic crossreactivity was surprising.[13,14]

Recombinant peptides produced from truncated portions of the HSP70-encoding gene were used for epitope mapping, and it was shown that the C-terminal domain of the *S. mansoni* and *S. japonicum* HSP70 contained the immunodominant epitopes; no other antibody activity was detected in patient sera against the remainder of the HSP70 molecule, although it is possible to elicit an immune response to other portions of the molecule when purified or recombinant HSP70 is used as an immunogen (as distinguished from its immunogenicity during the course of natural infections). Furthermore, the C-terminal immunodominant epitopes of the HSP70 peptides were immunologically distinct and showed no crossreactivity between *S. mansoni* and *S. japonicum.*[14]

FIGURE 4 shows the sequence comparison between the C-terminal domains of *S. mansoni* and *S. japonicum* HSP70, as well as the sequence of the human and *Drosophila* HSP70 in this same region. The immunodominance and unique immunologic reactivity of the C-terminal domain of the HSP70 molecule have since been documented in a variety of bacterial, protozoan, and helminthic infections. In most cases, the C-terminal is so distinct as to provide a signature for the infecting organism and sometimes the infecting strain.[15] In those cases where it has been examined, the immunodominant response is confined to the C-terminal part of the protein, suggesting a unique presentation of the antigen during infection.

Why is this interesting? Heat-shock proteins are amongst the most highly conserved proteins known in biology. HSP70 is only one of a number of heat-shock proteins; in general all of the members of the HSP family are highly conserved over a wide range of prokaryotic and eukaryotic species. They are universally made in response to a variety of stress conditions including heat, oxidant, and chemical shock. After cataloguing the presence and expression of these HSPs in many systems, researchers are just beginning to discover something about the roles of these proteins in cellular function. Heat-shock protein expression generally protects the cell in the sense that its induction allows the cell to survive after the stress is imposed; a functional role in gene regulation has been suggested: for example, HSP90 may be involved in steroid hormone receptor interactions and selective transcription. It has been suggested that HSPs are involved in protein transport, HSP70 being characterized in *Saccharomyces*

```
Sm   ERALTKDNNLLGKFELSGIPPAPRGTPQIEVTFDIDANGILNVSAVDKGTGK
Sj   **TM**************C*******V**********************A***
Hs   ***M**********R*************V*****************T*TKDS***
Dm   ***M******A**T*D************V*********L**********KEMS***

Sm   QNKITITNDKGRLSKEEIERMVADADKYKAEDEKQRDRVASKNSLESYVYTMKQQVEG
Sj   E*****************D**INE*****S*****KN*IC***********S***S***
Hs   A*****************QE*E*******V**E*******A****AFN**AFN***SA**
Dm   AKN***K********QA**D***NE****AD****H*Q*IT*R*A*******NV**S**Q

Sm   E-LKEKIPESDH-QVIISKCEDTISWLDVHQSAEKHETESKREELEKVCAPIITKVYQ
SJ   DEM*D**S***RKNRIL****E**R*M*NN*L***E*F*E*KS*******M****AMNR
Hs   EG**G**S*A*KKK*-LD**QEV*****ANTL***D*F*H**K***Q**N***SGL**
Dm   APA-G*LD*A*K-NSVLD**NE**R***SHTT***E*FDH*H***TRH*S**M**MH*

Sm   -AGG---------MPGGMHEAS--GAGGSG---------------KGPTIEEVD
Sj   -***---GVPSG*****---P--****G*----------------*********
Hs   -***------G-G-***-FG*Q-GPK****-----------------S********
Dm   Q--*AA---------**-PG*NCGQAGGF*GY-------------S********
```

FIGURE 4. Amino acid sequence comparisons between the C-terminal domains of HSP70 of *Schistosoma mansoni* (Sm), *Schistosoma japonicum* (Sj), *Homo sapiens* (Hs), and *Drosophila melanogaster* (Dm). The amino acid sequence was deduced from the nucleotide sequence (reviewed in Ref. 14). *Asterisks* denote regions of identity with the *S. mansoni* sequence. The *dashes* indicate that there are no intervening amino acids in the HSP70 of that species. The human and *Drosophila* sequences are from Hunt and Morimoto.[18]

cerevisiae as a molecular chaperone that escorts proteins across membranes, specifically the endoplasmic reticulum. HSPs are also purported to be involved in the coating and uncoating of clathrin-coated pits, in protein folding, and in protein aggregation (reviewed in Ref. 16). In sum, the HSPs seem to be conserved throughout biological systems because of their crucial and pervasive functions in the synthesis and assembly of macromolecular protein arrays—and from their pervasiveness in infections it would appear that they may also be somehow involved in the immunologic interplay between host and parasite.

In the example of antigenic variation of trypanosome VSGs, antibody reactions elicited against these antigens will result in antibody-mediated lysis of the parasite or, in the case of the chlamydia MOMPs, interfere with infection and penetration of host cells. One may therefore surmise that the antigenic diversity of these molecules provides a strategy whereby the parasite evades the host immune system and likewise that the response of the host has provided the selective pressure that has resulted in the evolution of these complex mechanisms. The antigenic diversity of the HSPs cannot be so easily explained. For the most part these are intracellular proteins, often confined to the cell nucleus, and their conservation of sequence and function across great evolutionary distances argues that they are crucial in cell biology. The extent of conservation of sequence would suggest that HSPs would either be poor immunogens or that antibodies made against these proteins would result in crossreactivity across species lines and thus contribute to autoimmunity. Antigenic diversity amongst the HSP70s of infectious organisms is confined to a highly variable C-terminal domain of the protein which constitutes the immunodominant epitope in infections; the remainder of the polypeptide is highly conserved and in the case of schistosomes, at least, antibodies have not been detected which react with the conserved portion of the molecule. Since it is possible to elicit an antibody response to the entire HSP70 sequence if the polypeptide is used as an immunogen, the restricted response to the C-terminal domain during infection seems to reflect a unique feature of the parasite-host interplay that remains to be discovered.

CONCLUSIONS

Antigenic variation and diversity of parasite antigens has generally been assumed to reflects the parasite's response to the host immune system. However, the diversity in HSP70s would suggest that our view of antigenic variation is perhaps too narrow. A wider view of the phenomenon might provide more important clues to understanding parasite cell biology in relation not only to the host's immune defenses, but also to the entire interplay between parasite and mammalian systems. It may be, for example, that the diversity of HSPs reflects a more fundamental role for these proteins in antigen recognition and presentation in both host and parasite rather than simply a "smokescreen" response by the parasite to decrease the efficacy of host immune surveillance. Viewed in this manner, perhaps the identity of other parasite antigens recognized during the course of infection will elucidate other classes of molecules which are important in the establishment and persistence of infection. In this context, HSPs are representative of other classes of antigens which are not found on the surface of the parasite but rather are intracellular or otherwise internalized within the parasite. Examples of these abound as recombinant DNA libraries are screened with infection sera: glutathione S-transferase, aldolase, glyceraldehyde-3-phosphate dehydrogenase, myosin, and paramyosin—metabolic enzymes and structural proteins that, when seen by the host immune system, or used as a protective antigen in model systems, are able to confer some degree of protection against infection.

Many lessons may be gleaned from the analysis of antigenic variation and diversity in parasite systems. The plasticity of the parasite genome and its inherent capacity for genetic diversity and variability were not anticipated in the first rush of enthusiasm for producing vaccines by recombinant genetic techniques. Antigenic diversity reflects the problems encountered by the parasite in establishing persistent infections and, as such, is a mirror of the immune challenge to parasite survival. More than this reflection, however, the molecular analysis of this complex phenomenon underscores the need for alternative targets for vaccinology. These targets are likely to be revealed only by studying the cell biology of the parasite itself and by developing a comprehension of the requirements of the parasite for survival in the host. Understanding the cell biology of parasitic organisms ought certainly to provide strategies for extending the natural repertoire of the immune system to cope with disease.

REFERENCES

1. VICKERMAN, K. & A. G. LUCKINS. 1969. Nature **244:** 1125
2. TURNER, M. J. 1982. Advan. Parsitol. **21:** 69.
3. LEVADITI, C. & J. MCINTOSH. 1910. Bull. Soc. Pathol. Exp. **3:** 368.
4. BORST, P. & G. A. M. CROSS. 1982. Cell **29:** 291.
5. SEGAL, E., E. BILLYARD, M. SO, S. STORZBACH & T. F. MEYER. 1985. Cell **40:** 293.
6. PLASTERK, R. H. A., M. I. SIMON & A. G. BARBOUR. 1985. Nature **318:** 257.
7. NASH, T. E. 1989. Exp. Parasitol. **68:** 238.
8. MACGOWAN, C., W. WOLLISH, L. ANDERSON & J. H. LEECH. 1988. J. Exp. Med. **168:** 1307.
9. GRAYSTON, J. T. & S.-P. WANG. 1975. J. Infect. Dis. **132:** 37.
10. STEPHENS, R. S., R. SANCHEZ PESCADOR, E. A. WAGEF, C. INOUYE & M. URDEA. 1987. J. Bacteriol. **169:** 3879.
11. STEPHENS, R. S., G. MULLENBACH, R. SANCHEZ-PESCADOR & N. AGABIAN. 1986. J. Bacteriol. **168:** 1277.
12. YUAN, Y., Y.-X. ZHANG, N. G. WATKINS & H. D. CALDWELL. 1989. Infec. Immun. **57:** 1040.
13. HEDSTROM, R., J. CULPEPPER, V. SCHINSKI, N. AGABIAN & G. NEWPORT. 1988. Molec. Biochem. Parasitol. **29:** 275.
14. HEDSTROM, R., J. CULPEPPER, R. HARRISON, N. AGABIAN & G. NEWPORT. 1987. J. Exp. Med. **165:** 1430.
15. NEWPORT, G., J. CULPEPPER & N. AGABIAN. 1988. Parasitol. Today **4**(11): 306-312.
16. PELHAM, H. 1988. Nature **332:** 776-777.
17. STEPHENS, R. S., C.-C. KUO, G. NEWPORT & N. AGABIAN. 1985. Infec. Immun. **47:** 713.
18. HUNT, C. & R. I. MORIMOTO. 1985. Proc. Natl. Acad. Sci. USA **82:** 6455.

Strategies for Vaccine Development: Schistosomiasis

ADEL A. F. MAHMOUD

Department of Medicine
Case Western Reserve University, and the
University Hospitals of Cleveland
Cleveland, Ohio 44106

INTRODUCTION

Schistosomiasis is the only worm infection to be discussed at this symposium. It is a fitting subject since the recipient of the L. H. Frohlich Award this year is Kenneth S. Warren, a physician and an investigator who dedicated most of his scientific career to studies of several aspects of this global health problem.

Human infection with several species of schistosomes accounts for considerable worldwide morbidity and mortality. The causative organisms are unique among infectious agents in many biologically and clinically relevant aspects. The most important of these are those that have a direct impact on strategies for the development of vaccines, and include the inability of schistosomes to multiply within the mammalian host and the slow rate of acquisition of infection in the population of endemic areas. The fundamental strategic questions in approaching the subject of immunity and its induction in schistosomiasis are:

1. Does immunity exist in infected humans?
2. Can resistance be induced in experimental animals?
3. Is it possible to isolate and characterize defined protective antigen(s) against this multicellular pathogen?
4. What are the effector mechanisms of immunity?
5. And, more importantly, is a vaccine needed as a part of the strategy to control schistosomiasis?

The purpose of this presentation is to examine the scientific basis for our understanding of the first four questions and to conclude with closing comments on the need for anti-schistosome vaccines. No attempt will be made to review the literature exhaustively since several publications cited below have recently appeared that have covered selected aspects of the subjects outlined above.

PROTECTIVE IMMUNITY IN HUMANS

Attempts to explain the features of age-specific variations in intensity of schistosome infection in communities living in endemic areas have centered on the following features:

1. Immunity is specifically acquired in infected individuals at a slow rate and may be dependent on intensity of infection or other host factors.[1,2]
2. The rise and decline in intensity of infection in populations of endemic areas parallel those observed in water contact studies; therefore, these changes may be ecologically rather than immunologically based.
3. The assumption that egg production by adult female worms is constant may be questioned. Older worms and worm aggregation in hosts with heavy infection have been demonstrated to produce fewer eggs, and therefore the decline in egg counts in older infected individuals may not reflect actual decrease in worm populations.[3]
4. Certain chronic stages of schistosome infection in humans may result in enough pathologic and fibrotic changes in the gut or urinary tract to alter the numbers or proportion of eggs passing in stools or urine.
5. Finally, the general arguments outlined above need to be appreciated with the host factors in mind. It has been demonstrated that susceptibility to infection and acquisition of specific immunity may be related to some genetic factors. Suggestions that this may be the case in human populations have also been reported.[4]

The acquisition of specific acquired resistance to schistosomiasis in humans is supported by *in vitro* studies demonstrating a multiplicity of effector mechanisms against the larval stage of the parasite.[5] In addition, follow-up study of infected persons after therapeutic cure of schistosomes indicates patterns suggestive of acquired resistance. The question, however, may not be of major significance in view of the repeated and successful results in induction of resistance in experimental animals. For several decades, it has been known that irradiated cercariae or schistosomulae induce significant resistance in mice and rats. Further investigations demonstrated that similar degrees of resistance may be induced in subhuman primates and cattle. A program to immunize cattle in the Sudan using irradiated organisms has been in effect for several years and has shown promising results. The positive outcome of these experiences with irradiated organisms is a realization that immunization against schistosomes can be achieved. The drawback is the limited supply if we have to use irradiated organisms in large-scale programs. This success, however, resulted in an aggressive program for obtaining and exploring immunization strategies based on isolating and characterizing defined antigens.

APPROACHES TO ANTI-SCHISTOSOME VACCINES

Over the past 10-15 years, most procedures available in modern immunology and molecular biology have been used to induce and examine the basis for resistance against schistosomiasis in experimental animals. These procedures include:

1. Crude parasite preparations;
2. Protective monoclonal antibodies;
3. Immunologically and biochemically defined parasite antigens or enzymes; and
4. Anti-idiotypic antibodies.

Crude Parasite Preparations

Attempts to induce resistance to schistosome infection in experimental animals by using crude parasite extracts have had inconsistent outcomes. Recently, however, investigators in two laboratories have systematically examined the potential protective effect of crude preparations.[6–8] TABLE 1 summarizes the results obtained in our laboratories.[6] In these studies, "freeze-thaw" schistosomula injected subcutaneously with or without BCG induced significant resistance. The next step was to identify components in the freeze-thaw preparation of larval schistosomes that may be involved in induction of resistance. Because of the simplicity of the humoral immune response in animals injected with freeze-thaw organisms, gel slices corresponding to the immunologically recognized 97-kD and 68-70-kD antigens were used (TABLE 2). Both produced significant protection and were biochemically and immunologically characterized further.

TABLE 1. Induction of Resistance by Freeze-Thaw Schistosomula after Subcutaneous Injection into CF_1 Mice

Experiment	No. of Mice in Each Group	Mean No. of Schistosomula Recovered (±SD)		% Protection (p value)
		Control	FT Schistosomula	
1	5	146 ± 18	114 ± 6	22% (p < 0.001)
2	5	190 ± 19	100 ± 10	47% (p < 0.001)
3	6	112 ± 4	88 ± 7	27% (p < 0.001)
4	5	105 ± 12	77 ± 5	29% (p < 0.001)
5	5	189 ± 12	121 ± 4	36% (p < 0.001)
6	9	145 ± 13	86 ± 5	41% (p < 0.001)
Mean of six experiments		148 ± 36	98 ± 17	34% (p < 0.020)

NOTE: Each animal was injected subcutaneously with ~freeze-thaw 2,000 organisms at days 1 and 14 and then exposed to 500 cercariae percutaneously on day 28. Recovery of lung schistosomula was performed on day 5 after challenge.

Drs. James, Sher and their colleagues worked on characterization of the 97-kD potential protective schistosome antigen.[9,10] They identified the antigen to be schistosome paramyosin and examined its protective effect when injected alone or in conjunction with BCG, We have used biochemical procedures to isolate schistosome paramyosin and have examined its protective potential (TABLE 3).[6] These studies confirm that crude schistosome antigens can be used as potential vaccines and that the host humoral immune response may be used to identify antigens of considerable

TABLE 2. Induction of Resistance by Schistosomula Membrane Extract and Schistosome Proteins

Experiment	Parasite Preparation	No. of Mice in Each Group	Mean No. of Schistosomula Recovered (± SD)		% Protection (p value)
			Control	Immunized	
1	1% Trixon X-100 extract of 5,000 schistosomula	5	159 ± 9	115 ± 11	27% ($p < 0.02$)
2	Gel slice with 97-kD protein	4	166 ± 13	117 ± 12	30% ($p <$ 001)
3	Gel slice with 97-kD protein	6	174 ± 8	91 ± 11	48% ($p < 0.001$)
4	Gel slice with 97-kD protein	9	145 ± 13	86 ± 5	41% ($p < 0.001$)
5	Gel slice with 68-70-kD protein	6	174 ± 8	91 ± 8	48% ($p < 0.001$)

NOTE: Each animal was injected subcutaneously with various doses of antigen on days 1 and 14 and then exposed to 500 cercariae percutaneously on day 28. Recovery of lung schistosomula was performed on day 5 after challenge. Control animals in experiment 1 received PBS and control animals in experiments 2-5 received polyacrylamide gel slice without protein. Animals in experiment 2 received only one dose of antigen and were then challenged on day 14.

TABLE 3. Induction of Resistance by Paramyosin Purified from Adult *S. mansoni*

Experiment	Preparation	No. of Mice in Each Group	Mean No. of Adult Worms Recovered (± SD)	% Protection (*p* value)
1	PBS	8	19 ± 7	
	Paramyosin	7	9 ± 6	53% ($p < 0.01$)
2	PBS	8	24 ± 10	
	Paramyosin	8	13 ± 10	46% ($p < 0.05$)
3	PBS	8	38 ± 8	
	Paramyosin	8	29 ± 8	24% ($p < 0.05$)
	BCG	7	29 ± 5	
	[a,b]Paramyosin + BCG	7	18 ± 7	52% ($p < 0.01$)

NOTE: Each animal was injected subcutaneously with 5 μg of paramyosin in 100 μl of PBS on days 1 and 14 and then exposed to 100 cercariae on day 28. Mice were perfused after 6 weeks to assess adult worm burden. Control mice (eight in each group) received 100 μl of PBS alone.

[a] Immunization with paramyosin + BCG when compared with BCG alone was significantly protective (38%, $p < 0.02$).

[b] Immunization with paramyosin + BCG when compared with immunization with paramyosin alone was significantly protective (38%, $p < 0.05$).

promise. Furthermore, we utilized immunoelectron microscopy to localize paramyosin in the tegument and cyton of adult worms.[11]

Protective Monoclonal Antibodies

Several laboratories have reported the production and testing of monoclonal antibodies that upon adoptive transfer result in partial acquired protection (TABLE 4).[12–16] Although monoclonal antibodies themselves are not of practical value in inducing resistance in humans, their protective effect confirmed the importance of the host humoral response in acquired immunity. Furthermore, these immunologic tools pro-

TABLE 4. Summary of Adoptive Transfer of Resistance by Potentially Protective Monoclonal Antibodies as Reported by Several Laboratories

Antibody	Species Protected	% Protected
AB1	Rat	53-62
AB3	Rat	50-76
Anti-KLH	Rat	48
Anti-P28AB	Rat	65
Anti-28K	Mouse	50
31-3B6	Mouse	27

vided for the first time the opportunity to isolate and characterize specific schistosome antigens that may be candidates for use as vaccines.

Defined Parasite Components

We will illustrate the use of monoclonal antibodies to isolate and characterize schistosome protective antigens by studies reported from our group.[17] It has to be recognized, however, that several other antigens (TABLE 5) and biochemically purified proteins such as glutathione transferase have also been reported to be partially protective.

Our studies were initiated by purifying the schistosome antigen that corresponds to the protective monoclonal antibody 31-3B6. Immunoaffinity purification resulted in the isolation of a 68-kD antigen that migrated as a single band on SDS-polyacrylamide gel electrophoresis followed by silver staining. The purified antigen resulted in significant protection when injected into outbred or inbred mice (TABLE 6). The most significant aspect of our results was that no adjuvant was needed. Further characterization of the resistance induced by the 68-kD antigen was achieved by examining optimal dose, duration of protection, nature of immune response in immunized animals, and, more importantly, the lack of sensitization to granuloma formation. In a recent study, we also examined the humoral response to 68-kD antigen in human populations infected with *S. mansoni* and found that in a subset the antibody responses were inversely correlated with fecal egg excretion.[18] Current efforts are concentrated on obtaining its encoding DNA sequences.

Induction of resistance to schistosomes using defined antigens allows a more systematic analysis of the host immune response in immunized animals. Recently the immune response to three synthetic peptides that were constructed to correspond to areas in the recombinant P28 protective schistosome antigen was reported.[9] The results of the study show that in immunized rats, the B-and T-cell responses were differentially induced by the different peptides. Furthermore, the IgG subclass induced was dependent on the peptide used for immunization. The biological relevance of some of these humoral responses was confirmed by demonstrating that antibodies cytotoxic to schistosomula *in vitro* were induced by the 24-43 peptide; these studies employed eosinophils as effector cells. This approach may be essential for the production of subunit vaccines and in enhancing their immunogenicity.

Anti-idiotypic Antibody Vaccines

An anti-idiotypic antibody vaccine was prepared using the partially protective monoclonal antibody 31-3B6.[20] The anti-idiotype antibody was used to immunize outbred mice against subsequent infection with *S. mansoni.* A mean of 41% protection as measured by schistosomula recovery from the lungs and 43% protection as measured by adult worm recovery were obtained. The protection was dependent on the number of injections of the anti-idiotypic antibody, its location, and the use of adjuvant. These results and the more recent report that anti-anti-idiotypic IgE antibodies were successfully used to confer protection[21] indicate the feasibility of this approach to vaccination.

TABLE 5. Summary of Protective Schistosome Parasite Antigens as Reported by Several Laboratories

Size (kD)	Species Protected	% Protection
26	Rat	40-60
38	Rat	53-63
38	Mouse	50
68	Mouse	24-66
97	Mouse	60-77

EFFECTOR MECHANISMS OF IMMUNITY

Our knowledge of the effector components of the host immunologic and inflammatory protective mechanisms in many infectious diseases is limited, but we know to a great extent the factors contributing to protection against schistosome infection. The original observations concerned the role of specific antibodies as a component of the

TABLE 6. Effect of Subcutaneous Administration of Two Doses of Immunoaffinity-Purified 68,000 MW Antigen on Recovery of Lung-Stage Schistosomula and Adult Worms of *S. mansoni*

			No. of Worms Recovered			
Experiment	Strain of Mice	Dose of Antigen	In lungs (5 days)	% Reduction	In portal circulation (8 weeks)	% Reduction
1	CF_1	0	169 ± 5[a]		158 ± 6[a]	
		1 μg	97 ± 4[b]	43	112 ± 11[b]	30
2	CF_1	0	213 ± 10[a]		35 ± 3[c]	
		1 μg	99 ± 9[b]	54	27 ± 1[b]	24
3	CF_1	0	145 ± 6[a]		32 ± 3[c]	
		0.5 μg	84 ± 8[b]	42	24 ± 2[b]	25
4	CF_1	0	NT[d]		24 ± 3[c]	
		0.5 μg			16 ± 3[b]	33
5	BALB/c	0	NT		70 ± 4[c]	
		0.5 μg			23 ± 3[e]	66
6	BALB/c	0	NT		21 ± 5[c]	
		1 μg			15 ± 3[f]	30

[a] Challenged with 500 cercariae.

[b] Significant difference from control group, $p < 0.05$; data reported are mean ± SEM for 6 to 10 mice in each group.

[c] Challenged with 100 cercariae.

[d] NT = not tested.

[e] Significant difference from control group, $p < 0.001$.

[f] Difference from control, NS, $p < 0.10$; overall, for combined BALB/c immunized vs. control groups (experiments 5 and 6), $p < 0.001$.

protective immunologic responses; adoptive transfer of resistance by serum from mice with chronic *S. mansoni* infection has been demonstrated.[2] Over the past 15 years, the role of eosinophils as the major effector cell of antibody-dependent cellular cytotoxicity was characterized both *in vitro* and *in vivo.*[22] Other contributory cells such as mononuclear phagocytes, T lymphocytes, and, more recently, platelets have been demonstrated to contribute to host protective mechanisms.[5] In other studies, the role of activated macrophages, whether induced specifically or nonspecifically, has been clearly demonstrated.[23]

What is important in developing vaccination strategies is that we know a lot about the host protective mechanism. Our knowledge is rudimentary, however, in regard to what specific parasite antigens are involved in stimulating these responses.

CONCLUDING COMMENTS

Experience to date indicates that immunity to a multicellular organism such as a schistosome is inducible in experimental animals. Protection is only partial and may be enhanced by adjuvants, but is never complete. Whether such a degree of induced protection, if achieved in humans, will make a difference in the prevalence and intensity of infection in infected populations remains to be seen. What is clear is an urgent need for vaccines to complement our control strategies. The remarkable progress in our knowledge of the nature of protective responses to schistosomes and the structure and determinants of resistance in the candidate vaccines should allow a rational approach to the next developmental steps.

REFERENCES

1. WARREN, K. S. 1973. Regulation of the prevalence and intensity of schistosomiasis in man: Immunology or ecology. J. Infect. Dis. **127:** 595.
2. BUTTERWORTH, A. E. 1987. Potential for vaccines against human schistosomes. *In* Bailliere's Clinical Tropical Medicine and Communicable Diseases. Vol. 2: Schistosomiasis. A. A. F. Mahmoud, Ed.: 465-483. Bailliere Tindall, Philadelphia, PA.
3. STURROCK, R. F. 1987. Biology and ecology of human schistosomes. *In* Bailliere's Clinical Tropical Medicine and Communicable Diseases.: 249-266 (see Ref. 2).
4. ABDEL SALAM, E., A. ABDEL KHALIK, A. ABDEL MEGUID, W. BARAKAT & A. A. F. MAHMOUD. 1986. Association of HLA class I antigens (A1, B5, B8 and CW2) with disease manifestations and infection in human schistosomiasis mansoni in Egypt. Tissue Antigens **23:** 142-146.
5. CAPRON, A., J. P. DESSAINT, M. CAPRON, J. H. OUMA & A. E. BUTTERWORTH. 1987. Immunity to schistosomes: Progress towards vaccine. Science **238:** 1065-1072.
6. FLANIGAN, T. P., C. H. KING, R. R. LETT, J. NANDURI & A. A. F. MAHMOUD. 1989. Induction of resistance to *Schistosoma mansoni* infection in mice by purified parasite paramyosin. J. Clin. Invest. **83:** 1010-1014.
7. JAMES, S. L. 1985. Induction of protective immunity against *Schistosoma mansoni* by a nonliving vaccine is dependent on the method of antigen presentation. J. Immunol. **134:** 1956-1960.
8. JAMES, S. L. 1986. Induction of protective immunity against *Schistosoma mansoni* by a nonliving vaccine. III. Correlation of resistance with induction of activated larvicidal macrophages. J. Immunol. **136:** 3872-3877.

9. PEARCE, E. J., S. L. JAMES, J. DALTON, *et al.* 1986. Immunochemical characterization and purification of Sm-97, a *Schistosoma mansoni* antigen monospecifically recognized by antibodies from mice protectively immunized with a nonliving vaccine. J. Immunol. **137:** 3593-3600.
10. PEARCE, E. J., S. L. JAMES, S. HIENY, *et al.* 1988. Induction of protective immunity against *Schistosoma mansoni* by vaccination with schistosome paramyosin (Sm97), a nonsurface parasite antigen. Proc. Natl. Acad. Sci. USA **85:** 5678-5682.
11. MATSUMOTO, Y., G. PERRY, R. J. C. LEVINE, R. BLANTON & H. AIKAWA. 1988. Paramyosin and actin in schistosomal tegument. Nature **333:** 76-78.
12. ZODDA, D. M. & S. M. PHILLIPS. 1982. Monoclonal antibody-mediated protection against *Schistosoma mansoni* infection in mice. J. Immunol. **129:** 2326.
13. HARN, D. A., M. MITSUYAMA & J. R. DAVID. 1984. Anti-egg monoclonal antibodies protect against cercarial challenge in vivo. J. Exp. Med. **159:** 1371.
14. SMITH, M. A., J. A. CLEGG, D. SNARY & E. J. TREJDOSIEWICZ. 1982. Passive immunization of mice against *Schistosoma mansoni* with an IgM monoclonal antibody. Parasitology **84:** 83.
15. GRZYCH, J. M., M. CAPRON, H. BAZIN & A. CAPRON. 1982. In vivo and in vitro effector function of rat IgG2a monoclonal anti-*S. mansoni* antibodies. J. Immunol. **129:** 2739.
16. HAZDAI, R. T., F. LEVI-SCHAFFER, V. BRENNER, S. HOROWITZ, Z. ESHHAR & R. ARNON. 1985. Protective monoclonal antibody against *Schistosoma mansoni:* Antigen isolation, characterization and suitability for active immunization. J. Immunol. **135:** 2772.
17. KING, C. H., R. F. LETT, J. NANDURI, S. EL IBIARY, P. A. S. PETERS, G. R. OLDS & A. A. F. MAHMOUD. 1987. Isolation and characterization of a protective antigen for adjuvant-free immunization against *Schistosoma mansoni.* **139:** 4218-4224.
18. KING, C. H., S. EL IBIARY, M. EL NAWAWI, J. SAWYER, A. GRIFFIN, A. EL HAWEY & A. A. F. MAHMOUD. 1989. Intensity of *Schistosoma mansoni* infection in a human population is inversely correlated with antibody response to SMW68, a protective parasite antigen. J. Infect. Dis. In press.
19. ANRIAULT, C., H. GRAS-MASSE, I. WOLOWCZUK *et al.* 1988. Analysis of T and B cell epitope of the *Schistosoma mansoni* P28 antigen in the rat model by using synthetic peptide. J. Immunol. **141:** 1687-1694.
20. KRESINA, T. F. & G. R. OLDS. 1989. Anti-idiotypic antibody vaccine in murine schistosomiasis mansoni comprising the internal image of antigen. J. Clin. Invest. **83:** 912-920.
21. VELGE-ROUSSEL, C. VER WAERDE, J. M. GRZYCH *et al.* 1989. Protective effect of anti-antidiotypic IgE antibodies obtained from an IgE monoclonal antibody specific for a 26-kilodalton *Schistosoma mansoni* antigen. J. Immunol. **142:** 2527-2632.
22. MAHMOUD, A. A. F. 1981. The ecology of eosinophils in schistosomiasis. J. Infect. Dis. **145:** 613-622.
23. ELLNER, J. J. & A. A. F. MAHMOUD. 1982. Phagocytes and worms: David and Goliath revisited. Rev. Infect. Dis. **4:** 698-714.

Strategies for the Development of Vaccines for Typhoid Fever, Shigellosis, and Cholera

SAMUEL I. MILLER[a] AND JOHN J. MEKALANOS

Department of Microbiology and Molecular Genetics
Harvard Medical School
Boston, Massachusetts 02115

Enteric fevers and diarrheal diseases are major causes of morbidity and mortality throughout the developing world.[1] Traditional approaches to the development of vaccines for bacterial diseases include the parenteral injection of purified components or killed organisms.[2] These methods require technologically advanced preparation and are relatively expensive despite their proven benefits. Live oral vaccine strains have several advantages over parenteral vaccines: low cost, ease of administration, and simple preparation.

The development of live vaccines has been limited by lack of understanding of the pathogenesis of disease on a molecular level. Candidate live vaccine strains require nonrevertable genetic alterations that affect the virulence of the organism, but not its induction of an immune response. Work defining the mechanisms of toxigenesis of *Vibrio cholerae* has made it possible to create live vaccine strains based on deletion of the toxin genes.[3,4] We will discuss below recent studies that have begun to define the molecular basis of *Salmonella typhimurium* macrophage survival and virulence. This may lead to the development of a live oral *Salmonella typhi* vaccine that can be used as a carrier for heterologous antigens. This approach has the advantage that immunity to multiple diseases could be generated with a single vaccine strain. Attenuated *Salmonella typhi* would deliver heterologous antigens directly to the immune effector cell, the macrophage, and generate cell-mediated as well as humoral immune response.[5]

VIRULENCE MECHANISMS AND IMMUNITY IN *SALMONELLA* DISEASE

Salmonella species cause a spectrum of clinical disease that includes enteric fevers and acute gastroenteritis.[1] Infections with *Salmonella* species are more common in immunosuppressed persons.[6] *S. typhi,* the bacterium that causes typhoid fever, can only infect man.[1] The narrow host specificity of *S. typhi* has resulted in the extensive

[a] Present address: Infectious Disease Unit, Massachusetts General Hospital, Boston, Massachusetts 02114.

use of *S. typhimurium* infection of mice as a laboratory model of typhoid fever.[7] Although the natural history of salmonellosis is understood, little is known about the molecular basis of *Salmonella* pathogenesis.

Salmonella infections are acquired by oral ingestion. The organisms, after traversing the stomach, replicate in the small bowel.[5] *Salmonella* are capable of invasion of the intestinal mucosal cells, and *S. typhi* can pass through this mucosal barrier and spread via the Peyer's patches to the lamina propria and regional lymph nodes.[5] Colonization of the reticuloendothelial cells of the host then occurs after bacteremia. The ability of *S. typhi* to survive and replicate within the cells of the human reticuloendothelial system is essential to its pathogenesis.[1,5,7]

Immunity to *Salmonella typhi* involves humoral and cell-mediated immunity[8] and is obtainable by vaccination.[9] Much of what we know about immunity is based on prior human vaccine studies and murine typhoid.

Serum antibody to *Salmonella* antigens is important to survival in murine typhoid.[10] Antibody is largely directed to the lipopolysaccharide, flagellar proteins, O antigen, and H antigen.[10] *Salmonella typhi* has an additional unique polysaccharide capsule on its surface, termed the Vi antigen.[11] Antibody against Vi antigen likely facilitates phagocytosis since organisms with a polysaccharide capsule are typically resistant to phagocytosis in the absence of specific antibody. Chronic carriers of *S. typhi,* who are asymptomatic and excrete the organism, can be identified by high antibody titers against Vi antigen.[11] Recently human field trials demonstrated significant protective efficacy against *S. typhi* infection after intramuscular vaccination with partially purified Vi antigen.[12] Antibody-dependent enhancement of *S. typhi* killing by T cells has been demonstrated in individuals who received a live *S. typhi* vaccine, indicating that these antibodies may be necessary for the host to generate a cell-mediated immune response.[13] These data imply that antibody-mediated cytotoxicity or opsonization is important to immunity to *S. typhi.* The cell-mediated immune response is also important in typhoid immunity[7,14] since killed vaccines that do not induce this immune response are not protective in man.[15]

From 1964 to 1972 several field trials of killed vaccines prepared by heat-phenolization and acetone-drying documented that typhoid immunity can be achieved by vaccination.[16–18] Approximately 70% of individuals in endemic areas who received killed vaccines were protected from subsequent typhoid. But these vaccine preparations had an unacceptable level of local and systemic reactions.[16–18] The main disadvantage of a killed vaccine is it may not contain antigens only expressed within the host.

LIVE VACCINES IN *SALMONELLA* DISEASE

A large body of work in animal models has documented the superiority of live versus killed bacterial vaccines.[19] Most preliminary work for the development of live attenuated *S. typhi* vaccines is based on work in mouse models using *S. typhimurium.* After *S. typhimurium* ingestion, mice develop a disease similar to typhoid fever with hepatosplenomegaly and fever leading to death.[7,20] The LD_{50} for Balb/c mice infected with *S. typhimurium* by intraperitoneal injection is fewer than 20 organisms.[7,20] The pathophysiology of mouse typhoid is similar to that of human disease, as the essential feature is *S. typhimurium* survival within mouse phagocytes.

S. typhimurium rough colony mutants, which have defective lipopolysaccharide O side chains, are avirulent for mice. This prompted Germanier in the 1970s to perform studies of *S. typhimurium* rough mutants (LPS-deficient) as vaccines in mice.[21] Strains with mutation in the *galE* gene gave superior protection over that afforded by other types of rough mutants.[22] There is evidence that antibody to lipopolysaccharide (LPS) is important for immunity and that *galE* mutants, unlike most rough mutants, are capable of making intact LPS when grown on galactose.

Germanier's work led to the development and testing in man of a *galE* mutant of *S. typhi*, strain Ty21a,[23] as a live vaccine. Ty21a was found to be safe in large field trials and provided protection against typhoid fever similar to that induced by more toxic killed vaccines.[24] However, in some trials in which a single dose was administered no significant protection was induced.[25] Ty21a colonizes humans very poorly, as evidenced by the fact that the organism cannot be recovered from the stools of volunteers even 48 hours after challenge.[26] The Ty21a strain was generated by chemical mutagenesis and it has other genetic defects, in addition to the *galE* mutation, which result in auxotrophic requirements that are not satisfied by the addition of defined nutrients to minimal media.[27] Recently a *Salmonella typhi* strain with a defined mutation in *galE* was administered to humans and was found to be virulent.[28] Thus, the molecular basis for the avirulence of Ty21a is unknown. Strains generated by chemical mutagenesis have the additional disadvantage of usually being point mutations and therefore subject to a high rate of reversion. While Ty21a was safe, it colonized the intestine poorly and grew poorly in the laboratory. The pioneering studies with Ty21a demonstrated the safety and the potential efficacy of a live oral bacterial vaccine for typhoid fever.

Bacon, Burrows, and Yates demonstrated in the early 1950s that auxotrophic mutants of *S. typhi* in pathways of aromatic amino acid and purine biosynthesis were avirulent for mice.[29] Stocker and his colleagues were the first to apply modern genetic techniques to construct defined, nonreverting strains with mutations in these pathways and to investigate their role in virulence. Stocker's elegant studies documented that *S. typhimurium* strains deleted in *aroA* are avirulent and immunogenic in mice.[30] Mutants in *aroA* cannot synthesize the central precursor chorismic acid, and thus will not grow in laboratory media in the absence of aromatic amino acids, *para*-aminobenzioc acid (PABA), and 2,3-dihydroxybenzoate (DHB). These metabolites are not available within the host and *aroA* mutants are starved for these compounds. These mutant organisms, when administered intraperitoneally, did protect animals against subsequent challenge by virulent wild-type *Salmonella*.[30]

A strain of *S. typhi* deficient in *aroA* and *purA* (which makes the organism auxotrophic for purines) is now being investigated in humans. Volunteer trials show that this organism can be safely administered and generates some cell-mediated response.[13] However, the organism generates little antibody to *S. typhi* antigens and poorly colonizes humans.[13] It remains to be seen whether this organism is protective in man, but the early results are not encouraging.[31]

The aforementioned studies seem to document that there are metabolites that are not available to *Salmonella* in the host. It may be that limiting the organism in these pathways is too crippling for the generation of immunity by administration of a live vaccine orally. These studies have not defined specific virulence properties involved in survival and growth of the organism in the macrophage.

Curtiss and his colleagues have recently found that *S. typhimurium* mutants with defects in the *crp* regulatory gene encoding cAMP binding protein or in the *cya* gene encoding adenylate cyclase are avirulent and can provide some protection as a live vaccine in mice.[32] This is a promising system based on the idea of inhibiting the expression of many bacterial genes by inactivating regulatory genes. The *crp* and *cya* gene products are involved in catabolite repression and thus regulate the expression of many genes involved in carbohydrate metabolism, as well as the synthesis of flagella, outer membrane proteins, and fimbria. These strains could revert to a virulent state because the genes regulated by *cya* and *crp* that are required for virulence have not been deleted. These genes may escape regulatory gene product control by mutations in their promoters and express a normal virulent phenotype. The alterations of surface proteins in these mutants may also effect colonization of the host and the induction of immunity (e.g., macromolecular structures like flagella and fimbriae are highly antigenic and therefore preferred targets of the immune system).

GENETIC ANALYSIS OF *SALMONELLA* VIRULENCE

None of the above approaches has elucidated the genes and gene products involved in the essential feature of *Salmonella* pathogenesis, macrophage survival. Strains deleted for genes involved in survival within the macrophage could be superior as live vaccines. Studies discussed below may provide an approach that should allow the definition of the molecular basis of *Salmonella* pathogenesis and the development of such a vaccine strain.

Recent work by Heffron and his collaborators has addressed the problem of *Salmonella* survival within the macrophage. They performed transposon mutagenesis of *Salmonella typhimurium* and screened organisms for the inability to survive in mouse macrophages.[33] There was good correlation between poor survival and avirulence. Those that were characterized included auxotrophs for purine and amino acid biosynthesis, and mutants deficient in oxidative stress response.[33]

Recent work in many laboratories, including ours, has documented that bacterial virulence factors are often coordinately regulated by environmental stimuli.[34] Two major bacterial pathogens, *Vibrio cholera* and *Bordetella pertussis,* have regulatory genes that control the expression of many virulence factors in response to environmental signals.[34] We began to search for a regulatory gene that might control the expression of genes encoding proteins necessary for macrophage survival. Strains with mutations in regulatory genes that respond to nitrogen limitation (*ntrA*)[35] and oxygen stress (*oxyR*),[36] conditions that are proposed to exist within the phagocytic vacuole, have no measurable virulence defect when injected into Balb/c mice.[60] We tested mutations in the *phoP* genetic locus, responsible for the synthesis of a periplasmic acid phosphatase, because of the presumed acidic environment of the phagocytic vacuole. Strains with *phoP* mutations have marked virulence attenuation.[60] We have been reassured that an intact *phoP* locus is essential for virulence by the recent observation by Heffron's group that strains with mutations that map to the *phoP* locus and are deficient in the production of acid phosphatase are among those identified as unable to survive in mouse macrophages.[34,61]

Further work has defined the *phoP* locus as part of a regulatory system in *Salmonella typhimurium* that dramatically attenuates the ability of the organism to cause murine typhoid and death in Balb/c mice.[60] Transposon insertions in the *phoP* genetic locus raise the LD_{50} of *S. typhimurium* for Balb/c mice from 20 to 5×10^5 organisms administered intraperitoneally.[34,60] The *phoP* locus is required for the synthesis of a periplasmic acid phosphatase.[37] *Salmonella typhimurium* strains deleted only for the acid phosphatase structural gene, termed *phoN,* are as virulent as wild-type organisms for Balb/c mice.

Using the transposon Tn*phoA* we have recently isolated a mutant strain with a transposon insertion in a gene (termed *pagC* for phoP-activated gene) that requires *phoP* for expression.[60] Bacteria secrete proteins through the cytoplasmic membrane by use of an amino terminal signal sequence. The *phoA* gene fusion approach is based on the fact that the normally periplasmic enzyme alkaline phosphatase, encoded by *phoA,* must be localized extracytoplasmically to be active.[38] Export and enzyme activity can be restored by fusing a restriction fragment containing a truncated *phoA* gene (lacking secretion signals) to portions of genes encoding signal sequences of heterologous proteins. Manoil and Beckwith have extended the utility of this approach by inserting a similar *phoA* restriction fragment near one end of Tn5 to create a transposon, designated Tn*phoA,* that can randomly generate gene fusions to *phoA* upon insertion into the chromosome.[39] Broad host range plasmid vectors containing Tn*phoA* developed by Taylor and Mekalanos[40] allow random mutagenesis and generation of Tn*phoA* fusions in *Salmonella.* The hybrid proteins expressed by such gene fusions display phosphatase activity only if the target gene contains a signal sequence.[39] When a population of bacteria is mutagenized with Tn*phoA,* colonies with fusions of *phoA* to genes that contain these export signals display a blue phenotype when plated on the chromogenic substrate XP.[39] Because such exported proteins represent the most frequent classes of proteins recognized to be involved in bacterial pathogenesis, the use of Tn*phoA* provides a strong enrichment for insertion mutations in virulence genes.

This *Salmonella typhimurium* strain with a *pagC* mutation likely are inactivated for the *phoP*-regulated gene product as these strains are attenuated for virulence by at least 1,000-fold.

As stated above, Heffron's group has also demonstrated a virulence defect in strains with mutations in the *phoP* locus by showing that they were among a number of strains isolated by their inability to survive in macrophages. This group has also shown that *phoP* mutants are more sensitive to killing by a low molecular weight cationic fraction from human neutrophils.[61] This fraction contains the cationic proteins termed defensins, which are known to have antibacterial activity.[41,61] These results, combined with the above data, suggest that *phoP* mutants are avirulent because of the inability to synthesize a regulated gene product specifically required to evade and survive the mammalian immune system. These mutations could be important for understanding the molecular basis of typhoid fever as well as the pathogenesis of the diarrheal disease caused by *S. typhimurium* in man.

We have also cloned the DNA encoding the *phoP* locus and determined its DNA sequence, direction of transcription, and deduced amino acid sequence. There is marked similarity between the deduced amino acid sequence of PhoP and other bacterial regulatory proteins, such as OmpR,[42] NtrC,[35] and PhoB,[43] that control the synthesis of numerous gene products in response to environmental signals. These proteins are one component (regulator) of what has become known as two-component regulatory systems.[44] In these systems, two gene products are required for regulation, a sensor such as NtrB that in conditions of nitrogen limitation functions as a kinase to phosphorylate the transcriptional activator NtrC.[45] This covalent modification of the transcriptional activator leads to the synthesis of gene products, like glutamine synthetase, essential to the organism in nitrogen limitation.[45] The genes encoding these two proteins are located in the same operon.[35,42–44] The members of the family have protein sequence similarities. The sensors have a carboxy terminal domain similarity that is thought to correspond to the kinase domain. The transcriptional activators all have amino terminal similarity that corresponds to a phosphate acceptor domain. Some of the transcriptional activators have additional carboxy terminal similarity that is thought to correspond to DNA binding and polymerase activation domains.[44] The deduced amino acid sequence of PhoP has similarity to OmpR in both domains, suggesting that it might be a member of a two-component regulatory system. It is interesting that the amino terminus of ToxR, which is necessary for DNA binding and transcriptional activation of the cholera toxin promoter, has homology with the carboxyl terminal domains of OmpR and PhoP that may be involved in gene activation.[46]

The DNA sequence of the *phoP* locus reveals that this system is a two-component regulatory system located in a single operon. The deduced amino acid sequence of PhoP shows it to be a 234-amino-acid protein with similarity to the members of the two-component family in both the amino and carboxyl terminal domains. The greatest similarity is to OmpR with PhoB and VirG being the next similar because they are members of the family with similarity in the phosphate acceptor domain as well as the transcriptional activator domain. Immediately 3′ to the termination codon of *phoP* is a start codon for the synthesis of a protein we term PhoQ. Strains with transposon insertions in either gene inactivate phosphatase activity and are avirulent for mice. DNA sequence analysis of this open reading frame indicated that it encodes a 487-amino-acid membrane protein whose topology predicts that it is a membrane protein with a periplasmic and cytoplasmic domain. Additionally Tn*phoA* fusions in this gene have alkaline phosphatase activity. Analysis of the predicted *phoQ* gene product demonstrates that it is the second member (the sensor) of the PhoP regulatory system. This protein has extensive cytoplasmic (carboxyl terminus) similarity to proteins such as EnvZ, and NR I, which are sensor kinase members of two component regulators.

Ames previously characterized the regulation of the acid phosphatase of *Salmonella typhimurium* and demonstrated that unlike the *E. coli* alkaline phosphatase (*phoA*) that is controlled by the *phoR/phoB* regulatory system, it was not regulated specifically by low phosphate.[36] Rather, induction of acid phosphatase production correlated with starvation conditions and was maximally 3-5-fold. Of interest in line with these data *phoP* can not complement a *phoB* mutation in *E. coli,* nor can *phoB* complement a *phoP* mutation in *Salmonella,* when on a multicopy plasmid. It is possible that another unidentified signal may produce more dramatic effects in the Phop/PhoQ regulon. We have demonstrated that several gene fusions to different *pag* genes have increased expression in media of low pH by a factor of 2-3-fold. We hope to further characterize the environmental signals that activate this regulon since it may reveal information about the *Salmonella* environment in the macrophage.

We have interested efficacy of strains with *phoP* mutations as vaccines against mouse typhoid. These strains afford partial protection to subsequent challenge with wild-type organisms. Specifically, survivors of a LD_{50} challenge have a 1,000-fold increase in LD_{50} when challenged with wild-type organisms. Our future studies will focus on the characterization of the virulence proteins regulated by PhoP that appear necessary for virulence. We believe that this analysis could lead to the development of a *Salmonella* vaccine that has stable mutations in several genes regulated by PhoP. We will study the ability of strains with such mutation to protect mice against enteric fever, and we hope in the future to study the effect of similar mutation in *S. typhi* as vaccine candidates in man.

MULTIVALENT LIVE VACCINES UTILIZING *SALMONELLA* AS A CARRIER

The potent immunogencity of live *Salmonella* has sparked interest in the development of the organism as a carrier for other protein antigens. The capacity of this organism to elicit humoral and cell-mediated immunity, the oral mode of administration, and the ease of genetic manipulation are factors in favor of this idea. The advantage of induction of a specific intestinal immune response is an attractive idea for protection against mucosal infections such as cholera, toxigenic *E. coli,* rotavirus, and polio.

This thinking has led investigators to express *E. coli* enterotoxin and *Shigella* surface antigens (LPS) expressed from plasmids inserted into Ty21a and to demonstrate the development of an immune response to these heterologous antigens.[47,48] *S. typhimurium aroA* mutants have been engineered to express *E. coli* antigens from plasmids, and a serum- and gut-associated IgA and IgG response was documented in animals.[49] Recently the bacterial intracellular protein beta-galactosidase was expressed on a plasmid in an *aroA* mutant of *S. typhimurium.*[49] An antibody response was elicited, indicating that intracellular proteins expressed in *Salmonella* are recognized by the immune system. More importantly, as tested by mouse foot pad injections, delayed-type hypersensitivity was also induced. Therefore the practicality of developing both a humoral and cellular immune response to heterologous proteins of different origin seems possible.

In regard to using *Salmonella* carrier vaccines to immunize against cholera and shigellosis, several additional recent advances have been made. The TCP pilus of *V. cholerae* has been identified as the major colonization factor in both mice[50] and humans.[51] The major subunit of this pilus (TcpA) has been expressed in *S. typhimurium,*[52] and this approach to vaccination against cholera can be investigated in animal models.

Although the role of Shiga toxin in the pathogenesis of shigellosis is unknown, it remains an attractive vaccine component that might augment the immunity induced by live, attenuated *Shigella* vaccines that boost immunity to the invasive factors of this organism.[53,54] The Shiga-like toxin of *E. coli* has been shown to be virtually identical to Shiga cytotoxin of *S. dysenteriae.*[55,56] In this regard, site-directed mutations in the Shiga-like toxin A subunit have been constructed that have identified a glutamic acid residue as being important for its enzymatic activity.[57] Introduction of the genes for such "genetically detoxified" versions of Shiga toxin, diphtheria toxin,[58] and pertussis toxin[59] into a *Salmonella* carrier vaccine is the logical next step toward a multivalent vaccine for many of the great neglected diseases that exist under the volcano of the Third World.

REFERENCES

1. HOOK, E. & R. GUERRANT. 1980. Salmonella infections. *In* Harrison's Principles of Internal Medicine, 9th ed.: 641-648. McGraw Hill. New York.
2. PLOTKIN, S. L. & S. A. PLOTKIN. 1988. A short history of vaccination. *In* Vaccines.: 1-8. W. B. Saunders. Philadelphia, PA.
3. MEKALANOS, J. J., D. J. SWARTZ, G. D. N. PEARSON, N. HARFORD, F. GROYNE & M. DEWILDE. 1983. Cholera toxin genes: Nucleotide sequence, deletion analysis, and vaccine development. Nature **306:** 551.
4. LEVINE, M. M., J. B. KAPER, D. HERRINGTON, G. LOSONSKY, J. G. MORRIS, M. L. CLEMENTS, B. TALL & R. HALL. 1988. Volunteer studies of deletion mutants of *Vibrio cholerae* 01 prepared by recombinant techniques. Infect. Immun. **56:** 161-167.
5. HORNICK, R. B. *et al.* 1970. Typhoid fever: Pathogenesis and immunological control. I, II. N. Engl. J. Med. **283:** 686-739.
6. CELUM, C. L. *et al.* Incidence of salmonellosis in patients with AIDS. 1987 J. Infect. Dis. **156:** 998-1001.
7. CARTER, P. B. & F. M. COLLINS. 1984. The route of enteric infection in normal mice. J. Exp. Med. **139:** 1189-1203.

8. MURPHY, J. R. *et al.* 1987. Characteristics of humoral and cellular immunity to *Salmonella typhi* in residents of typhoid-endemic and typhoid-free regions. J. Infect. Dis. **156:** 1005-1009.
9. EDELMAN, R. & M. M. LEVINE. 1986. Summary of an international workshop on typhoid fever. Rev. Inf. Dis. **8:** 329-349.
10. BLANDEN, R. V. *et al.* 1966. Mechanisms of acquired resistance in mouse typhoid. J. Exp. Med. **124:** 585-600.
11. LANATA, C. F. *et al.* 1983. Vi serology in detection of chronic *Salmonella typhi* carriers in an endemic area. Lancet **2:** 441-443.
12. ACHARYA, I. L. *et al.* 1987. Prevention of typhoid fever in Nepal with the Vi capsular polysaccharide of *Salmonella typhi:* A preliminary report. N. Engl. J. Med. **317:** 1101.
13. LEVINE, M. M. *et al.* 1987. Safety, infectivity, immunogenicity and *in vivo* stability of two attenuated auxotrophic mutant strains of *Salmonella typhi,* 541Ty and 543Ty, as live oral vaccines in humans. J. Clin. Invest. **79:** 888-902.
14. DUPONT, H. L. *et al.* 1971. Immunity in typoid fever: Evaluation of a live streptomycin-dependent vaccine. Antimicrob. Agents Chemother. **45:** 236-239.
15. COLLINS, F. M. & P. B. CARTER. 1972. Comparative immunogenicity of heat-killed and living oral *Salmonella* vaccines. Infect. Immun. **41:** 742-750.
16. ASHCROFT, M. T. *et al.* 1967. A seven-year field trial of two typhoid vaccines in Guiana. Lancet **ii:** 1056-60.
17. YUGOSLAV TYPHOID COMMISSION. 1964. A controlled field trial of the effectiveness of acetone-dried and inactivated and heat-phenol-inactivated typhoid vaccines in Yugoslavia. Bull. WHO **30:** 623-30.
18. POLISH TYPHOID COMMITTEE. 1966. Controlled field trials and laboratory studies on the effectiveness of typhoid vaccines in Poland 1961-1964. Bull. WHO **34:** 211-222.
19. GERMANIER, R. 1972. Immunity in experimental salmonellosis. III. Comparative immunization with viable and heat inactivated cells of *Salmonella typhimurium.* Infect. Immun. **5:** 792-797.
20. HORMAECHE, C. E. 1979. Natural resistance to *Salmonella typhimurium* in different inbred mouse strains. Immunology **37:** 311-318.
21. GERMANIER, R. 1970. Immunity in experimental salmonellosis. I. Protection induced by rough mutants of *Salmonella typhimurium.* Infect. Immun. **2:** 309-315.
22. GERMANIER, R. & E. FURER. 1971. Immunity in experimental salmonellosis II. Basis for the avirulence and protective capacity of *gal*E mutant of *Salmonella typhimurium.* Infect. Immun. **4:** 663-673.
23. GERMANIER, R. & E. FURER. 1975. Isolation and characterization of *gal*E mutant Ty21a of *Salmonella typhi:* A candidate strain for a live oral vaccine. J. Infect. Dis. **141:** 553-558.
24. LEVINE, M. M. *et al.* 1987. Large scale field trial of Ty21a a live oral typhoid vaccine in enteric coated capsule formation. Lancet **1:** 1049-1052.
25. LEVINE, M. M. *et al.* 1987. Field trials of efficacy of attenuated *Salmonella typhi* oral vaccine strain Ty21a. *In* Proceedings of the International Symposium on Bacterial Vaccines. J. Robbins, Ed. Praeger. New York.
26. GILMAN, R. H. *et al.* 1977. Evaluation of UDP galactose 4-epimeraseless mutant of *Salmonella typhi* as a live oral vaccine. J. Infect. Dis. **136:** 717.
27. GERMANIER, R. & E. FURER. 1983. Characterization of the attenuated oral vaccine strain *S. typhi* Ty21a. Dev. Biol. Stand. **53:** 3-7.
28. HONE, D. M. *et al.* 1988. A *galE via* (Vi antigen-negative) mutant of *Salmonella typhi* Ty2 retains virulence in humans. Infect. Immun. **56:** 1326-1333.
29. BACON, G. A. *et al.* 1951. The effect of biochemical mutation on the virulence of *B. typhosum:* The loss of virulence of certain mutants. Br. J. Exp. Pathol. **32:** 85.
30. HOISEITH, S. K. & B. A. D. STOCKER. 1981. Aromatic dependent *Salmonella typhimurium* are non-virulent and effective as live vaccines. Nature **291:** 238-241.
31. STOCKER, B. A. D. 1988. Auxotrophic *Salmonella typhi* as live vaccine. Vaccine **6:** 141-145.
32. CURTISS, R., III & S. M. KELLY. 1987. *Salmonella typhimurium* deletion mutants lacking adenylate cyclase and cyclic AMP receptor protein are avirulent and immunogenic. Infect. Immun. **55:** 3035-3043.

33. FIELDS, P. J. *et al.* 1986. Mutants of *Salmonella typhimurium* that cannot survive within the macrophage are avirulent. Proc. Natl. Acad. Sci. USA. **83:** 5189-5193.
34. MILLER, J. F., J. J. MEKALANOS & S. FALKOW. 1988. Coordinate regulation and sensory transduction in the control of bacterial virulence. Science. In press.
35. KUSTU, S., K. SEI & J. KEENER. 1986. *In* Regulation of Gene Expression—25 Years on. Society for General Microbiology, I. Booth & C. F. Higgins, Eds.: 139-154. Cambridge University Press.
36. CHRISTMAN, M. F. *et al.* 1985. Positive control of a regulon for defenses against oxidative stress and some heat-shock proteins in *Salmonella typhimurium.* Cell **41:** 753-762.
37. KIER, L. D., R. M. WEPPLEMAN & B. N. AMES. 1979. Regulation of nonspecific acid phosphatase in Salmonella: *phoN* and *phoP* genes. J. Bacteriol. **138:** 155-161.
38. BROCKMAN, R. W. & L. A. HEPPEL. 1968. On the localization of alkaline phosphatase and cyclic phosphodiesterase in *E. coli.* Biochemistry **7:** 2554-2562.
39. MANOIL, C. & J. BECKWITH. 1985. Tn*phoA:* A transposon probe for protein export signals. Proc. Natl. Acad. Sci. USA. **82:** 8129-8133.
40. TAYLOR, R. K., C. MANOIL & J. J. MEKALANOS. 1989. Broad host range vectors for the delivery of Tn*phoA:* Use in analysis of virulence determinants of *Vibrio cholerae.* J. Bacteriol. **171:** 1870-1878.
41. GANZ, T., M. E. SELSTED, D. SZKLARNEK, S. S. L. HARTWIG, K. DAHER & R. I. LEHRER. 1985. Defensins: natural peptide antibiotics of human neutrophils. J. Clin. Invest. **76:** 1427-1435.
42. COMEAU, D. E., K. IKENAKA, K. TSUNG, & M. INOUYE. 1985. Primary characterization of the protein products of the *E. coli ompB* locus: Structure and regulation of synthesis of the OmpR and EnvZ proteins. J. Bacteriol. **164:** 578-584.
43. MAKINO, K., H. SHINAGAWA, M. AMEMURA & A. NAKATA. 1986. Nucleotide sequence of the *phoR* gene, a regulatory gene for the phosphate regulon of *E. coli.* J. Mol. Biol. **192:** 549-556.
44. RONSON, C. W., B. T. NIXON & F. M. AUSUBEL. 1987. Conserved domains in bacterial regulatory proteins that respond to environmental stimuli. Cell **49:** 579-581.
45. NINFA, A. J. & B. MAGASANIK. 1986. Covalent modification of the *glnG* product, NR_I, by the *glnL* product, NR_{II}, regulates the transcription of the *glnALG* O operon in *E. coli.* Proc. Natl. Acad. Sci. USA **83:** 5909-5913.
46. MILLER. V. L., R. K. TAYLOR & J. J. MEKALANOS. 1987. Cholera toxin transcriptional activator ToxR is a transmembrane DNA binding protein. Cell **48:** 271-279.
47. CLEMENTS, J. D. & E. S. MORSHIDY. 1984. Construction of a potential live oral bivalent vaccine for typhoid fever and cholera-*E. coli* related diarrhea. Infect. Immun. **46:** 564.
48. TRAMONT, E. C. *et al.* 1984. Safety and antigenicity of typhoid-*Shigella sonnei* vaccine (strain 5076-1c). J. Infect. Dis. **149:** 133.
49. DOUGAN, G. *et al.* 1987. Live oral *Salmonella* vaccines: Potential use as carriers of heterologous antigens of the immune system. Parasite Immunol. **9:** 151-160.
50. TAYLOR, R., V. L. MILLER, D. FURLONG & J. J. MEKALANOS. 1987. Use of gene fusions to identify a pilus colonization factor coordinately regulated with cholera toxin. Proc. Natl. Acad. Sci. USA **84:** 2833-2837.
51. HARRINGTON, D. A., R. H. HALL. G. LOSONSKY, J. J. MEKALANOS, R. K. TAYLOR & M. M. LEVINE. 1988. Toxin, toxin-coregulated pili, and the *toxR* regulon are essential for *Vibrio cholera* pathogenesis in humans. J. Exp. Med. **168:** 1487-1492.
52. TAYLOR, R., C. SHAW, K. PETTERSON, P. SPEARS & J. MEKALANOS. 1988. Safe live *Vibrio cholerae* vaccines. Vaccine **6:** 151-154.
53. FORMAL, S. B., L. S. BARON, D. J. KOPECKO, O. WASHINGTON, C. POWELL & C. A. LIFE. 1981. Construction of a potentially bivalent vaccine strain: Introduction of *Shigella sonnei* form I antigen genes into the *galE Salmonella typhi* Ty21a typhoid vaccine strain. Infect. Immun. **34:** 746.
54. LINDBERG, A. A., A. KARNELL, B. A. D. STOCKER, S. KATAKURA, H. SWEIHA & F. P. REINHOLT. 1988. Development of an auxotrophic oral live *Shigella flexneri* vaccine. Vaccine **6:** 146-150.
55. CALDERWOOD, S. B., F. AUCLAIR, A. DONOHUE-ROLFE, G. T. KEUSCH & J. J. MEKA-

LANOS. 1987. Nucleotide sequence of the shiga-like toxin genes of *Escherichia coli.* Proc. Natl. Acad. Sci. USA **84:** 4364-4368.

56. STROCKBINE, N. A., L. R. M. MARQUES, J. W. NEWLAND, H. W. SMITH, R. K. HOLMES & A. D. O'BRIEN. 1988. J. Bacteriol.
57. HOVDE, C. J., S. B. CALDERWOOD, J. J. MEKALANOS & R. J. COLLIER. 1988. Evidence that glutamic acid 167 is an active-site residue of Shiga-like toxin I. Proc. Natl. Acad. Sci. USA **85** 2568-2572.
58. BARBIERI, J. T. & R. J. COLLIER. 1987. Expression of a mutant full-length form of diphtheria toxin in *E. coli.* Infect. Immun. **55:** 1647-1651.
59. BURNETTE, W. N., W. CIEPLAK, V. L. MAR, K. T. KALJOT, H. SATO & J. M. KEITH. 1988. Pertussis toxin S1 mutant with reduced enzymatic activity and a conserved protective epitope. Science **242:** 72-74.
60. MILLER, S. I., A. KUKRAL & J. MEKALANOS. A two component regulatory system (*phoP* and *phoQ*) controls *Salmonella typhimurium* virulence. Proc. Natl. Acad. Sci. USA **86:** 5054-5058.
61. FIELDS, P. I., E. A. GROISMAN & F. HEFFRON. 1989. A *Salmonella* locus that controls resistance to microbicidal proteins from phagocytic cells. Science **243:** 1059-1062.

New Strategies for Leprosy and Tuberculosis and for Development of Bacillus Calmette-Guérin into a Multivaccine Vehicle

BARRY R. BLOOM AND WILLIAM R. JACOBS, JR.

Department of Microbiology and Immunology
Albert Einstein College of Medicine
Bronx, New York 10461

Tuberculosis and leprosy remain major problems in the developing world. The World Health Organization estimates that 10 million new cases of tuberculosis occur each year, with 3 million annual deaths.[1] In the United States, there are 20,000 cases, and for the first time in 32 years, the number is increasing.[2] For example, the incidence of tuberculosis in New York City rose by 17% in the past year.[3] Worldwide, one-fifth of AIDS patients present first with tuberculosis, now regarded as a sentinel for AIDS in Africa. Half of the population in the developing world is infected with *Mycobacterium tuberculosis* and conversion to HIV-positivity increases risk for tuberculosis 30-fold or possibly more.[4] Tuberculosis is the only communicable disease besides AIDS likely to spread from HIV-positive to HIV-negative individuals within the community, and represents an explosive threat in both the urban areas of the developed countries and in regions of Africa where AIDS is most prevalent.

Although *M. leprae* was the first major human bacterial pathogen described in 1873, it remains the one of few human pathogens that has not been grown successfully in culture. Leprosy afflicts ten to thirteen million people, resulting in deformity in 30 percent.[5] There is generally a long latency, averaging 5 years, between infection and manifestation of clinical disease, and it is likely that the transmission occurs in many individuals before there is clear evidence or awareness of disease.

Throughout time and in virtually every culture, leprosy has engendered a unique horror and fascination. There is a unique stigma associated with leprosy, largely due to the deformities associated with untreated disease, and the challenge is to overcome that stigma by scientific means. The immunologic fascination derives from the fact that leprosy is not a single clinical entity, but rather comprises a clinical and immunologic spectrum.[6,7] At one end of the spectrum, tuberculoid leprosy, patients develop high levels of cell-mediated immunity that ultimately kills and clears the bacilli in tissues, albeit often with concomitant immunologic damage to the nerves. At the opposite end, patients with lepromatous leprosy exhibit a selective immunologic unresponsiveness to antigens of *M. leprae* and the organisms inexorably multiply in the macrophages and Schwann cells of the skin, often to very high numbers (e.g., 10^{10} bacilli/g tissue). As shown in FIGURE 1, the major parameter that varies across the spectrum is the state of patients' cell-mediated immunity; patients with tuberculoid leprosy have strong cell-mediated immunity, while those with multibacillary lepro-

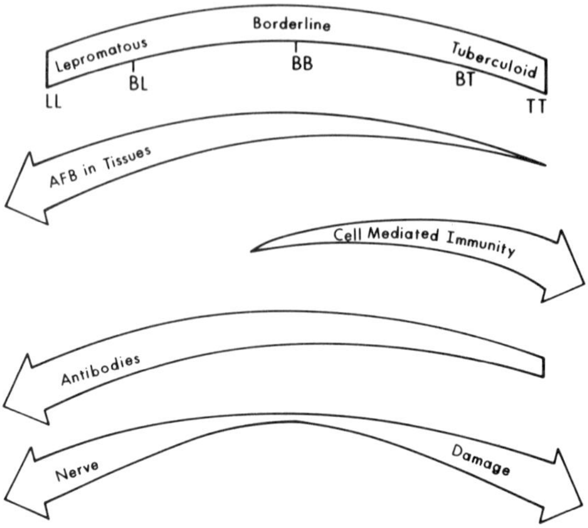

FIGURE 1. The spectrum of leprosy. LL = lepromatous leprosy: BL = borderline lepromatous leprosy; BB = borderline leprosy; BT = borderline tuberculoid leprosy; TT = tuberculoid leprosy.

matous leprosy are selectively unresponsive to antigens of *M. leprae.* Although antibodies reactive with *M. leprae* antigens are found throughout the spectrum, the highest levels occur at the multibacillary, lepromatous end of the disease, strongly suggesting that protection against the leprosy bacillus requires specific cell-mediated immunity. In endemic areas or within families of lepromatous patients, it is likely that large numbers of persons are infected with the leprosy bacillus, but because of their development of appropriate immune responses, the vast majority are protected from any of the obvious manifestations of the disease. It will be important to understand why the vast majority of exposed individuals fail to develop clinical disease, and why, of that minority who do develop clinical leprosy, a proportion, which varies in different parts of the world, becomes immunologically unresponsive and develops the lepromatous form of the disease. Unfortunately, there is currently too little information on genetic or environmental risk factors of the host or possible genetic differences in the pathogen to explain the variability.

There are few infectious diseases for which the pathogenesis has been better described than for tuberculosis,[8] yet many fundamental questions remain unanswered. Once again, the vast majority of persons infected with *M. tuberculosis* develop appropriate cell-mediated immunity, as reflected in the classical positive delayed-type hypersensitivity tuberculin test, and do not develop disease. In exogenous infections, bacilli seed small lesions in the lung which, in most individuals, then heal. In individuals destined to developed clinical disease, there appears to be a hematogenous spread of *M. tuberculosis* from the initial site of infection to the more highly oxygenated regions of the lung, namely the apices, resulting in the primary complex, sometimes with plural effusion. There, in the absence of treatment, the lesions can usually be contained, but the viable organisms probably never eliminated, by a cell-mediated immune response. Or tuberculosis may progress to other organs such as the meninges in children, with a devastating course. The fatality rate from untreated tuberculosis remains 50 percent in the developing world, and in only 30 percent does cure occur spontaneously.[9]

Even among those who recover, there is the life-long possibility of post-primary pulmonary tuberculosis, caused by reactivation of the early infection; this can occur up to 50 years later. It is this endogenous reactivation that is so devastating in patients infected with *M. tuberculosis* who become infected with HIV.

THE PROBLEM OF SPECIFIC IMMUNOLOGIC UNRESPONSIVENESS

Because of the centrality of immunologic tolerance to an understanding of the nature of immunoregulation, the mechanism of the unresponsiveness in lepromatous leprosy has long been of interest in our laboratory.[10] The unresponsiveness to *M. leprae* antigens *in vitro* and *in vivo* is specific for *M. leprae*; most lepromatous patients are fully capable of responding to killed *M. tuberculosis* antigens, many of which are serologically highly cross-reactive. Thus, T lymphocytes of lepromatous patients are incapable of recognizing a set of common or related antigens when they are expressed by the leprosy bacillus, but are able to do so when they are expressed by the tubercle bacillus. To explain this paradox we proposed that one or a small number of unique antigens associated with *M. leprae* may be able to engender suppressor T cells which are capable of suppressing either the function or expansion of clones of helper T cells that activate macrophages to resist infections. In more than 250 patients tested, greater than 80 percent of lepromatous patients were found to have T cells that, when stimulated by *M. leprae* antigens, induced suppression of both mitogen and specific antigen responses *in vitro*. We have characterized the phenotype of those cells as CD8+, CD3+, HLA-DR+, FcR+, 9.3-.[11] Further, our collaborators, R. Modlin and T. Rea, provided evidence that T cells of the suppressor phenotype predominate in lepromatous lesions, whereas cells of the T helper phenotype predominate in tuberculoid lesions.[12] Recently, it has been possible to derive T-cell clones directly from lepromatous lesions that retained suppressor activity *in vitro*. With them we established that these human CD8+ suppressor cells expressed T-cell receptor α, β [13] and were genetically restricted by MHC class II antigens.[14]

CHEMOTHERAPY AGAINST LEPROSY AND TUBERCULOSIS

For many years, it was acceptable to treat leprosy with a single, inexpensive bacteriostatic drug, dapsone. Recently, as might be expected from long-term treatment (>5 years) with a single drug, primary and secondary dapsone-resistance has emerged in many countries. The THELEP Committee of WHO has recommended that multidrug therapy, consisting of the bactericidal drug rifampicin, together with clofazimine and dapsone, be used to treat leprosy.[15] The effectiveness has been dramatic, and this combination offers the possibility of shorter-term, more effective treatment (albeit still taking a year), which in turn has an enormous beneficial effect on compliance. Possible new therapeutic agents, including the fluoroquinolones,[16] offer the prospect of shortening multidrug therapy even further.

It has long been recognized that multidrug chemotherapy was important in the treatment of tuberculosis. The regimen presently still recommended (TABLE 1) requires at least one year of continuous treatment, and costs only $15, but, except for reducing mortality, it is basically only 10% more effective in terms of cures than is no treatment. Recently, in light of the current crisis of tuberculosis as a consequence of HIV infection, particularly in Africa, a more effective short-term chemotherapy regimen consisting of rifampicin, pyrazinamide, and isoniazid, possibly supplemented with clofazimine, for two months, has been introduced that is 90% effective in trials in Africa, and has increased compliance. Despite the increased cost of short-term chemotherapy, its effectiveness in reducing transmission makes it significantly more cost-effective.[17] The progress in increasing effectiveness of chemotherapy and reduction in duration of treatment offers the possibility that new drugs may be added that could reduce treatment to a matter of 2-3 months, and, it is hoped, lower the cost, which would profoundly enhance the effectiveness of chemotherapy in the Third World. While the scientific advantages of the short-term and new chemotherapy are clear, nonetheless the ethical dilemma remains. In a world where many countries cannot afford or deliver a treatment that costs only $15 per patient, is it reasonable to expect that a more effective treatment costing $45 can be implemented?

TABLE 1. Chemotherapy of Tuberculosis

Treatment	Mortality	Cure	Cost
None	50%	32%	(a lifetime)
Standard (2SHT/10HT)	10%	40%	$15
Short-Course (2HRP/4HR)	5%	95%	$45

ABBREVIATIONS: H = isoniazid; S = streptomycin; T = thiacetazone; R = rifampicin; P = pyrazinamide.

VACCINES AGAINST LEPROSY

Chemotherapy is expensive and, in a disease with a latency between infection and clinical symptoms estimated to average 5 years, is most often implemented only after significant transmission of infection has occurred. Is there reason to believe that effective vaccines could be developed against tuberculosis and leprosy? Curiously, it is little recognized that bacillus Calmette-Guérin (BCG) vaccine given to protect against tuberculosis is the most widely utilized vaccine in the world today.[18] BCG is an attenuated strain derived in 1908 during repeated passage of virulent bovine tubercle bacilli (*M. bovis*). A summary of the results of 8 major trials of BCG against tuberculosis (TABLE 2) indicates that its effectiveness against pulmonary tuberculosis has varied dramatically, ranging from 80% protection to nil, in different parts of the world, and even within different regions in the United States. An increasing body of data indicates, however, that BCG vaccination of newborn infants provides very significant protection in several geographic regions against tuberculosis meningitis, a major killer of children.[19] Similarly, the protection by BCG against leprosy has been analyzed in four major trials (TABLE 3), and some degree of protection was engendered in each, although once again the efficacy varied tremendously in different regions of

TABLE 2. Summary of Major Controlled BCG Vaccine Trials against Tuberculosis

Area	No. of Subjects/ Age at Vaccination	Year Started	Follow-Up (years)	Percent Protection
1. South India (Chingleput)	113,000 (all ages)	1968	15	nil
2. Georgia (USA)	4,839 (5 to 19 yr)	1947	20	nil
3. Georgia/Alabama	34,767 (5+ years)	1950	20	6
4. South India (Madanapalle)	10,877 (All ages)	1950	16-21	20
5. Puerto Rico	77,972 (0-20 yr)	1949	18-20	29
6. Chicago (USA)	3,381 (newborns)	1937	12-23	73
7. Western U.S. (Indians)	3,008 (0-19 years)	1936	9-11	75
8. England (Medical Research Council)	32,282 (14-15 yr)	1950	18-20	77

Adapted from data provided to WHO by Drs. G. Comstock and P.E.M. Fine.

the world. The reasons for the varied effectiveness of BCG against tuberculosis and leprosy in different geographical regions remain puzzling, but might be related to exposure to environmental mycobacteria, differences in host responsiveness, or genetics of different isolates. Nonetheless, these results encourage us to try to understand the circumstances in which BCG is most effective and, using modern technology, to try and improve on it.

In the case of leprosy, the unique challenge is how to produce a better vaccine than BCG for a pathogen, *M. leprae,* that cannot be grown in culture. The first breakthrough that made the study of the immunology and biochemistry of *M. leprae* possible was the discovery that the bacillus could be grown in very large numbers in the nine-banded armadillo. With the support of the IMMLEP program of WHO, methods were developed for preparing large numbers of highly purified bacilli from the armadillo. The second breakthrough was the development of the first new vaccine

TABLE 3. Vaccine Trials of BCG against Leprosy[a]

Area	No. of Subjects/ Age at Vaccination	Year Started	Follow-up (yr)	Percent Protection
Burma	28,220 (0-14 yr)	1964	9	20
South India (Chingleput)	210,337 (all ages)	1968	5-10	30
New Guinea	5,000 (all ages)	1962	10	44
Uganda	16,150 childhood contacts	1960	8	80

[a] Adapted from : FINE P. E. M. 1985. Ethiop. Med. J. **23:** 179.

against leprosy by Dr. J. Convit of Caracas, Venezuela—a combined vaccine of killed *M. leprae* plus live BCG.[20] The first application of this combined vaccine was immunotherapeutic, namely, to treat patients with lepromatous leprosy. The concept was to overcome the patients' unresponsiveness and to engender specific cell-mediated immunity, leading to clinical upgrading of their lesions, and, it was hoped, cure. More recently, two cultivable mycobacteria discovered in India, the ICRC bacillus and *Mycobacterium* "*w*" have been used in similar immunotherapeutic studies in lepromatous patients, with very similar findings.[21,22] The results in TABLE 4 are of interest since they represent the first example of the breaking of specific immunologic unresponsiveness in man by means of immunologic intervention. At the present time, there are perhaps a quarter of a million persons undergoing preventive vaccine trials against leprosy in Venezuela, Malawi, and India, but it will take 5-10 years before the results of these trials can be assessed.

TABLE 4. Protein Antigens of *M. leprae*

Molecular Size (kDa)	Recognized by Monoclonal Ab	Recognized by Human Ab	Recognized by Human T Cells	Stress-Related
71	+	−	+	+
65	+	+	+	+
50	−	−	+	−
36	+	+	+	−
35	+	−	+	−
32	−	+	−	−
28	+	−	−	−
18	+	+	+	+
16	−	−	+	−
12	+	−	−	+
7	−	−	+	−

We have had the opportunity to collaborate with Dr. Convit and his colleagues in examining, in blinded experiments, suppression and antigen-specific T-cell responses of 10 patients with lepromatous leprosy both prior to and after successful immunotherapy with BCG + *M. leprae*.[23] The results revealed that the *in vitro* suppression that was initially found disappeared in all patients who responded to immunotherapy, providing laboratory evidence that the vaccine was affecting the immune response.

It could be argued that the immunotherapeutic efficacy of the Convit and Indian vaccines depends on the fact that they are immunizing against a related organism, but that there is no general principle associated with these immunotherapeutic vaccines. That view is challenged by recent studies of Convit and his colleagues,[24] in which patients with localized cutaneous leishmaniasis, a chronic ulcerating disease caused by protozoal parasites which persist for many months, and more severe forms of leishmaniasis[25] were cured by three immunizations with a combined vaccine of live BCG + killed *L. mexicana* promastigotes. Thus BCG has adjuvant properties in man capable of overcoming unresponsiveness in both leprosy and in leishmaniasis.

The Search for Protective Antigens

For pathogens in which cell-mediated immunity is important, two presumptions are commonly made that are not supported by the known facts and are probably incorrect, namely that: (1) parasite surface antigens are likely to be most important for protection; and (2) any antigen or epitope recognized by T cells or T-cell clones is probably a protective one. In the case of intracellular pathogens, particularly viruses, it has become clear that there is no need for protective antigens to be surface antigens of the pathogen, since antigenic determinants (epitopes) that are presented to T cells are processed by antigen-presenting cells and selected by their major histocompability antigens for expression on the surface of the antigen-presenting cell itself.[26] For example, internal antigens of viruses are found to be the major targets for cytotoxic T cells.[27]

In order even to address the second presumption, namely, that there are antigens that simulate T cells or T-cell clones from patients and contacts that could be protective, one first had to overcome the unique challenge that the leprosy bacillus poses—that is, how to obtain antigens from a pathogen that cannot be grown *in vitro* to test. The identification and preparation of significant amounts of antigens that might be candidates for immunodiagnosis or protection really awaited the development of recombinant DNA technology, monoclonal antibodies, and T-cell cloning. Genomic DNA libraries from both *M. leprae* and *M. tuberculosis* were made in λgt11 recombinant expression vectors; indeed they were the first libraries made in this vector from any pathogen.[28,29] DNA from most organisms containing high guanine-cytosine ratios, like the mycobacteria, is generally not expressed well in *E. coli.* By virtue of the fact that DNA inserted into λgt11 produces fusion proteins with β-galactosidase, it has been possible to isolate genes from many different antigens of *M. leprae* and *M. tuberculosis* (TABLE 5). The identification of these antigens has been greatly facilitated by the establishment of WHO Monoclonal Antibody and Gene Banks of the IMMLEP and IMMTUB programs, which make the reagents available to qualified investigators all over the world.

Of particular interest is the unexpected finding that several antigens have sequence homologies with highly conserved "stress" or "heat-shock" proteins (*hsp*) found in other bacteria and in mammalian cells.[30,31] Since there is approximately 50% amino acid identity between the mycobacterial stress proteins and their human counterparts, this finding has potentially important implications. For example, *hsp* could be involved in the etiology of certain autoimmune diseases. In rheumatoid arthritis T cells responding to the BCG 65kDa *hsp* have been reported in joints and blood, and it has been suggested that some bacterial infections could trigger a response to conserved epitopes in the *hsp* such that T cells now cross-react with epitopes on *hsp* in inflamed joints, even in the absence of the bacterial antigen.

The other issue that is raised is whether protective immunity to bacterial and protozoal pathogens is engendered predominately by highly conserved antigens, such as *hsp*, or by unique species-specific antigens and epitopes. One line of reasoning argues that in infectious diseases, such as leprosy and tuberculosis, only one person in a thousand infected with the pathogen (i.e., is lepromin- or PPD skin test-positive) develops clinical disease because cross-reactions to conserved antigens and *hsp* of environmental bacteria to which everyone is exposed have stimulated protective immunity. The alternative view would hold that since tuberculosis remains a major health problem and since BCG is not fully protective against tuberculosis, the antigens critically required for protection are likely to be those specific to the pathogen, and not found on BCG or environmental organisms. This issue is a general one and can only be critically resolved when sets of both unique and conserved antigens and epitopes can be identified and tested for protection in appropriate animal models.

A prior concern is the nature of protective immunity to intracellular pathogens like *M. leprae.* The earliest immunologic correlations with the spectrum of leprosy showed that resistance to infection by pathogenic mycobacteria was largely, if not solely, a function of cell-mediated immunity rather than antibodies. Yet two key questions remain: What type of cellular immune responses are necessary and sufficient for resistance? Does one need only T helper cells and lymphokine production, or are cytotoxic T cells of either the CD8 or CD4 subsets required? It is clear that patients with lepromatous leprosy that cannot activate CD4+ T helper cells to produce lymphokines, including interferon-γ, are unable to develop protective immunity. However, recent data in experimental animal models indicate that, in addition to CD4 T helper cells, cytotoxic T cells may be essential for protection.[32] T cell receptor γ, δ cells similarly may have a role to play in granuloma formation and protection.[45]

The nature of antigens involved in protection against mycobacterial disease is not known. In practical terms, recombinant DNA libraries are currently being screened for additional antigens recognized by various T-cell subsets. Screening recombinant expression libraries by T cells is a challenge of general significance beyond antigens relevant only to leprosy and tuberculosis, and crucial to understanding resistance to virtually all infectious agents. It is gratifying that the most imaginative of approaches

TABLE 5. Potential Advantages of BCG as a Multivaccine Vehicle

1. BCG has been used in more than 2.5 billion people since 1948, with a very low frequency of serious complications.
2. BCG is the only vaccine, other than oral polio, recommended by the WHO to be given at birth.
3. BCG requires only a single immunization that can engender cell-mediated immunity to tuberculoproteins for 5-50 years.
4. BCG is the most effective known adjuvant for induction of cell-mediated immunity in animals and man.
5. BCG costs $0.55 per dose.

developed thus far for attacking this problem have been developed in the studies of T-cell responses to mycobacterial antigens. One approach has been to use *in vitro* lymphocyte transformation assays using primary T cells or T-cell clones from patients or healthy contacts with high levels of cell-mediated immunity to screen electrophoretically separated components of mycobacterial extracts (1D and 2D T-cell Western blots) and to assess which of the antigens is recognized by them.[33] Then, if antibodies can be made to those T cell antigens, or oligonucleotides corresponding to partial amino acid sequences, the recombinant libraries can be screened for antigens recognized by T cells. Using a limiting dilution analysis of *M. leprae* antigen-responsive T cell precursors, we observed that the majority of human antigen-reactive CD4 T cells ($1/10^3$ in blood and 1/20 in lesions) recognize antigens different from most of those identified by monoclonal antibodies, specifically antigens associated with highly purified mycobacterial cell walls.[34] This is of particular interest since it has long been known that the adjuvant activity of mycobacteria is associated with cell walls,[35] and we have recently demonstrated that highly purified cell walls are immunogenic.[29] This suggests that an effective subunit mycobacterial vaccine containing cell walls could be developed for use in populations in which immunization with live vaccines would be of concern due to widespread HIV infection.

DEVELOPMENT OF A RECOMBINANT BCG MULTIVACCINE VEHICLE

BCG presents unique advantages for developing a recombinant polyvalent vaccine vector expressing antigens for a wide variety of pathogens, particularly those for which cell-mediated immunity is important in protection. Such a vaccine could be achieved if genes encoding protective antigens from a variety of pathogens could be introduced and stably expressed in the BCG cell. Regrettably, knowledge of the genetics of mycobacteria has been virtually nonexistent. We therefore set out to develop genetic systems employing a molecular genetic approach. The introduction of recombinant DNA molecules into mycobacteria requires: (1) an efficient means of introducing foreign DNA into the mycobacterial cell; (2) recombinant DNA vectors that can replicate and be stably maintained in the mycobacterial host; and (3) expression of genes encoding selectable phenotypes for identifying mycobacterial cells containing recombinant DNA. Because of the slow generation time of BCG (24 hours compared with 20 minutes for *E. coli*), our initial studies were initiated with a fast-growing, nonpathogenic *Mycobacterium smegmatis*. Because it requires weeks to grow BCG vaccine strains or *M. tuberculosis*, the fundamental decision we made was to develop "shuttle" vectors that could exchange DNA between mycobacteria and the much more tractable *E. coli*. These shuttle vectors would permit us to carry out many genetic manipulations in *E. coli* and then to transfer those recombinant vectors into the mycobacteria.

Two basic strategies exist for stably introducing the foreign DNA into bacterial cells: (1) integration of the foreign genes of interest into the mycobacterial chromosomes by a phage-based recombination event or by homologous recombination, where they can be replicated as part of the chromosome; or (2) introduction of the foreign genes on an extrachromosomal, autonomously replicating vector (i.e., a plasmid). Because no mycobacterial plasmids containing selectable markers for mycobacteria existed, we initially screened a variety of plasmids useful in *Streptomyces* and *Bacillus* for their ability to transform *M. smegmatis*. To date, these attempts have failed totally.

To address the possibility that our failure was due to an inability of DNA to penetrate the cell wall and complex lipid coat into the cells, we developed methods for transfecting mycobacterial cells with mycobacteriophage DNAs. By adapting methods for producing spheroplasts, we were able to introduce phage DNA into mycobacterial cells with high efficiency (10^5 plaque-forming units per microgram of phage DNA). When *Streptomyces* plasmids were introduced under the same conditions, transformation was still not achieved, indicating that the problem lay in: (1) the inability to introduce "foreign" DNA molecules into mycobacterial hosts because of the degradation of "foreign" DNA by a host restriction system: (2) the lack of an origin of replication that functioned in mycobacteria; (3) the failure to express the selectable marker gene in mycobacteria: or (4) our inability to reconstitute or regenerate bacterial cell walls from spheroplasts. Using mycobacteriophages as vectors, we were able to analyze and overcome these potential problems.

Phage-Based Strategy

Mycobacteriophages represent excellent candidates as recombinant DNA vectors for mycobacteria, since many phages are known that infect and replicate in a wide range of both fast-growing and slow-growing mycobacterial species. To construct mycobacteriophage vectors, we utilized the observation that mycobacterial genes are not well expressed in *E. coli.*[36] Therefore we could clone, into *E. coli* plasmids, mycobacteriophage DNA that would produce lytic phage if expressed in mycobacteria; and yet, these fragments would be unexpressed in *E. coli* and thus not lyse the *E. coli* cell. We named such constructs "shuttle phasmids" because they would replicate in *E. coli* as plasmids and in mycobacteria as phages (FIG. 2). In addition, when we introduced the recombinant phasmid DNA by transfection directly into a fast-growing *Mycobacterium,* such as *M. smegmatis,* the recombinant DNA molecules would then be packaged into mycobacteriophage particles. It then became possible to introduce the recombinant DNA in these phage particles produced by the rapidly growing species by phage infection of slow-growing species of mycobacteria, such as BCG, at high efficiency. If mycobacteriophages that were temperate and nonlytic could be found, it should be possible, then, to introduce and stably express recombinant DNA in mycobacterial cells by lysogeny. We successfully utilized a cosmid cloning strategy and mycobacterial transfection to produce *E. coli*-mycobacteria shuttle phasmids, using the mycobacteriophage TM4 and the cosmid pHC79. These recombinant phasmids were shown to be capable of infecting both *M. smegmatis* and BCG vaccine substrains, thereby introducing recombinant DNA into both slow-growing and fast-growing mycobacteria for the first time.[37] Success was not altogether sweet, however, because the initial phage used, TM4 (which had been chosen because it was reported a temperate phage isolated from *M. avium*), was lytic and killed *M. smegmatis* and BCG. Consequently, we were obliged to start again and screen a panel of mycobacteriophages to identify some that are truly temperate and stably lysogenize *M. smegmatis.* One such phage, L1, had been previously reported to be temperate. We confirmed the observations that it was capable of making *M. smegmatis* cells resistant to superinfection, as would be expected for a lysogen. In addition, we were able to demonstrate,

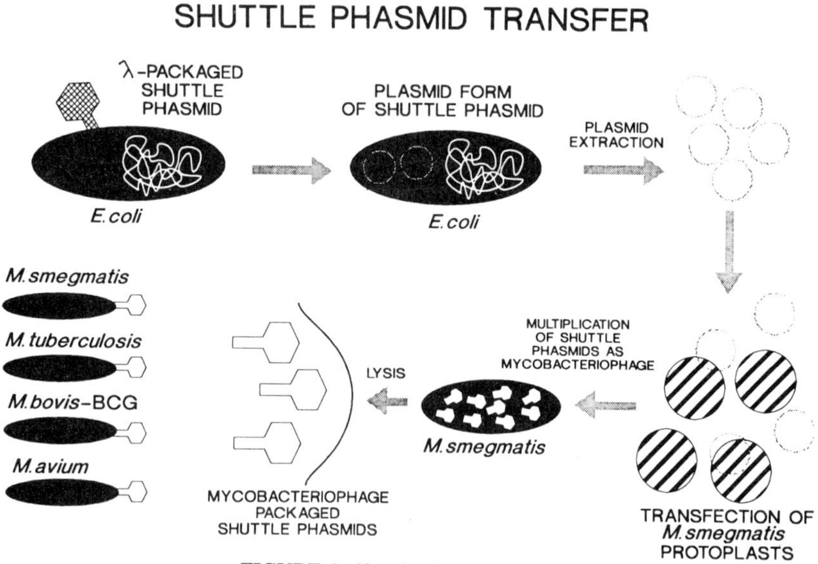

FIGURE 2. Shuttle phasmid strategy.

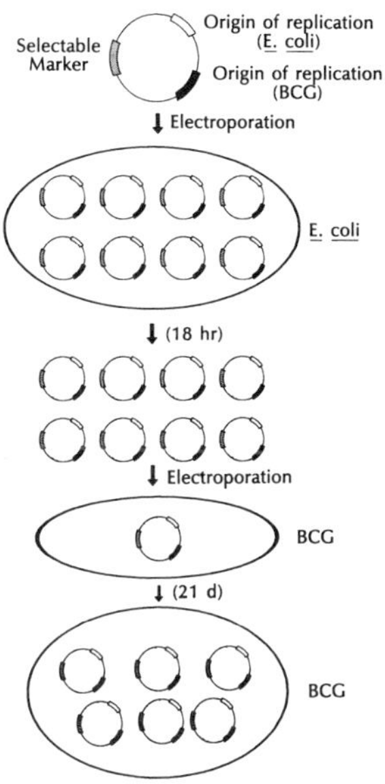

FIGURE 3. Shuttle plasmid strategy.

by Southern blot analysis, that the L1 prophage integrates in a site-specific fashion into the *M. smegmatis* chromosome as its means of establishing lysogeny, the first such demonstration for a mycobacteriophage.[38] We thus had, for the first time, the ability to introduce recombinant DNA into mycobacterial cells in a stable manner. We were able to clone into one such L1-shuttle plasmid a gene encoding kanamycin resistance and established that this gene conferred kanamycin resistance to mycobacterial cells. This established the kanamycin-resistance gene and kanamycin as the first selectable marker gene system for the mycobacteria. Overall these studies established lysogeny as one potentially useful means to intrude and express foreign genes in mycobacteria.

Plasmid-Based Strategy

Plasmid genetic systems extend the capability of phages by offering increased cloning capacity, ease of DNA manipulation, and possibly increased copy number of the vector. Because of the lack of any mycobacterial plasmids containing a selectable marker, and because of our failure to transform mycobacteria using plasmids developed in other genera, we constructed, in collaboration with T. Kieser and A. Jekkel, a hybrid plasmid by ligating a full-length *E. coli* plasmid, pIJ666, containing a gene for kanamycin resistance, randomly into a cryptic mycobacterial plasmid, pAL5000, originally isolated from *M. fortuitum*[38] (FIG. 3). When the library containing these inserts was transformed by electroporation into *M. smegmatis* or BCG vaccine substrains, transformants resistant to kanamycin were found (FIG. 4). Isolated plasmids from

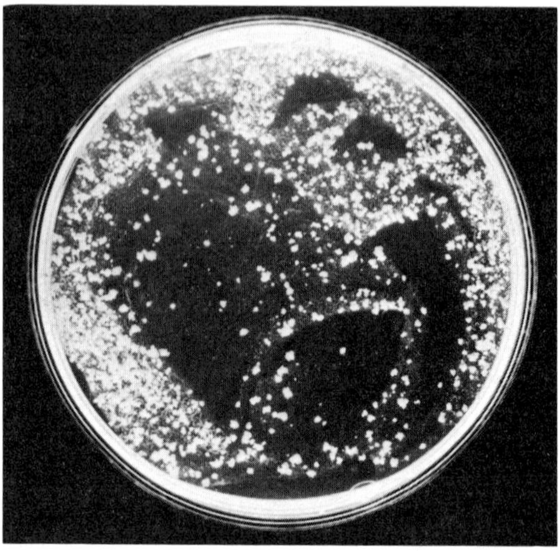

pYUB13

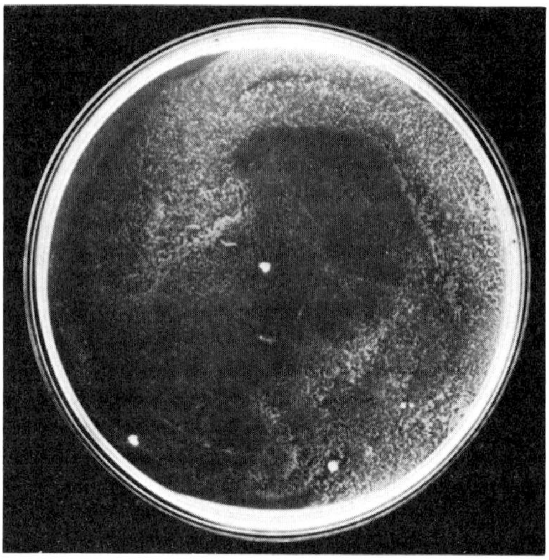

No DNA

FIGURE 4. Transformation of BCG with a recombinant shuttle plasmid. (*Top*) the Pasteur BCG substrain transformed with shuttle plasmid, pYUB 12, containing the gene from Tn903 for kanamycin-resistance, and plated on medium containing kanamycin. (*Bottom*) mock-transformed BCG plated on medium containing kanamycin.

the transformants had the ability to replicate and transform both *E. coli* and mycobacteria. Further analysis of these transformants should indicate the mycobacteria plasmid DNA sequences required for replication (replicon). Conditions have now been developed as well for permitting transformation by the hybrid plasmids of several BCG vaccine substrains at high efficiency (10^4 transformants/μg DNA).[38,39]

PERFECTING A RECOMBINANT BCG VECTOR

Much remains to be done to develop BCG into a useful multivaccine vehicle. To develop optimally effective vaccines, we will need to optimize the expression of the foreign antigens in BCG and define, in molecular terms, the important parameters for immunization of animals and humans. To achieve these goals, we will have to accumulate much additional basic knowledge of mycobacterial molecular biology and genetics.

Optimization of the Expression of Foreign Antigens

Ideally, we would like to express in BCG any open reading frame of DNA derived from any foreign antigen. The first necessity will be to identify mycobacterial expression sequences. Mycobacteria contain high G-C DNA and, while related to gram-positive organisms, may have special DNA sequences useful for expressing foreign genes. We are constructing reporter genes (e.g., genes containing β-galactosidase) to identify mycobacterial promoters that can be used to transcribe genes encoding foreign antigens. In addition, we will need to define and characterize the sequences necessary for efficient translation in the mycobacteria. Using this information, we should be able to construct a series of expression vectors that permit us to clone any open reading frame downstream from efficiently expressed transcriptional and translational elements. It may be necessary to develop regulated expression systems that will allow for expression of the foreign antigens in defined periods of growth of the BCG cell in the mammalian host in order to optimize immune response.

Stabilizing Foreign Genes in Mycobacteria

Optimal expression of foreign antigens will require that the recombinant DNA constructs encoding the expressed foreign antigens be retained during growth of the BCG in the mammalian host. To ensure that these recombinant constructs are not lost, we must develop systems that select against the loss of the recombinant DNA. In general, antibiotic resistance genes are inappropriate selectable markers for human vaccine vectors. We have begun to develop insertional mutagenic strategies that will allow us to isolate auxotrophic mutations in the BCG chromosome. A well-defined stable mutation and a complementing gene cloned on a plasmid offer alternative selection systems for stabilizing plasmid vectors. Such a system has been used successfully to stably maintain recombinant plasmids in *Salmonella* vaccine strains *in vivo.*[40]

Alternatively, foreign antigen genes could be placed in the BCG chromosome by using mycobacteriophage site-specific integration systems or homologous recombination in BCG. The advantage of this strategy is that the foreign genes are introduced into the host chromosome and may not require continuous selection; a disadvantage is that only a single copy can be introduced.

Optimal expression of foreign antigens in BCG will require that expressed proteins themselves be stably maintained in the BCG cell. It is clear that expression of some foreign genes in *E. coli* is limited by enzymes of the host capable of degrading foreign proteins selectively. It has been possible to stabilize expression by developing mutants in the host proteolytic enzymes in many instances in *E. coli*,[41] and similar approaches may be useful to increasing stability of expression of foreign antigens in BCG.

Optimizing the Immunization Potential of Expressed Foreign Antigens: Targeting the Recombinant Antigens Produced to be Secreted or Expressed in the Cell Wall

We have established that major antigen(s) in *M. leprae* and *M. tuberculosis* recognized by T helper cells reside in the cell wall and that purified cell walls are immunogenic.[31,42] To increase immunogenicity, particularly for developing antibodies, and to prevent foreign proteins from becoming toxic to the BCG it may be advantageous to include mycobacterial signal sequences that will permit a significant portion of recombinant proteins to be secreted from the recombinant BCG vector. An equally compelling immunologic reason for developing recombinant BCG that can secrete introduced antigens derives from the elegant demonstration by Bevan and associates[43] that in order to generate MHC Class I restricted cytotoxic T lymphocytes (CTL) it is obligatory for the antigen to be present in the cytoplasm of the antigen presenting and target cells. Targeting of recombinant antigens to the cell wall is attractive because of the high immunogenicity and adjuvanticity of mycobacterial cell walls. In addition, because of possible concerns with introducing live vaccines in populations with a high prevalence of HIV seropositivity, nonliving, but highly immunogenic recombinant cell wall subunit vaccines provide a useful alternative to live vaccines. (It should be noted that there is little evidence at present that vaccination with BCG has increased the risk of untoward complications in such high-risk populations). Overall, the recently developed genetic tools for studying and manipulating mycobacteria suggest that the limiting factor in development of recombinant BCG multivaccine vehicles will be biological problems, such as the nature of protective antigens and development of high levels of specific immune responses (e.g., antibodies or cytotoxic T cells) rather than genetic ones.

FUTURE POSSIBILITIES

We are currently at the advantageous stage in which many of the initial technical hurdles have been overcome and it is possible to entertain a number of fantasies about possible experiments. While it is tantalizing to think about these possibilities, one must acknowledge that our ability to undertake the experiments to be described means that we are rapidly approaching the time of "reality testing."

Culturing M. leprae

One of the fantasies that these genetic approaches suggest is the possibility of making *M. leprae*, which has not successfully been grown in culture, into a cultivable organism that can be biochemically studied and genetically manipulated. By virtue of the fact that it grows within macrophages and in Schwann cells in the infected host, we know that it is functionally auxotrophic, and capable of growth given appropriate environmental conditions. Our strategy will be to prepare DNA libraries representing all the genes of a cultivable mycobacterium and transform *M. leprae* with these libraries. If only one or a small number of genes is required to enable *M. leprae* to grow, by simply selecting for growing transformed colonies we might obtain a rapidly growing strain of *M. leprae*, and, it is hoped, as a result be able to identify the genes required for growth. It might then be possible to produce large amounts of *M. leprae* inexpensively in culture for use as a killed vaccine. In addition, it might be possible to examine genetically the factors required for virulence of the leprosy bacillus.

Designing New Drugs for Leprosy

To assay candidate anti-leprosy drugs or vaccines presently requires the arduous procedure of inoculating *M. leprae* from tissue biopsies into the mouse footpad and waiting 9 months until sufficient growth occurs to enable visual counting of bacilli. Drugs are administered during this long period of infection and the efficacy in diminishing the number of *M. leprae* in the footpads is assessed after 9 months for each experiment. The genetic system thus far developed in mycobacteria suggests that, after identifying appropriate target enzymes for antimycobacterial drugs to be tested, it may be possible to isolate *M. leprae* genes encoding those enzymes by a variety of approaches. By then replacing the homologous genes in a rapidly growing cultivable mycobacterium with the *M. leprae* gene encoding the putative drug target, it should then be possible to develop a rapid (1-4-day) assay for screening new or modified drugs for efficacy in blocking the *M. leprae* enzyme and inhibiting growth of the recombinant test strain expressing that *M. leprae* enzyme.

Strategy for Producing a New Anti-Tuberculosis Vaccine

Our basic strategy would first be to identify virulence genes of *M. tuberculosis*. This might best be done by preparing a genomic library in a mycobacterial shuttle vector containing DNA (approximately 40-kb inserts) from a virulent isolate of *M. tuberculosis*. We would stably transform an avirulent isolate (e.g., H37Ra) derived from that virulent strain with the cosmid library. Then mice would be infected with the transformed mycobacteria. Transformants that express the virulence genes should kill their murine host. By culturing the mycobacteria from mice that died, we would recover the recombinant organisms expressing the virulence genes. It should then be possible to characterize the inserted mycobacterial genes in the cosmids, or in smaller subclones derived from them, to gain insight into the nature of the genes involved in virulence.

The second step would be to delete the set of virulence genes, if they are not essential for survival, in *M. tuberculosis*. One could insertionally "mutagenize" the *M. tuberculosis* virulence genes in *E. coli*, for example, by passing the plasmid containing it through a strain containing a transposon with an appropriate selectable marker. The mutagenized gene would then be reintroduced into *M. tuberculosis* and colonies expressing the selectable marker would be grown out in which the wild-type virulence gene in *M. tuberculosis* had been replaced by the mutagenized virulence gene by homologous recombination.

If a clever selectable marker were chosen to create the mutation, after selecting *for* the marker to obtain the mutagenized gene, one could then select *against* the selectable marker, resulting in growth essentially only of organisms that had a deletion in the virulence gene and which could no longer revert to virulence. Finally, one would immunize experimental animals with the avirulent deletion mutant of *M. tuberculosis* to see whether it was fully avirulent and effective in protection against challenge with virulent strains of *M. tuberculosis.*

General Strategy for Developing Vaccines for Any Pathogen That is Lethal for Mice

The ultimate fantasy is a new vaccine strategy based on the premise that recombinant BCG would be such a potent vaccine that even small number of organisms expressing protective antigens for a foreign pathogen would engender a protective immune response. One would simply create a cDNA or genomic expression library of the pathogen and transform BCG with the library. One would immunize mice with pools of the transformed recombinant BCG and challenge with lethal infection of the pathogen in question. All the mice should die except those receiving BCG transformants expressing protective antigens. One would simply isolate the recombinant BCG from the survivors, and carry out a "sib-selection,"[44] that is, sequential dilutions of the pool of mycobacteria, until individual transformed BCG clones are obtained that protect against challenge. Only then would one need to characterize the gene. The beauty of this strategy, if it were feasible, is that one would have created a new vaccine before having to invest in the molecular biological study of the protective antigen gene.

CONCLUSIONS

Tuberculosis and leprosy are devastating diseases in which cell-mediated immunity is required for resistance. Each one now can be controlled by multi-drug chemotherapy, although that is expensive and requires long periods of treatment for which compliance is a major problem. Through recombinant DNA technology and modern immunology, major antigens recognized by T cells are being identified that may be important for developing new diagnostic tests and candidate vaccines. Because BCG vaccine is currently the world's most widely used vaccine, and is one of the safest and least expensive and a uniquely effective adjuvant, efforts have been made to develop a genetic system in mycobacteria that permits the introduction and expression of foreign genes in BCG vaccine substrains. We have recently developed successful strategies for expressing foreign genes in BCG by integration of recombinant temperate mycobacteriophages (lysogeny) and by plasmid transformation. In the case of leprosy, since there is no animal reservoir known to be involved in transmission to man, as was the case with smallpox, the hope is to develop an effective vaccine that will eradicate the disease from the face of the earth. The possibility is being pursued that a more effective anti-tuberculosis vaccine than BCG itself can be constructed in a recombinant BCG by introduction of specific antigens of *M. tuberculosis* recognized by appropriate T-cell populations. Finally, the use of recombinant BCG vaccines expresssing protective antigens from many infectious agents for which cell-mediated immunity is required for resistance gives hope for a novel multivaccine vehicle capable of being given at birth and simultanously immunizing against several infectious diseases.

REFERENCES

1. JOINT INTERNATIONAL UNION AGAINST TUBERCULOSIS AND WORLD HEALTH ORGANIZATION STUDY GROUP, 1982. Tuberculosis control. Tubercle **63:** 157-169.
2. CENTERS FOR DISEASE CONTROL. 1987. Tuberculosis final data—United States 1986. Mortal. Morbid. Wkly. Rep. **36:** 817-820.
3. NEW YORK CITY DEPARTMENT OF HEALTH. 1988. Tuberculosis in New York City—1986.: 30-33. New York Lung Association, New York.
4. SELWYN, P., D. HARTEL, V. LEWIS, L. SCHOENBAUM, S. VERMUND, R. KLEIN, A. WALKER & G. FRIEDLAND. 1989. A prospective study of the risk of tuberculosis among IV drug useres with HIV infection. N. Engl. J. Med. **320:** 545-550.
5. BLOOM, B. R. & T. GODAL 1983. Selective primary health care: Strategies for control of disease in the developing world. V. Leprosy. Rev. Infect. Dis. **5:** 765-779.
6. BLOOM, B. R. & V. MEHRA. 1984. Immunological unresponsiveness in leprosy. Immunol. Rev. **80:** 5-28.
7. HASTINGS, R. C., ED. 1985. Leprosy. Churchill Livingstone. Edinburgh and New York.
8. RICH, A. R. 1951. The Pathogenesis of Tuberculosis. Charles C Thomas. Springfield, IL.
9. LEOWSKI, J. 1988. The Role of Short-Course Chemotherapy in National Tuberculosis Control Programmes in Developing Countries. WHO/TB/88.156. World Health Organization. Geneva.
10. BLOOM, B. R. 1986. American Association of Immunologists—Presidential Address: Learning from leprosy: A perspective on immunology and the Third World. J. Immunol. **137:** i-x.
11. MEHRA, V., J. CONVIT, A. RUBINSTEIN & B. R. BLOOM. 1982. Activated suppressor T cells in leprosy. J. Immunol. **129:** 1946-1951.
12. MODLIN, R. L., J. MELANCON-KAPLAN, P. BARNES, S. M. M. YOUNG, J. CONVIT, T. H. REA & B. R. BLOOM. 1988. Learning from lesions: Patterns of tissue inflammation in leprosy. Proc. Natl. Acad. Sci. USA **85:** 1213-1217.
13. MODLIN, R. L., M. B. BRENNER, M. S. KRANGEL, A. D. DUBY & B. R. BLOOM. 1987. T cell receptors of human suppressor cells. Nature **329:** 541-545.
14. MODLIN, R. L., H. KATO, V. MEHRA, E. E. NELSON, X.-D. FAN, T. H. REA, P. K. PATTENGALE & B. R. BLOOM. 1986. Genetically restricted suppressor T cell clones derived from lepromatous leprosy lesions. Nature **322:** 459-461.

15. WORLD HEALTH ORGANIZATION. 1987. Tropical Disease Research: A Global Partnership.: 119-121. WHO. Geneva.
16. GROSSET, J. 1988. Int. J. Leprosy **56:** 259-264.
17. BARNUM, H. N. 1986. Cost savings from alternative treatment of tuberculosis. (World Bank Reprint Series No. 427.) Soc. Sci. Med. **23:** 847-850.
18. UNITED NATIONS CHILDREN'S FUND (UNICEF). 1987. The State of the World's Children, 1987. Oxford University Press. Oxford.
19. WORLD HEALTH ORGANIZATION. 1986. Efficacy of infant BCG immunization. WHO Weekly Epidemiological Record **28:** 216-218, 1986.
20. CONVIT, J., N. ARANZAZU, M. ULRICH, M. E. PINARDI, O. REYES & J. ALVARADO. 1982. Immunotherapy with a mixture of *Mycobacterium leprae* and BCG in different forms of leprosy and in Mitsuda-negative contacts. Int. J Lepr. **50:** 415.
21. DEO, M. G., C. V. BAPAT, V. BHALERAO, R. M. CHATURVEDI, R. G. CHULAVALA & W. S. BHATKI. 1983. Anti-leprosy potentials of the ICRC vaccine: A study in patients and healthy volunteers. Int. J. Lepr. **51:** 540.
22. CHAUDHURI, S., A. R. FOTEDAR & G. P. TALWAR. 1983. Lepromin conversion in repeatedly lepromin negative B1/LL patients after immunization with autoclaved *Mycobacterium* w. Int. J. Lepr. **51:** 159-168.
23. MEHRA, V., J. CONVIT, A. RUBINSTEIN & B. R. BLOOM. 1982. Activated suppressor T cells in leprosy. J. Immunol. **129:** 1946-1951.
24. CONVIT, J., A. RONDON, M. ULRICH, B. R. BLOOM, P. L. CASTELLANOS, M. E. PINARDI, M. CASTES & L. GARCIA. 1987. Immunotherapy versus chemotherapy in localized cutaneous leishmaniasis. Lancet **i:** 401-404.
25. CONVIT, J., P. L. CASTELLANOS, M. ULRICH, M. CASTS, A. RONDON, M. E. PINARDI, N. RODRIGUEZ, B. R. BLOOM, S. FORMICA, L. VALECILLOS & A. BRETAA. Immunotherapy of localized, intermediate and diffuse forms of american cutaneous leishmaniasis. J. Infect. Dis. In press.
26. SCHWARTZ, R. H. 1985. T-lymphocyte recognition of antigen in association with gene products of the major histocompatibility complex. Annu. Rev. Immunol. **3:** 237-261.
27. TOWNSEND, A. R. M., F. M. GOTCH & J. DAVEY. 1985. Cytotoxic T cells recognize fragments of the influenza nucleoprotein. Cell **42:** 457-467.
28. YOUNG, R. A., B. R. BLOOM, C. M. GROSSKINSKY, J. IVANYI & R. W. DAVIS. 1985. Dissecting Mycobacterium tuberculosis antigens using recombinant DNA. Proc. Natl. Acad. Sci. USA. **82:** 2583-2587.
29. YOUNG, R. A., V. MEHRA, D. SWEETSER, T. M. BUCHANAN, J. CLARK-CURTISS, R. W. DAVIS & B. R. BLOOM. 1985. Genes for the major protein antigens of Mycobacterium leprae. Nature **316:** 450-452.
30. SHINNICK, T. M., M. H. VODKIN & J. C. WILLIAMS. 1988. The *Mycobacterium tuberculosis* 65-kilodalton antigen is a heat shock protein which corresponds to common antigen and to the *Escherischia coli* GroEL protein. Infect. Immun. **56:** 446-451.
31. YOUNG, D., R. LATHIGRA, R. HENDRIX, D. SWEETSER & R. A. YOUNG. 1988. Stress proteins are immune targets in leprosy and tuberculosis. Proc. Natl. Acad. Sci. USA. **85:** 4267-4270.
32. KAUFMANN, S. H. E. 1988. Immuol. Today **9:** 168-174.
33. LAMB, J. R. & D. B. YOUNG. 1987. A novel approach to identification of T cell epitopes in *Mycobacterium tuberculosis* using human T lymphocyte clones. Immunology **60:** 1-5.
34. MELANCON-KAPLAN, J., S. WU HUNTER, M. MCNEIL, C. STEWART, R. L. MODLIN, T. REA, J. CONVIT, P. SALGAME, V. MEHRA, B. R. BLOOM & P. J. BRENNAN. 1988. Immunological significance of Mycobacterium leprae cell walls. Proc. Natl. Acad. Sci. USA. **85:** 1917-1921.
35. RIBI, E., D. L. GRANGER, K. C. MILNER, K. YAMAMOTO, S. M. STRAIN & R. PARKER. 1982. Immunology **46:** 297-305.
36. JACOBS, W. R., M. A. DOCHERTY, R. CURTISS, III & J. E. CLARK-CURTISS. 1986. Expression of a *Mycobacterium leprae* genes from a *Streptococcus mutans* promoter in *Escherichia coli* K-12. Proc. Natl. Acad. Sci. **83:** 1926-1930.
37. JACOBS, W. R. JR., M. TUCKMAN & B. R. BLOOM. 1987. Introduction of foreign DNA into mycobacteria using a shuttle plasmid. Nature **327:** 532-536.

38. Snapper, S. B., L. Lugosi, A. Jekkel, R. E. Melton, T. Kieser, B. R. Bloom & W. R. Jacobs, Jr. 1988. Lysogeny and transformation in mycobacteria: Stable expression of foreign genes. Proc. Natl. Acad. Sci. USA. **85:** 6987-6991.
39. Lugosi, L., W. R. Jacobs, Jr. & B. R. Bloom. Genetic transformation of BCG. Tubercle. In press.
40. Nakayama, K., S. M. Kelly & R. Curtiss, III. 1988. Construction of an Asd^+ expression-cloning vector: Stable maintenance and high level expression of cloned genes in a *Salmonella* vaccine vector strain. Bio/Tech **6:** 693-697.
41. Goldberg, A. L. & A. C. St. John. 1976. Intracellular protein degradation in mammalian and bacterial cells. Annu. Rev. Biochem. **45:** 747-803.
42. Melancon-Kaplan, J., S. Wu Hunter, M. McNeil, C. Stewart, R. L. Modlin, T. Rea, J. Convit, P. Salgame, V. Mehra, B. R. Bloom & P. J. Brennan. 1988. Immunologicasl significance of Mycobacterium leprae cell walls. Proc. Natl. Acad. Sci. USA. **85:** 1917-1921.
43. Moore, M. W., F. R. Carbone & M. J. Bevan. 1988. Introduction of soluble protein into the Class I pathway of antigen processing and presentation. Cell **54:** 777-785.
44. Cavalli-Sforza, L. L. & J. J. Lederberg. 1956. Isolation of pre-adaptive mutants in bacteria by sib-selection. Genetics **41:** 367.
45. Modlin, R. L., C. Pirmez, F. M. Hofman, V. Torigian, K. Uyemura, T. Rea, B. R. Bloom & M. B. Brenner. 1989. Lymphocytes bearing antigen-specific $\gamma\delta$ T-cell receptors accumulate in human infectious disease lesions. Nature **339:** 544-548.

Molecular Aspects of *Theileria parva* and Approaches to Vaccine Development for Animals[a]

ONESMO K. OLE-MOIYOI,[b] ANITA NAYAR,[b] KEITH IAMS,[b] ANTHONY J. MUSOKE,[b] AND TILAHUN YILMA[c]

[b]*International Laboratory for Research on Animal Diseases*
P.O. Box 30709
Nairobi, Kenya

[c]*Department of Veterinary Microbiology and Immunology*
University of California, Davis
Davis, California 95616

BACKGROUND

Theileria parva is a tick-transmitted, obligate intracellular protozoan parasite which causes an acute and often fatal form of theileriosis, East Coast fever (ECF), in large areas of eastern and central Africa. *T. annulata,* which usually infects B cells, causes a related disease of cattle or domestic buffalo around the Mediterranean and in vast areas of Asia including India, southern Russia, and China. The mammalian-infective stage of the parasite, the sporozoite, is injected into vector attachment sites during tick feeding. In *Rhipicephalus appendiculatus,* the vector for *T. parva,* rapid feeding does not occur until the third to fifth day of tick attachment, during which time the host target leukocytes will have been attracted into the vector attachment site.

Although *T. parva* sporozoites enter a variety of bovine leukocyte populations engaging a receptor/ligand-like passive endocytotic process, the parasite appears to survive in, and induce proliferation of, mostly T cells *in vivo.*[1,2] The sporozoites of *T. parva* develop in the salivary glands of the tick vector and are morphologically identical to sporozoites or merozoites of *Plasmodium* spp. in having a surface coat and subcellular organelles such as micronemes and rhoptries. The process of *T. parva* sporozoite entry into target cells has several features of interest which have been well characterized.[1] First, the process is rapid and is not ultrastructurally directional, unlike what has been shown to be the case for sporozoites or merozoites of *Plasmodium.* Second, entry of target cells occurs at 0°C, suggesting that metabolic energy requirement may be minimal.[1] This suggestion is complemented by observations showing

[a]This is ILRAD publication number 794. The work on rinderpest was supported by Cooperative Agreement DAN-4178-A-00-6040-00 from the United States Agency for International Development (USAID) of the State Department.

that even dead sporozoites will enter bovine lymphocytes. Third, shedding of the sporozoite surface coat occurs around junctions of close apposition between the parasite and host cell plasma membranes. This process creates progressive invagination of the parasite into the host-cell cytoplasm. Fourth, shortly after entry, rapid dissolution of the host cell plasma membrane surrounding the sporozoite occurs concurrent with the diminution of the electron-dense material contained in rhoptries and micronemes. Parasitophorous vacuole formation does not, therefore, occur and, although lysosomal-like organelles have been observed in lymphocytes around the sporozoite shortly after the latter's interioration, such structures disperse.[1] The efficiency of host cell membrane dissolution by *T. parva* sporozoites relative to the speed of lysosome formation by a cell may thus serve to define the host cell types in which theilerial sporozoites can survive. Within the T cell, the sporozoite differentiates into a multinucleate schizont. Studies on merogony in *T. parva* suggest that the schizont undergoes fission to release merozoites, which reacquire rhoptries, micronemes, and a surface coat before leaving the lymphocyte to enter the circulation, where infection of erythrocytes occurs.

Cattle infected with *T. parva* develop a granulocytopenia early in the disease. The intralymphocytic schizont induces blastogenesis of what appear to be mostly T cells *in vivo.* Lymphocytolysis occurs generally around the second or third week of infection and animals usually die of massive pulmonary edema. The etiology of this syndrome is unknown, although the role of complement activation with release of anaphylatoxins in granulocytopenic animals is likely to contribute to this process. Transmission of piroplasm-infected erythrocytes to the tick vector completes the mammalian phase of the parasite's life cycle.

IMMORTALIZATION OF BOVINE LYMPHOCYTES

One of the most unique features of *Theileria* is that the parasite induces blastogenesis and clonal expansion of lymphocytes.[3] *T. parva*-infected lymphocytes exhibit cellular pleiomorphism and short doubling times (16–25 hr). Although such parasitized cells retain expression of most of their differentiation antigens, surface phenotype alterations have been detected using monoclonal antibodies, which react with a variety of leukocyte differentiation antigens or bovine CD analogues (Ref. 2; Conrad *et al.*, unpublished observations). These features are characteristic of transformed cells. However, the disease is completely curable by administration of appropriate drugs, such as Parvaquone (2-cyclohexyl-3-hydroxy-1, 4-naphthoquinone; Wellcome Research, Nairobi, Kenya). Because of the reversibility of this process, the use of the terms theileria-induced "cellular proliferation" or "reversible transformation" is preferred to using just the term "transformation." The latter is misleading since it suggests a neoplastic etiology.

In attempts to identify the molecular mechanisms associated with theileria-induced proliferation, we compared protein kinase activities in membrane and soluble fractions prepared from cloned and uncloned bovine lymphocytes before and after infection with a variety of *T. parva* stocks isolated from various parts of Kenya including Muguga, Mariakani, Marikebuni; one from Uganda; and one stock from Zimbabwe (Boleni).[4,5] All theileria-infected cells had markedly enhanced (4.5- to 11-fold) incorporation of ^{32}P into protein substrates as assessed by nuclease-resistant TCA-precipitable radioactivity.[6] The enzyme that phosphorylated these proteins was cyclic nucleotide-independent, Ca^{2+}/calmodulin- and Ca^{2+}/phosphoinositide-insensitive.

The activity of the theileria-associated kinase was also not susceptible to inhibition by a variety of commercially available kinase inhibitors including derivatives of methylpiperazine, isoquinolinesulphonamides, and tosyllysylchloromethylketone (TLCK).

In order to determine the target amino acid residues for the kinase(s) associated with theileria infections, cloned IL-2-dependent bovine lymphocytes[7,8] or concanavalin A blasts in log phase growth, were metabolically labeled in parallel with the same cell clones after infection with various *T. parva* stocks. Particulate (100,000 $\times$ *g*) and supernatant fractions from these cells were analyzed by SDS-PAGE in order to identify infection-specific proteins. *In vitro* kinase assays were also performed using the 100,000 $\times$ *g* particulate and supernatant fractions as source of both enzyme and substrates. Partial alkaline hydrolysates of whole-cell particulate fractions, obtained as described by Martensen,[6] were analyzed on Dowex ion-exchange resins or by HPLC or by thin-layer electrophoresis; these analyses revealed no differences between the trace amounts of phosphotyrosine detectable in normal or in theileria-infected cells. Similarly, when a group of protein substrates, which only appeared in association with theileria infections, were electroeluted from gels, dialyzed, and then subjected to alkaline hydrolysis, no phosphotyrosine was detected on HPLC ion-exchange resins (ole-MoiYoi *et al.,* submitted for publication). On the other hand, acid hydrolysates of the same protein bands revealed radioactivity which co-eluted with cold phosphoserine or phosphothreonine internal standards. The dominant kinase that phosphorylated theileria-specific substrates was thus not a tyrosine kinase, but rather a serine/threonine-specific kinase. Further analyses of the specificity of this enzyme(s) suggest that the phosphotransferase in theileria-induced lymphocyte proliferation has the characteristics of casein kinase II (Ref. 9; ole-MoiYoi *et al.,* submitted for publication).

POSSIBLE MECHANISMS OF THEILERIA-INDUCED LYMPHOPROLIFERATION

The modulations of a large number of important cellular processes including signal transduction, cellular differentiation, and transformation are mediated by a variety of post-translational modifications. Prominent among these are phosphorylation/dephosphorylation. Evidence has recently been presented to amply implicate a large number of retrovirally transduced protein kinases in cellular transformation. The majority of these protein kinases are tyrosine-specific.[10,11] Cells proliferate in response to external as well as internal signals. Indeed the interaction between polypeptide hormones or growth factors with their respective membrane receptors has been shown to involve activation of receptor-associated kinases (for review see Ref. 12). The intracellular events that follow activation of growth-factor receptor kinases, which must involve cytoplasmic and nuclear signal transduction leading eventually to DNA replication and cellular division, are unknown. However, the products of some oncogenes have been shown to have sequence homologies with some growth factors, membrane receptors or to be localized in the cytoplasm or nucleus. Indeed transcription of some proto-oncogenes has been shown to occur in response to stimulation of cells by growth factors.[13] It is thus envisaged that uncontrolled cellular growth may occur if any molecule in a cellular mitogenic pathway ceases, because of structural alterations, to respond to regulatory physiological signals or if such a molecule is produced constitutively.[12]

An intracellular parasite, such as *Theileria,* may induce cellular proliferation by activation of an intracellular mitogenic pathway, thereby eliminating the need to involve exogenous growth signals. We used IL-2-dependent bovine lymphocytes as controls in our studies for the identification of protein kinases activated in theileria-infected lymphocytes. This approach would eliminate intracellular pathways activated by IL-2. The fact that we see such vast differences of the casein kinase II-like enzymes at the functional and antigenic levels between the IL-2-dependent control lymphocytes and theileria-infected cells suggests that the former may not engage a pathway of which casein kinase II is a constituent. It is indeed of great interest that brisk activation of casein kinase II occurs in response to insulin or epidermal growth factor[14] and that substantial production of this enzyme occurs during differentiation of 3T3-L1 adipocytes.[15] The products of the cell cycle control genes in yeast[16] and their human homologue *CDC*2Hs[17] have striking similarities in primary structure to the catalytic domains of casein kinase II.[18] Studies of the molecular mechanisms engaged by *Theileria* to reversibly transform bovine lymphocytes would be of interest and may elucidate fundamental processes involved in post-receptor pathways engaged in growth signal transduction.

CURRENT MANAGEMENT: INFECTION AND TREATMENT

The work of Lowe,[19] Barnett,[20] and Wilson[21] suggested that the severity of ECF in susceptible cattle depended on the number of organisms being introduced at the time of infection. Thus a low number of organisms induced mild infection while a high number produced severe disease. Later, titration experiments in susceptible cattle infected with triturated tick suspensions as a source of parasites provided further proof for this hypothesis.[22,23] These findings encouraged workers to initiate immunization experiments based on this hypothesis and on the observation that animals that recover are solidly immune to re-infection with a homologous stock. However, using low numbers of parasites did not produce mild disease consistently, since on a number of occasions severe reactions were observed, indicating that this, as a method of immunization, was unsuitable. Alternative procedures had therefore to be sought.

Attention was then focused on the effect of broad-spectrum antibiotics, such as tetracyclines, on the parasites. Initial experiments conducted by Neitz[24,25] demonstrated that cattle could be immunized by administering tetracyclines at the time of infection and continuing drug therapy over a prolonged period. Similar results were obtained by Brocklesby and Bailey,[26] who administered oral tetracyclines over a period of 28 days to animals that were undergoing infection with ECF. Although both groups of workers recommended the use of tetracyclines to protect valuable exotic stock against ECF, the method proved unpopular because of the high cost of tetracyclines and its prolonged administration, which necessitated employment of trained personnel.

Later, Cunningham *et al.*[27] and Brown *et al.*[28] improved on this method by inoculating animals with four doses of *N*-pyrrolidinomethyl tetracycline at 5 mg/kg body weight, over a period of 3 days, starting from the day of infection. These workers also used sporozoite suspensions of defined infectivity, rather than ticks, to induce ECF. This regime gave excellent chemoprophylactic coverage against ECF, but was still cumbersome. Further improvement of the method was achieved with a formulation of a long-acting oxytetracycline, which, when delivered at 20 mg/kg simultaneously with *Theileria parva* sporozoites, resulted in the production of homologous immunity.[29] One major disadvantage of this improved regime was that the tetracycline formulation was not adequate for a number of stocks, necessitating prolongation of the treatment for as long as six days with administration of the drug at 5 mg/kg.

Another complication of the infection and treatment method, in general, is that of the existence of a diversity of parasite stocks. Some *T. parva* stocks appeared to confer broader protection than others, thus giving rise to the concept of a "master" *T. parva* which could be used to protect against all others.

Recent evidence employing DNA probes has clearly revealed a great deal of genomic diversity within and amongst *T. parva* stocks.[30] Whether such diversity, detected using repetitive DNA sequences, will correlate with relevant (protective antigens) phenotypic differences between parasite strains remains to be established. The identification of a master strain has thus remained elusive. As a practical approach, it was decided that a combination of immunogenic strains from different geographical regions are being used to provide a wider coverage against ECF. In practice this idea has proved successful in a number of field trials.[31,32] The duration of immunity induced by infection and treatment appears to be long lasting and does not differ in any way from that developed after natural infection and recovery.

Finally there are a number of new drugs on the market for the treatment of clinical ECF. These include paravaquone, an analogue of menoctone (Naphthoquinone; Wellcome Laboratories); halofuginone lactate (Terit, Hoechst AG, West Germany), and a new naphthoquinone, Buparvaquone (Wellcome Laboratories). When these drugs were used in the infection and treatment protocol, only Buparvaquone appeared to hold any promise, and it has proved useful against stocks that were not controllable with long-acting tetracycline (Morzaria and Dolan, unpublished material.)

MECHANISMS OF IMMUNITY AND VACCINE DEVELOPMENT

Cattle that recover spontaneously from *T. parva* infections or after treatment become immune to homologous challenge, but may succumb to infection with heterologous stocks of *T. parva.* It is thought that the immunity that develops in these animals is cell-mediated (see Ref. 33 for review). This postulate, which is firmly engrained in the literature, seems to rest upon the observation that cytotoxicity restricted to syngeneic cells bearing schizonts appears soon after recovery from ECF and on rechallenge with a homologous stock.[34,35] In addition, cells sensitive against *T. parva* antigens, as measured by leukocyte migration inhibition,[36] have been reported. Indeed, class I MHC-restricted T-cell clones that appear to be *T. parva* stock-specific have been identified.[37] More recent data, however, have suggested a role for humoral antibodies in immunity to ECF[38,39] and have led to the postulate that the cell-mediated responses against the schizont act in concert with antibodies against the sporozoites. It was suggested that when sporozoites are deposited by ticks into the skin of immune animals they are killed by sporozoite-specific antibody-mediated processes and that those escaping the latter proceed to invade target cells and develop into schizonts, which could then be eliminated by cytotoxic cells.

In addition to the cellular and humoral responses, other antitheilerial activity, causing intracellular degeneration of schizonts in the sera of cattle recovering from *T. parva* infection, has been described.[40] Furthermore, increased numbers of macrophage-like cells have been identified in lymph nodes of cattle that have spontaneously recovered from ECF (Dolan, unpublished material). It has been suggested that these cells may secrete a factor or factors that could be responsible for anti-theilerial activity.

Further work is required to evaluate the possible role these factors could play in the recovery and establishment of immunity against ECF.

It has been possible to raise monoclonal and polyclonal antibodies against sporozoites of *T. parva.* Polyclonal antibodies from cattle recovering from *T. parva* infections as well as those from artificially infected animals have been purified and employed to identify relevant parasite surface antigens as well as for screening libraries of *T. parva* DNA constructed in expression bacteriophage lambda vectors according to established techniques.[41] The genes encoding these antigens are being sequenced and those regions encoding the antigenic domains recognized by sera of animals recovering from *T. parva* infections are being mapped.

With the gene coding for surface antigens at hand, it should be possible to test the feasibility of producing vaccines for theilerosis that are tailored to meet the economic and logistic problems of production and vaccination in developing nations.

A promising approach is to develop live-virus recombinant vaccines that express one or more of the relevant antigens of *T. parva.* Live, attenuated vaccines have advantages over inactivated, subunit and synthetic peptide vaccines because they replicate in the host and thereby "amplify" the antigen. However, they also have the following drawbacks: (1) one cannot often distinguish vaccinated animals from those animals that recovered from infection; (2) attenuated strains might revert to virulence in the vertebrate host or arthropod vector; (3) new strains of the agent may arise from the vaccine strain; and (4) the vaccine may induce disease in pregnant or debilitated animals. Many of these disadvantages could be overcome by the use of subunit or synthetic peptide vaccines, which also are advantageous because the immune system of the animal is stimulated with only the relevant antigens. The major problem with subunit and synthetic peptide vaccines, including inactivated vaccines, is that the antigenic mass cannot be greater than the amount of protein injected; there is no amplification of the antigen, for example, as in an attenuated live-virus vaccine.

Recombinant DNA technology has made it possible to insert and express heterologous genes in a variety of different viruses. Thus far, simian virus 40, bovine papillomavirus, adenovirus and members of the retrovirus family have been used most extensively as expression vectors. Although the relatively small size of these viruses facilitates genetic engineering, this property also restricts the amount of DNA that can be inserted into the viral genome. In addition, virus vectors usually have a limited host range and are defective, requiring either helper virus or special cell lines for replication. Furthermore, many of these vectors are oncogenic and therefore may be unsuitable for use as vaccines in humans and domestic animals. Disadvantages of these viral vector systems can be overcome by inserting and expressing foreign DNA in a virus, such as, vaccinia.

Vaccinia virus, a member of the poxvirus family, is a large double-stranded DNA virus that packages a complete transcription system and replicates in the cytoplasm of infected cells.[42] The virus has a wide host range including humans, cattle, horses, swine, sheep, goats, mice and monkeys, and a large genome that can accept heterologous genes. Recombinant DNA technology has developed convenient marker rescue techniques and plasmid sequences homologous to the virus DNA, allowing recombination within infected cells.[43]

There are a number of advantages to the vaccinia virus vector system. Like subunit vaccines, this system permits expression of single genes coding for immunogenic proteins. There is also amplification of the antigen, as for live-virus vaccines. It is possible to make a polyvalent vaccine expressing several genes representing various serotypes of the same agent or a number of unrelated agents. Rapid diagnostic kits can be developed to distinguish vaccinated animals from those exposed to the whole agent by infection. Such kits have been developed for vasicular stomatitis and foot-

and-mouth disease.[44] Finally, unlike many live vaccines, the lyophilized form of vaccinia virus is heat-stable, removing the need for refrigeration. This is a major advantage in carrying out a successful vaccination program in developing countries, which often lack cold-storage facilities.

To illustrate the potential for infectious vaccinia virus recombinant vaccines we will describe one that has just been developed for rinderpest. This disease is not only the single most important viral disease of livestock in developing countries, but it also has played a crucial role in the development of veterinary science. Rinderpest is an acute, febrile, highly contagious and fatal viral disease of ruminants, particularly cattle and buffalo. The disease is characterized by inflammation, hemorrhage, tissue necrosis and erosion of the gastrointestinal tract accompanied by bloody diarrhea, wasting, and death.[45]

The rinderpest virus (RPV) is enveloped and has a single-stranded RNA genome with a minus polarity. The virus is in the family Paramyxoviridae and is a member of the morbillivirus group, along with measles virus of humans, distemper virus of dogs and peste-des-petits-ruminants virus (PRRV) of goats and sheep. In paramyxoviruses, the hemagglutinin (HA) and fusion (F) surface proteins have been shown to provide protective immunity. One of us (T.Y.), with associates at the University of California, Davis, has propagated the highly virulent Kabete "O" strain of RPV in primary bovine kidney cells and characterized eight viral proteins.[46] The complete nucleotide sequences of both HA and F cDNA copies have been determined.[47,48] Standard procedures were used to construct vaccinia virus recombinants expressing the HA gene (vRVH) and the F gene (VRVF) of RPV.[49]

Immune response studies in cattle were assessed by serum neutralization (SN) assays[50] and by protection from challenge. Single and double vaccination experiments were conducted and the vaccine was found to be completely protective against 1000×, a normally lethal dose of RPV. The test animals exhibited no detectable illness and had a normal temperature of 101°F. All animals vaccinated with the recombinants produced SN antibodies to RPV. Pock lesions in all animals vaccinated with the recombinants were limited to the site of inoculation, and were healed completely by two weeks. All control animals developed high fever (108°F) and lesions typical of severe rinderpest by day 2 after challenge and died by day 6. As expected, control animals had no detectable antibody titer.[49]

Thus, this clearly demonstrates the potential of vaccinia virus recombinant vaccines to protect against a massive challenge dose of virus. It is important, however, that safety considerations be addressed before introducing live recombinant viruses into the environment. With this in mind, the recombinant vaccines with the attenuated strain (Wyeth) that had been used worldwide against smallpox were constructed. It has been demonstrated that insertional inactivation of the TK gene further attenuates this virus.[51] The use of lyphokine genes, such as interferon-gamma or interleukin-2, to enhance immune responses and to further attenuate vaccinia virus recombinant vaccines, is also being investigated.[52,53] It was recently demonstrated that expression of interleukin-2 prevented disseminated vaccinia virus infection in immunodeficient mice.[54]

Currently, the Plowright tissue culture vaccine (PTCV) is widely used for vaccination against rinderpest. However, there have been difficulties in sustaining the manufacture of this vaccine and in its delivery to the field. The need for skilled personnel, the lack of refrigeration facilities, and the vaccine's instability have also been disadvantageous. In contrast, the lyophilized form of recombinant vaccinia virus is heat-stable and is easily produced, transported and administered by scarification.

An effective vaccinia virus recombinant vaccine has thus been developed for one of the most devastating livestock diseases in Africa and Asia. The availability of this vaccine eliminates many of the economic and logistic problems of vaccine production, distribution, and administration in endemic areas. This encourages us to pursue similar strategies in developing vaccines for other livestock diseases.

ACKNOWLEDGMENTS

We would like to thank Yasmin Verjee, Catherine Nkonge, and Micheal Kibe for technical assistance in some of the experiments described herein. We also thank Mrs. Lucy Thairo for typing the manuscript. We are most grateful to Drs. C. L. Baldwin, W. C. Brown, P. C. Conrad, S. P. Morzaria, T. T. Dolan, W. I. Morrison and to Dr. Sally Owens for their helpful comments or for critical review of this manuscript.

REFERENCES

1. FAWCETT, D. W., S. DOXEY, D. A. STAGG & A. S. YOUNG. 1982. Eur. J. Cell Biol. **27:** 10-21.
2. BALDWIN, C. L., S. J. BLACK, W. C. BROWN, P. A. CONRAD, B. M. GODDEERIS, S. W. KINUTHIA, P. A. LALOR, N. D. MACHUGH, W. I. MORRISON, S. P. MORZARIA, J. NAESSENS & J. NEWSON. 1988. Infect. Immun. **56:** 462-467.
3. BROWN, C. G. D. 1983. *In In Vitro* Cultivation of Protozoan Parasites. J. B. Jensen, Ed.: 243-284. CRC Press. Boca Raton, FL.
4. MINAMI, T., P. R. SPOONER, A. D. ARVIN, J. G. R. OCAMA, D. A. E. DOBBELEARE & T. FUJINAGA. 1983. Res. Vet. Sci. **35:** 334-340.
5. IRVIN, A. D., D. A. E. DOBBELEARE, D. M. MWAMACHI, T. MINAMI, P. R. SPOONER & J. G. R. OCAMA. 1983. Res. Vet. Sci. **35:** 341-346.
6. MARTENSEN, T. M. 1984. Meth. Enzymol. **107:** 3-23.
7. BROWN, W. C. & D. J. GRAB. 1985. J. Immunol. **133:** 3184-3189.
8. MORRISON, W. I., B. M. GODDEERIS & A. J. TEALE. 1987. Eur. J. Immunol. **17:** 1703-1709.
9. HATHAWAY, G. M. & J. A. TRAUGH. 1982. Curr. Topics Cell. Regul. **21:** 101-127.
10. HUNTER, T. & J. A. COOPER. 1985. Annu. Rev. Biochem. **54:** 897-930.
11. BISHOP, J. M. 1985. Cell **42:** 23-38.
12. HELDIN, C-H. & B. WESTERMARK. 1984. Cell **37:** 9-20.
13. KELLEY, K., B. H. COCHRAN, C. P. STILES & P. LEDER. 1983. Cell **35:** 603-610.
14. SOMMERCORN, J., J. A. MULLIGAN, F. J. LOZEMAN & E. G. KREBS. 1987. Proc. Natl. Acad. Sci. USA **84:** 8834-8838.
15. SOMMERCORN, J. & E. G. KREBS. 1987. J. Biol. Chem. **262:** 3839-3843.
16. LORINCZ, A. T. & S. I. REED. 1984. Nature **307:** 183-185.
17. LEE, M. G. & P. NURSE. 1987. Nature **327:** 31-35.
18. SAXENA, A., R. PADMANABHA & C. V. C. GLOVER. 1987. Mol. Cell. Biol. **7:** 3409-3417.
19. LOWE, H. J. 1953. Annual Report of the Department of Veterinary Science and Animal Husbandry.: 7. Tanganyika Territory.
20. BARNETT, S. F. 1957. Bull. Epizoot. Dis. Afr. **5:** 343-357.
21. WILSON, S. G. 1950. Parasitology **40:** 195-203.
22. CUNNINGHAM, M. P., C. G. D. BROWN, M. J. BURRIDGE, A. J. MUSOKE, R. E. PURNELL, D. E. RADLEY & J. SEMPEMBWA. 1974. Brit. Vet. J. **130:** 336-345.
23. RADLEY, D. E., C. G. D. BROWN, M. J. BURRIDGE, M. P. CUNNINGHAM, M. A. PEIRCE & R. E. PURNELL. 1974. Expt. Parasitol. **36:** 278-287.
24. NEITZ, W. O. 1953. Nature **171:** 34-35.

25. NEITZ, W. O. 1957. Onderst. J. Vet. Res. **27:** 275-430.
26. BROCKLESBY, D. W. & K. P. BAILEY. 1965. Bull. Epizoot. Dis. Afr. **13:** 161-168.
27. CUNNINGHAM, M. P., C. G. D. BROWN, M. J. BURRIDGE, A. D. IRVIN, R. E. PURNELL & D. E. RADLEY. 1973. Res. Vet. Sci. **15:** 263-265.
28. BROWN, C. G. D., D. E. RADLEY, M. P. CUNNINGHAM, I. M. KIRIMI, S. P. MORZARIA & A. J. MUSOKE. 1977. Tropenmed. Parasitol. **28:** 342-348.
29. RADLEY, D. E. 1981. *In Advances in the Control of Theileriosis* A. D. Irvin, M. P. Cunningham & A. S. Young, Eds.: 227-237. Martinus Nijhoff. The Hague.
30. CONRAD, P. A., K. IAMS, W. C. BROWN, B. SOHANPAL & O. K. OLE-MOIYOI. 1987. Mol. Biochem. Parasitol. **25:** 213-226.
31. UILENBERG, G., B. E. C. SCHRENDER, G., MPANGALA, R. S. SILAYO, W. TONDEUR, R. J. TATCHELL & H. J. N. SANGA. 1976. *In* Proceedings of the International Conference on Tick-borne Diseases and Vectors J. K. H. Wilde, Ed.: 307-311. Edinburgh.
32. UILENBERG, G., R. S. SILAYO, C. MPANGALA, W. TONDEUR, R. J. TATCHELL & H. J. N. SANGA. 1977. Z. Tropenmed. Parasitol. **28:** 499-506.
33. MORRISON, W. I. & B. M. GODDEERIS. 1989. Curr. Topics Microbiol. Immunol. In press.
34. ALLISON, A. C. & E. M. EUGUI. 1980. Am. J. Pathol. **101:** 114-118.
35. EUGUI, E. M. & D. L. EMERY. 1981. Nature **290:** 251-254.
36. MUHAMMED, S. I., L. H. LAUERMAN & L. W. JOHNSON. 1975. Am. J. Vet. Res. **36:** 399-402.
37. MORRISON, W. I., B. M. GODDEERIS, A. J. TEALE, C. L. BALDWIN, A. BENSAID & J. ELLIS. 1986. Immunol. Today **7:** 211-216.
38. MUSOKE, A. J., V. M. NANTULYA, F. R. RURANGIRWA & G. BUSCHER. 1984. Immunology **52:** 231-238.
39. MUSOKE, A. J., V. M. NANTULYA, G. BUSCHER, R. A. MASAKE & B. OTIM. 1982. Immunology **52:** 43-47.
40. DOLAN, T. T., D. A. STAGG & L. M. NJUGUNA. 1985. Int. J. Parasitol. **15:** 43-47.
41. YOUNG, R. A., V. MEHRA, D. SWEETSER, T. BUCHANAN, J. CLARK-CURTISS, R. W. DAVIS & B. R. BLOOM. 1985. Nature **316:** 450-452.
42. MOSS, B. 1974. *In* Comprehensive Virology, Vol. 3. E. Frankel-Conrat, Ed.: 405-474. Plenum. New York.
43. MACKETT, M., T. YILMA, J. ROSE & B. MOSS. 1985. Science **227:** 433-435.
44. WORKMAN, T., D. SHEN, L. WOODARD & T. YILMA. 1986. Am. J. Vet. Res. **47:** 1507-1512.
45. PLOWRIGHT, W. 1968. Virology Monographs 3: Rinderpest virus: 25-110. Springer-Verlag. Vienna and New York.
46. GRUBMAN, M. J., C. MEBUS, B. DALE, M. YAMANAKA & T. YILMA. 1988. Virology **163:** 261-266.
47. YAMANAKA, M., D. HSU, B. DALE, T. CRISP, M. GRUBMAN & T. YILMA. 1988. Virology **166:** 251-253.
48. HSU, D., M. YAMANAKA, J. MILLER, B. DALE, M. GRUBMAN & T. YILMA. 1988. Virology **166:** 149-153.
49. YILMA, T., D. HSU, L. JONES, S. OWEN, M. GRUBMAN, C. MEBUS, M. YAMANAKA & B. DALE. Science. In press.
50. YILMA, T., M. MACKETT, J. ROSE & B. MOSS. 1985. *In* Vaccinia Viruses as Vectors for Vaccine Antigens. G. V. Quinnan, Ed.: 187-200. Elsevier. New York.
51. BULLER, R. M. L., G. L. SMITH, K. CREMER, A. L. NOTKINS & B. MOSS. 1985. Nature **317:** 813-815.
52. YILMA, T., K. ANDERSON, K. BRECHLING & B. MOSS. *In* Vaccines 87: Modern Approaches to New Vaccines Including Prevention of AIDS. R. M. Chanock, H. Giensburg, R. Lerner & F. Brown, Eds.: 393-396. Cold Spring Harbor Laboratory. Cold Spring Harbor, NY.
53. ANDERSON, P. K., E. H. FENNIE & T. YILMA. 1988. J. Immunol. **40:** 3599-3604.
54. FLEXNER, C., A. HUGIN & B. MOSS. 1987. Nature **330:** 259-262.

Leishmaniasis and Malaria: DNA Probes for Diagnosis and Epidemiologic Analysis[a]

DYANN F. WIRTH,[b,c] WILLIAM O. ROGERS,[c] ROBERT BARKER,[c] HEITOR DOURADO,[d] LAKSAMI SUESEBANG,[e] AND BERNADINO ALBUQUERQUE[d]

[c] *Department of Tropical Public Health*
Harvard School of Public Health
Boston, Massachusetts 02115

[d] *Instituto de Medicina Tropical de Manaus*
Manaus, Amazonas, Brazil

[e] *Malaria Division*
Ministry of Public Health
Bangkok 10200, Thailand

Parasitic diseases are still prevalent in many parts of the world, causing both human suffering and economic loss. Major efforts to control and even eradicate parasitic diseases have met with some success (for example, elimination of malaria from the southern United States and Cuba), but in many developing tropical countries, parasitic diseases remain major health problems. Such diseases can pose a significant barrier to economic development, and their control is an important goal for improved world health. Intensive research is being devoted to the development of new control measures for many parasitic diseases. These control measures include development of vaccines and new chemotherapeutic agents as well as improved vector control strategies. Previous experience has demonstrated the need for extensive baseline information before the introduction of any control program and the need for continued monitoring of the control program in order to assess its effectiveness. These diseases have complex life cycles involving both vectors of transmission and often intermediate hosts, both of which have an impact on the transmission of disease and can affect the outcome of any control measure.

Recent developments in biotechnology, including the use of monoclonal antibodies and recombinant DNA, have provided new tools for the collection of information on these diseases and have the potential for providing both more extensive and detailed information on the parasite in the infected human and in insect vectors. This article focuses on the potential impact of these new methodologies on epidemiologic studies

[a]This work was supported by the UNDP/World Bank/WHO Special Programme for Research and Training in Tropical Diseases, the National Institutes of Health (Grants AI 21365 and AI 19392), and the John D. and Catherine T. MacArthur Foundation. D.F.W. is a Burroughs-Wellcome Scholar in Molecular Parasitology.

[b]To whom correspondence should be addressed.

of two parasitic diseases, leishmaniasis and malaria, for which new methods of detection, both in man and in insect vectors, have been developed. These diseases are caused by parasitic protozoa of different genera, *Leishmania* and *Plasmodium*, respectively, each of which has a unique life cycle. Each poses a separate set of problems for epidemiologic studies and for eventual control.

LEISHMANIASIS

Human leishmaniasis is caused by at least 14 different species and subspecies of the genus *Leishmania*. The clinical manifestations of the disease depend in part on the infecting *Leishmania* organism and fall into three general categories: simple cutaneous disease, which is often self-limiting; mucocutaneous disease, which involves the destruction of nasal tissue; and visceral disease, a systemic infection that is often fatal if untreated. In fact, the diseases share relatively few properties except that they are caused by organisms of the same genus and that, in humans, the parasite grows in the phagolysosomal vesicles of macrophages. Epidemiologic studies over the last 25 years have shown that, in general, leishmaniasis is a zoonotic disease; the parasite is transmitted to man from a reservoir mammalian host by a phlebotomus sandfly vector during a blood meal. Of the numerous *Leishmania* species, infective for mammals, only a subset can infect and cause disease in humans. Presumably, this selectivity is a combination of factors, including the intrinsic susceptibility of humans and the feeding habits of the sandfly. Enormous effort has been devoted to the isolation and characterization of *Leishmania* organisms that infect man and to the identification of the principal mammalian reservoirs and species of phlebotomus vector (for a review see Ref. 1). The result of many such studies has been the correlation of particular clinical manifestations with certain species or subspecies of the parasite (see TABLE 1 for summary).

The identification of *Leishmania* species is based on a variety of ecological, biological, biochemical, and immunologic criteria (for a review see Ref. 2). Each cultured isolate of the parasite has been analyzed by the use of one or more of these criteria and categorized as to species and subspecies. There remain certain controversies as to whether organisms isolated in distant geographic locations but sharing certain common properties belong to the same or distinct subspecies of *Leishmania*. For example, *L. mexicana garnhami*[3] isolated in Venezuela is very similar to *L. mexicana amazonensis* isolated in Brazil, as determined by isoenzyme profiles and monoclonal antibodies,[4–6] but there are conflicting results as to its growth characteristics in sandfly vectors.[7] Whether these organisms represent strains of the same subspecies or distinct subspecies cannot be resolved because there is no single generally accepted method for species identification in the genus *Leishmania*. This uncertainty complicates comparison of the epidemiology of the disease in distinct geographic locations and represents a potential limitation on the transfer of control measures from one geographic location to another. The World Health Organization has addressed this problem by establishing a set of reference strains for the various species and subspecies to be used for comparison and classification of new isolates.

The diverse nature of leishmaniasis clearly requires a diverse control program with specific targets for each focus of the disease. This will require more extensive collection of baseline data with regard to the infecting *Leishmania* species in humans, the relevant sandfly vector, and the principal mammalian reservoir of the particular species or

TABLE 1. Major Leishmania Species Causing Human Disease

Primary Geographic Disease[a] and Species	Location
Cutaneous Leishmaniasis	
L. Mexicana mexicana	Mexico, Central America
L. mexicana amazonensis	Brazil (Amazon region)
L. mexicana pifoni	Venezuela
L. major	Southern USSR, Middle East
L. tropica	Asia, southern Europe, northern and western Africa
L. braziliensis guyanensis	Northern, southern South America
L. braziliensis panamensis	Central America
L. braziliensis peruviana	Peru
Diffuse cutaneous disease	
L. mexicana amazonensis	Brazil (Amazon region)
L. aethiopica	Ethiopia and Kenya
Mucocutaneous disease	
L. braziliensis braziliensis	Western and northern South America
Visceral disease	
L. donovani	India
L. donovani infantum	Mediterranean area
L. chagasi	Northern South America

[a] Based on Marinkelle.[9]

subspecies. These data must be collected at each focus for proper implementation of any control program directed at either the sandfly vector or the mammalian reservoir. For control measures that involve identification and treatment of patients, accurate, rapid diagnosis of leishmaniasis must be achieved before treatment with relatively toxic chemotherapeutic agents is begun.[8]

One of the major problems in further analysis of the ecology and epidemiology of the disease is the extremely laborious task of identifying the parasite. All of the work documenting the species and subspecies of *Leishmania* is dependent on the isolation of the organism either directly in culture or after passage through a susceptible laboratory animal, most commonly the hamster. This has several limitations, namely, the number of samples that can be handled at any one time, the time it takes to grow the parasites and subsequently type them, and perhaps more important, the selection from an otherwise mixed population of parasites of those that grow either *in vitro* or in experimental animals. A method of direct identification of *Leishmania* parasites from lesions, sandfly vectors, and intermediate mammalian reservoirs is necessary if broader epidemiologic studies involving large numbers of samples are to be initiated.

Current diagnosis of leishmaniasis is achieved either by direct examination of a tissue biopsy or by means of a delayed-type hypersensitivity test referred to as the Montenegro test.[9] Neither of these methods is able to distinguish *Leishmania* species or subspecies, and the Montenegro test cannot distinguish current from previous infections. For certain forms of leishmaniasis, the most effective control measures may be the direct treatment of infected patients[10] and will require specific diagnosis of *Leishmania* species or subspecies from lesion material in order to design treatment regimens that minimize morbidity and mortality (for a review see Ref. 11). For example, cutaneous infection with *L. braziliensis* is often associated with subsequent mucocutaneous disease, and early diagnosis could facilitate treatment and perhaps reduce the frequency of mucocutaneous disease.

DNA Probes in the Diagnosis of Leishmaniasis

A new method based on DNA probes specific for the various *Leishmania* species was developed to provide a direct diagnosis of patients with leishmaniasis and to eliminate the need for culturing parasites before species identification.[12] This method allows direct diagnosis from lesion material without requiring isolation of the parasite. Such direct diagnosis of *Leishmania* species, which had not been possible with any of the existing methods, provides the basis for the clinical management of this disease. In the initial studies, the DNA probes, which were based on total kinetoplast DNA (kDNA), would differentiate the major species complexes in New World *Leishmania, L. mexicana,* and *L. braziliensis.* Subsequent experiments in which recombinant DNA methods were used resulted in the development of DNA probes that can differentiate species, subspecies, and even distinct isolates of the parasite.[12–17]

The basis for the DNA probes is the minicircle, which is a highly repeated small circular DNA molecule found within the mitochondria of the parasite. It has no apparent function and has an apparent high rate of DNA sequence divergence as measured by restriction-site polymorphism and DNA hybridization studies.[18–22] In the New World *Leishmania* sp., the kDNA minicircles isolated from *L. mexicana* do not share any sequence homology with those isolated from *L. braziliensis.*[12,13] These differences in DNA sequence have provided the basis for a DNA probe that can distinguish the two *Leishmania* species directly when material obtained from a lesion is applied to nitrocellulose.

These DNA probes have been used to diagnose leishmaniasis in patients from the Instituto de Medicina Tropical de Manaus[23] (TABLE 2). In each case, the results of the DNA probe were compared to standard diagnostic tests, including the Montenegro test (see above), histopathology, and culturing and subsequent characterization of the parasite. As can be seen in TABLE 2, the DNA probe detected the disease in 32 of the 43 patients who had positive results in the Montenegro test. This observation may mean that in some patients, the parasite density was below the detection limit of the assay, which, based on laboratory experiments, is as few as 50 organisms in a single spot on nitrocellulose. There are cases in which organisms were cultured from lesions that were originally negative. Another possibility is that the delayed-type hypersensitivity test detected either a previous infection or a cross-reacting antigen from another type of infection.[24] A third possibility is that the parasite in the lesion is of a type not recognized by the kDNA probe; however, every parasite that has been isolated from a lesion has reacted with either the *L. braziliensis* or *L. mexicana* kDNA probes.

The DNA probe clearly detects infections in more patients than can be detected by either histopathologic studies or culturing. Although this probably results from the greater sensitivity of the DNA probe in comparison to these other methods, it may also represent false positives in the DNA probe method. Because there is no

TABLE 2. Comparison of Diagnostic Tests for Leishmaniasis in Brazil

Diagnostic Test	No. of Patients
Montenegro-test-positive	43
Hybridization-positive	32
L. mexicana DNA probe	2
L. braziliensis DNA probe	30
Culture-positive	27
Histopathology	17

NOTE: Results from 57 patients examined at the *Leishmania* clinic of the Instituto de Medicina, Tropical de Manaus during January-February 1984. Each patient was given a Montenegro test and those with positive results on the test were given further diagnostic tests, which included a tissue biopsy (4 mm) taken directly from the lesion. This biopsy specimen was divided: one-half was placed directly in Schneider's growth medium and the other half touched to nitrocellulose. The remainder was processed for histopathologic study. The hybridization was performed by standard procedures as described.[12] The *L. mexicana* probe was a combination of DNA extracted from strain WR303 (*L. mexicana amazonensis*) and L11 (*L. mexicana mexicana*). The *L. braziliensis* probe was isolated from strain WR2903. All hybridization results were read independently by two people.

single "gold standard" for the detection of parasites, the exact determination of false positives is not possible. However, in ten cases in which histopathologic study failed to detect parasites and the result of the DNA probe was positive, the culturing of parasites clearly demonstrated their presence. The question of the false positive reaction with DNA probes has been tested experimentally. These kDNA probes did not hybridize with touch preparations of uninfected tissue from several animals and from a limited number of human lesions that subsequently proved not to be due to leishmaniasis. In addition, these DNA probes did not react with *Trypanosoma cruzi,* malaria, or *Escherichia coli.* Further evidence that the number of false positives with the kDNA probes is relatively low was obtained by testing duplicate touch preparations of each lesion with kDNA from both *L. mexicana* and *L. braziliensis.* In every case in which there was a reaction with the kDNA probe, it was specific for either *L. mexicana* or *L. braziliensis,* and the duplicate lesion showed no reaction above background. When parasites were isolated from these lesions and subsequently tested by kDNA hybridization, the original identification was confirmed. An alternative method of limiting the number of false positive reactions due to nonspecific binding of labeled DNA to tissue or blood is to perform *in situ* hybridization and examine each preparation under the microscope as suggested by Barker and coworkers.[15] This is a very time-consuming and expert process not easily adapted to large numbers of samples.

One of the limitations of the kDNA minicircle as a hybridization probe is that although it can distinguish the major species complexes of New World cutaneous leishmaniasis, the kDNA minicircle from each complex is homologous to all the subspecies and it is therefore impossible to distinguish subspecies.[12,13] This identification of subspecies is important clinically because certain manifestations of the disease are specific to the parasite subspecies and it is also important in the description of any intermediate host or insect vector carrying a particular subspecies. In addition, our work and the work of others has indicated that in the Old World *Leishmania* species causing cutaneous and visceral disease, kDNA sequence homology occurs among different species.[12,16,17,24–27] For example, kDNA isolated from *L. major* hybridizes with both of the other cutaneous species, *L. tropica* and *L. aethiopica* and with the visceral strain *L. donovani.*[17]

Therefore a new approach is required for the development of DNA probes that can distinguish subspecies in New World cutaneous leishmaniasis and differentiate the species complexes of the Old World isolates. Several groups have used recombinant DNA methods to develop such DNA probes with these narrower specificities (TABLE 3).[14–17,26,28–30] The method has been to clone restriction fragments of a kDNA minicircle and to use these cloned subfragments as more specific probes for species, subspecies, and even isolates. The general observation from this body of work is that within the minicircle population, there are DNA sequences that have undergone rapid sequence divergence and can thus serve to differentiate even closely related organisms.[28] In addition, we have shown that this sequence divergence can occur within a single minicircle. A nested set of deletions of a single cloned minicircle fragment from *L. mexicana amazonensis* was generated and then tested for hybridization specificity. The full-length minicircle had a similar specificity to total kDNA, and two deletions demonstrated species and isolate specific hybridization patterns.[30]

The next step for the utilization of DNA probes will be in the detection of infected insect vectors and intermediate hosts. Preliminary laboratory experiments show that parasites can be detected in infected sandflies that have been squashed directly on nitrocellulose.[31] This approach must now be tested in the field. Similarly, laboratory-based experiments have demonstrated that parasite infections can be detected in tissue touch preparations from animals experimentally infected;[12] however, both the intensity of the infection and the target tissue in natural hosts will be different and thus the DNA probe must be tested directly in field-extracted material. These will be compared with alternate methods developed for antigen detection in insect vectors and infected animals.[32,33]

The DNA probe method should be readily adaptable to field situations. Once the tissue biopsy or sandfly vector is obtained, it is applied directly to nitrocellulose or other solid supports and is stable in this form indefinitely. Thus samples could be collected from distant sites and returned for processing. The major disadvantage of this methodology is the requirement for a radioisotope. Alternative methods of labeling DNA, which are being developed and tested for such biological specimens, should be useful in field situations.

TABLE 3. Hybridization Specificities of Cloned Kinetoplast DNA Fragments

Source	Specificities	Reference
L. donovani	Species	28
L. infantum	Species	28
L. donovani	Visceral complex	16
L. chagasi	Non-Indian visceral	16
L. major	Isolate	17
L. mexicana amazonensis	Species	30
	Subspecies	30
	Isolate	30
L. major	Isolate	14
L. tropica	Isolate	14
L. aethiopica	Isolate	14

MALARIA

Human malaria is caused by the four major *Plasmodium* species—*P. falciparum, P. vivax, P. malaria,* and *P. ovale.* In most parts of the world, the prevailing parasite species is *P. falciparum,* which causes the most severe form of the acute disease and is often fatal in children.[34] *Plasmodium vivax,* the next most prevalent disease is characterized by relapses caused by parasites that remain in the liver in a latent form. The parasite is transmitted by various species of the anopheline mosquito to the human host. The sporozoite, the infectious form of the parasite released from mosquito salivary glands, initiates the exoerythrocytic cycle in the liver. Subsequently developed merozoites invade erythrocytes, and the asexual cycle continues through the course of the infection. A subset of the infected erythrocytes develop into gametocytes, the form that can develop in mosquitoes, and results in disease transmission. There is no significant animal reservoir for this disease.

Malaria is among one of the major infectious diseases in the world, with acute clinical malaria affecting some 90 million to 100 million people per year according to the World Health Organization estimates.[35] In addition, there is a large reservoir of chronic infection. The World Health Organization estimates that more than 40% of the world's population is at risk of malaria infection and that some 365 million people live in areas where malaria endemicity has remained unchanged despite intensive world efforts at eradication of the disease.[35]

Elimination of malaria worldwide has proved to be a difficult goal, and thus current efforts are devoted to the control of malaria.[36] During the eradication program, several problems arose that will have an impact on any control program. Among these problems is the widespread resistance of anopheline vectors to insecticides,[37] and the emergence of *P. falciparum* strains resistant to chloroquine, the primary chemotherapeutic agent, and the subsequent development of multidrug-resistant parasite strains.[38] New approaches to control measures include improved conventional methods of vector control and chemotherapy and the development of innovative measures including vaccines for the malaria parasite and biological control of anopheline vectors.

The parameters of malaria transmission and disease prevalence have been studied for the last 40 years in many parts of the world. Mathematical models[39,40] of disease transmission have been developed on the basis of both entomological factors and human factors such as immunity (for a review see Ref. 41). In addition, epidemiologic studies have demonstrated an association of malaria prevalence with certain variants in erythrocytes, sickle cell trait,[42] glucose-6-phosphate dehydrogenase deficiency,[43] Duffy blood-group antigens,[44] and recently, alpha-thalassemia.[45] These studies have shown that malaria is a complex and dynamic disease that is varied throughout the world. Thus any control program must take into consideration the multiple factors that can affect malaria transmission and must measure these factors in each situation. For this to be achieved, it is imperative that new and efficient means of measuring both entomological and human factors on a large scale be implemented.

Detection of Malaria Infection

Both vaccine and future drug trials will require a sensitive and rapid method for detecting parasites. Currently, malaria infection is determined by the use of a thick smear stained with Giemsa. This method is both specific and sensitive for the diagnosis

TABLE 4. Comparison of DNA Probes Specific for *P. falciparum* in Thailand

Diagnostic Test Result	No. of Patients
Clinic-microscope-positive	121
DNA-positive	129
Clinic-negative	511
DNA-negative	503

NOTE: The patient population consisted of 632 patients examined at malaria clinics of the Malaria Division of the Thailand Ministry of Public Health in either Bangnamron or Chantiburi, Thailand in July 1985. Blood was collected by digital puncture into a heparinized capillary and treated as previously described.[47] Malaria thick smears were prepared in the routine manner for diagnosis at the clinic. A separate set of slides, with both thin and thick smears, was prepared and subsequently analyzed by malaria experts.[47]

of malaria, but has severe limitations when large numbers of samples must be handled in a timely fashion, as will be the case for the collection of baseline data for many of the vaccine trials and chemotherapy studies. A trained microscopist is required for each determination, and this is time-consuming, tiring, and potentially subject to reader bias, especially when large numbers of slides must be read in a short time period. Thus alternative methods for handling large numbers of samples are necessary.

DNA probes specific for human malaria have been developed by several groups,[46] and recent work by Barker *et al.*[47] has demonstrated that the DNA probe specific for *P. falciparum* can be used to detect malaria infection directly in finger-stick blood of infected patients. The DNA probes specific for *P. falciparum* are dispersed, highly repeated DNA sequences isolated from the *P. falciparum* genome using recombinant DNA technology. Both in laboratory and field testing, the pPF14 probe[47] is specific for *P. falciparum* and does not react with *P. vivax,* the other major human malarial parasite. The method compares favorably in sensitivity with routine microscopy, detecting parasite densities as low as 40 parasites per microliter of blood. As can be seen in TABLE 4, the DNA probe method detected *P. falciparum* infection in 129 of 632 patients compared with the 121 detected by routine examination of Giemsa-stained thick smears. Subsequent examination of duplicate slides by expert microscopists confirmed the DNA probe diagnosis in those patients missed by routine microscopy. The DNA probe method offers the advantage of a standardized procedure that can be used in batch fashion on large numbers of samples. An important feature of this method is that it is reproducible over a large number of samples and should be less subject to reader bias. In addition, in our recent work, we have been able to correlate the intensity of DNA hybridization with parasite density, and thus the DNA probes may also provide information on the intensity of infection. One limitation of the correlation of hybridization intensity with parasite density is the potential for variation in the number of repeated target sequences in different *P. falciparum* strains. The DNA probe method now must be tested in an epidemiologic study to assess its general usefulness.

DEVELOPMENT OF THE POLYMERASE CHAIN REACTION TO AMPLIFY DNA SIGNALS

Recent development of a method to amplify target DNA sequences has greatly enhanced the sensitivity of our DNA probes and will now allow the use of nonradioactive methods to detect target sequences. We have tested the polymerase chain reaction (PCR) developed by the Cetus Corporation and have been able to demonstrate a million-fold amplification of target DNA sequences in both the *Leishmania* sp. kDNA system and for *P. falciparum*- and *P. vivax*-specific DNA probes. In each case, the cloned target DNA has been sequenced and oligonucleotide primers based on this sequence have been used in the PCR reaction. Target DNA has been successfully amplified from purified DNA, tissue samples and blood samples and from formalin-fixed, paraffin-embedded tissue sections. In addition, we have been able to amplify sequences directly from infected insect vectors. This method is successful in the laboratory and should be readily adaptable to field use.

CONCLUSION

The application of new methods of biotechnology to the epidemiology of leishmaniasis and malaria is in its initial phases. The new tools offer distinct advantages with regard to specificity, sensitivity, and ease of use for large numbers of samples when compared to existing methods and have enormous potential for their contribution to new knowledge on the transmission and prevalence of these diseases. Before these methods are generally accepted for use, they must be extensively tested under field situations and modified to provide the relevant information important for epidemiologic analysis.

REFERENCES

1. LAINSON, R. 1983. Trans. Roy. Soc. Trop. Med. Hyg. **77:** 569; LAINSON, R. & J. J. SHAW. 1978. Nature (London) **273:** 595.
2. CHANCE, M. L. & B. C. WALTON, Eds. 1982. Biochemical Characterization of Leishmania, UNDP/World Bank/WHO. Geneva.
3. SCORZA, J. U., *et al.* 1979. Trans. Roy. Soc. Trop. Med. Hyg. **73:** 293.
4. MOMEN, H. & G. GRIMALDI. 1984. Trans. Roy. Soc. Trop. Med. Hyg. **78:** 701.
5. MILES, M. A., *et al.* 1980. Trans. Roy. Soc. Trop. Med. Hyg. **74:** 243.
6. LAINSON, R. 1983. Proceedings of the 3rd Venezuelan Congress of Microbiology and Symposium on Leishmaniasis, Bouquisimeto, Venezuela.
7. LAINSON, R. & J. SHAW. 1979. *In* Biology of Kinetoplastidae 2. W. H. R. Lunden & Evans, Eds.: 1-116. Academic Press. London.
8. PETERS, W., *et al.* 1983. J. Roy. Soc. Med. **76:** 540.
9. MONTENEGRO, 1926. An. Fac. Med. Univ. São Paulo **1:** 323.
10. MARINKELLE, C. J., 1980. Bull. World Health Organization **58:** 807.
11. DEANE, L. M. & G. GRIMALDI. 1985. Leishmaniasis, Chang & Bray, Eds. Elsevier. Amsterdam.
12. WIRTH, D. F. & D. MCMAHON-PRATT. 1982. Proc. Natl. Acad. Sci. USA **79:** 6999.
13. BARKER, D. C. & J. BUTCHER. 1983. Trans. Roy. Soc. Trop. Med. Hyg. **77:** 285.
14. KENNEDY, W. P. K. 1984. Mol. Biochem. Parasitol. **12:** 313.
15. BARKER, D. C., *et al.* 1985. Parasitology **91:** S139.
16. LOPES, U. G. & D. F. WIRTH. Mol. Biochem. Parasitol. In press.
17. WIRTH, D. F. & W. O. ROGERS. 1985. Rapid Detection and Identification of Infectious Agents. D. Kingsbury & S. Falkow, Eds. Academic Press. New York.
18. ENGLUND, P. T. 1979. J. Biol. Chem. **254:** 4895.
19. KIDANE, G. Z., D. HUGHES & L. SIMPSON. 1984. Gene **27:** 265.
20. JACKSON, P. R., *et al.* 1984. Am. J. Trop. Med. Hyg. **33:** 808.

21. STEINERT, M. & S. VANASSEL. 1980. Plasmid **3:** 7.
22. LOPES, U. G., *et al.* 1984. Parasitology **70:** 89.
23. ROGERS, W. O., *et al.* In preparation.
24. ASTON, D. C. & A. P. THORNLEY. 1970. Trans. R. Soc. Trop. Med. Hyg. **75:** 537.
25. ARNOT, D. F. & D. C. BARKER. 1981. Mol. Biochem. Parasitol. **3:** 47.
26. BARKER, D. C. & D. F. ARNOT. 1980. Eur. J. Cell Biol. **22:** 124.
27. SPITHILL, T. W., *et al.* 1984. J. Cell Biochem. **24:** 103.
28. LAWRIE, J. M., *et al.* 1985. Am. J. Trop. Med. Hyg. **34:** 257.
29. FRASCH, A. C. C., *et al.* 1985. Mol. Biochem. Parasitol. **4:** 163.
30. ROGERS, W. O. & D. F. WIRTH. In press.
31. PERKINS, P. & D. F. WIRTH. Unpublished observations.
32. MCMAHON-PRATT, D. & J. DAVID. 1981. Nature (London) **291:** 581; JAFFE, C. C., *et al.* 1984. J. Immunol. **133:** 440; MCMAHON-PRATT, D., *et al.* 1985. J. Immunol. **134:** 1935; FRANKENBERG, *et al.* 1985. Am. J. Trop. Med. Hyg. **34:** 266.
33. MCMAHON-PRATT, D., *et al.* 1983. Am. J. Trop. Med. Hyg. **32:** 1268.
34. COHEN, S. & P. H. LAMBERT. 1982. *In* Immunology of Parasitic Infections. S. Cohen & K. S. Warren, Eds.: 422. Blackwell. Oxford, England.
35. 1984. World Health Stat. Q., **37:** 130-161.
36. 1979. WHO Technical Report Series, No. 640.
37. 1980. WHO Technical Report Series, No. 655.
38. 1984. WHO Technical Report Series, No. 711.
39. MCDONALD, G. 1952. Trop. Dis. Bull. **49:** 813; MCDONALD, G., 1955. Proc. Roy. Soc. Trop. Med. **48:** 295.
40. BRUCE-CHWATT, J. A. 1976. Trop. Geograph. Med. **28:** 1-8; NAJERA, J. A. 1974. Bull. WHO **50:** 449-457.
41. MOLINEAUX, L. & G. GRAMICCIA. 1980. The Garki Project: 109-115. World Health Organization. Geneva.
42. HALDANE, J. B. S. 1949. 8th International Congress Genet.: 267-273 (Hereditas Suppl. **35**); WALKER, J. H. & L. J. BRUCE-CHWATT. 1956. Trans. Roy. Soc. Trop. Med. Hyg. **50:** 511; FLEMING, A. F., 1979. Ann. Trop. Med. Parasitol. **73:** 161.
43. LUZZATO, L., *et al.* 1979. Bull. WHO **50:** 195; LUZZATO, L. 1979. Blood **54:** 961.
44. MILLER, L. H., *et al.* 1976. N. Engl. J. Med. **295:** 302; MILLER, L. H., *et al.* 1978. Am. J. Trop. Med. Hyg. **27:** 1069.
45. FLINT, J., *et al.* Nature (London) **321:** 744.
46. FRANZEN, *et al.* 1984. Lancet **1:** 525; POLLACK, Y., *et al.* 1985. Am. J. Trop. Med. Hyg. **34:** 663; MCLAUGHLIN, E., *et al.* 1985. Am. J. Trop. Med. Hyg. **34:** 837.
47. BARKER, R. B., *et al.* 1986. Science **231:** 1434.

Trypanothione Reductase

NICHOLAS J. MURGOLO, ANTHONY CERAMI, AND
GRAEME B. HENDERSON

Laboratory of Medical Biochemistry
The Rockefeller University
New York, New York 10021

There are 20,000 new cases of African trypanosomiases reported each year and some 50 million people residing on a third of the African continent are at risk of infection.[1] In the case or Chagas' disease, the South American form (*T. cruzi*), no completely suitable drugs exist for prevention or treatment.[2] Chagas' disease is prevalent throughout Central and South America, where 16 to 18 million people are infected and 200,000 new cases are reported each year. There is also a great need for the development of new drugs for the treatment of leishmaniasis. A recent World Health Organization report noted that a major goal for African trypanosomiases is the identification of enzyme targets for drug intervention.[3] Trypanothione reductase presents one such target.

The role of glutathione as an intracellular protectant is of chemotherapeutic interest since trypanosomes lack adequate defenses against H_2O_2 and H_2O_2-related free radicals such as OH··.[2,4,5,6] The parasite must exist in an environment of high oxygen tension, so defense mechanisms against oxidative stress are crucial to development. In mammals and most other aerobes, the tripeptide glutathione plays a key role in the antioxidant defense process.[7] Glutathione reductase [EC 1.6.4.2], a flavoprotein disulfide reductase, acts to maintain a ratio of free thiol (reduced form) to disulfide (oxidized form) of about 300:1. Reduced glutathione protects against oxidative stress both nonenzymatically by free-radical scavenging through thiol/disulfide exchange and enzymatically by peroxide metabolism (FIG. 1). Examination of the mechanism of glutathione metabolism in trypanosomatids led to the discovery that they do not enzymatically reduce glutathione; instead glutathione is reduced via a nonenzymatic thiol/disulfide exchange with a cyclic spermidine-containing glutathione-based peptide, trypanothione, that is apparently unique to Kinetoplastida[8–10] (FIG. 2). The development of a protocol for the synthesis of trypanothione and related compounds has led to an examination of the substrate specificity of trypanothione reductase.[11,12]

Purification and characterization of trypanothione reductase from a variety of sources showed that trypanothione reductase and human erythrocyte glutathione reductase, which have many of the same physical characteristics, possess mutual exclusivity for their respective substrates.[13–15]

The sensitivity of the trypanothione system to the ornithine decarboxylase inhibitor DFMO[16,17] and arsenicals,[18] coupled with the development of futile redox cyclers,[19] demonstrates that trypanothione reductase is a unique trypanosomal enzyme that may be exploited for the development of novel trypanocidal agents.

Trypanothione reductase represents an ideal enzyme for the application of computer-assisted conformational analysis, given its high degree of homology with human erythrocyte glutathione reductase. An understanding of the differences in the binding

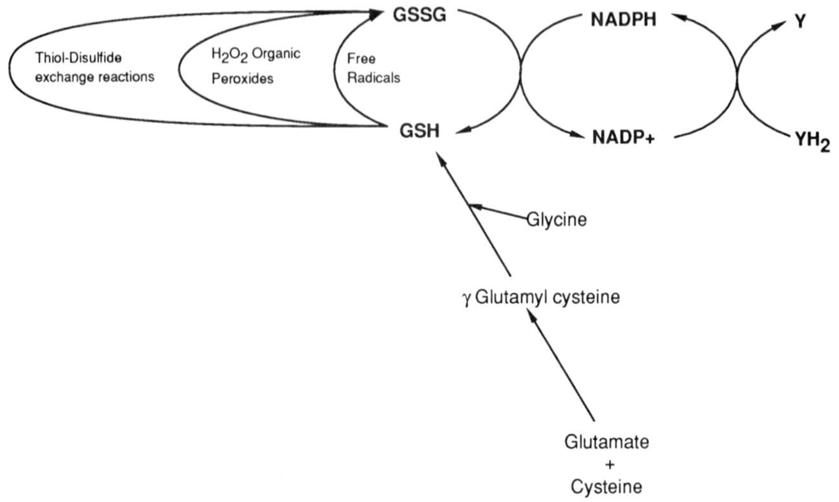

FIGURE 1. Protective functions of glutathione.

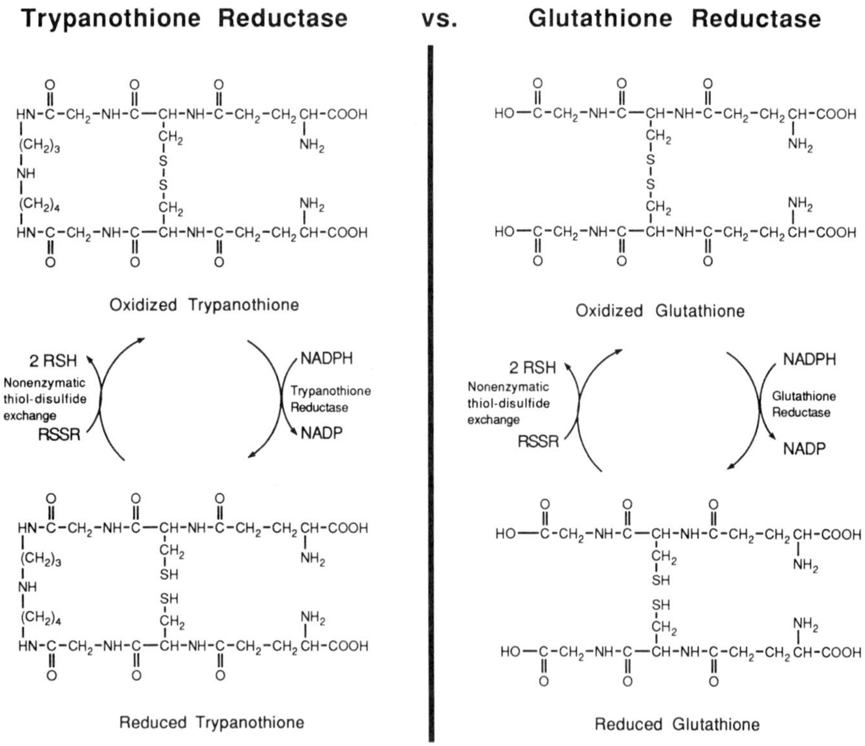

FIGURE 2. Comparison of reduction mechanisms.

of glutathione to glutathione reductase and trypanothione to trypanothione reductase will prove useful for the development of trypanocidal drugs. The technique of homology modeling, in which the backbone structure of a homologous enzyme of known crystal structure is used as a template for an enzyme of unknown conformation, has been outlined elsewhere.[20,21] The successful application of this technique to the modeling of the HIV protease from the crystal structure of Rous sarcoma virus protease, in which concurrent publication of the model structure and crystal structure of HIV protease by independent groups showed high similarity, demonstrates the validity of this technique.[22,23] The crystal structure of human erythrocyte glutathione reductase is known to a resolution of 1.54 angstroms[24] and its mechanism of catalysis has been studied.[25] From a sequence alignment of trypanothione reductase from *Trypanosoma congolenese* and human erythrocyte glutathione reductase[15] we have determined primary sequence identity of 41 percent. This rises to greater than 90% homology within 7 angstroms of the active site. A Chou and Fasman method of secondary structural analysis[26] shows greater than 60% overall homology, reflecting a higher degree of secondary structural homology than primary sequence would dictate (TABLE 1). Both enzymes are dimeric, have a monomer mass of about 50 kDa, possess an FAD cofactor,

TABLE 1. Relative Amounts of Secondary Structural Elements in Homology of Human Erythrocyte Glutathione Reductase (GR) and *Trypanosoma congolense* Trypanothione Reductase (TR)

Species	Percent α	Percent β	Percent Turn	Percent Coil
Overall GR	63.39	21.34	14.84	0.42
Overall TR	63.82	24.80	11.38	0.00
Δ Overall	0.43	3.46	3.47	0.42
Overlapping regions GR	65.76	21.77	12.47	0.00
Overlapping regions TR	63.04	26.30	10.66	0.00
Δ Overlapping regions	2.72	4.53	1.81	0.00

use NADPH as a pyridine nucleotide, and have comparable specific activity, K_m, and catalytic rates, as well as similar spectrophotometric properties. Previously the homology modeling technique has been applied to construct a model of *Escherichia coli* lipoamide dehydrogenase [EC 1.8.1.4] from glutathione reductase where primary sequence identity is 28 percent.[27] In the model of lipoamide dehydrogenase, as in our model of trypanothione reductase, the highest degree of primary sequence identity is within the active-site region.

We have constructed a homologous model for *Trypanosoma congolense* trypanothione reductase by using the crystal structure of human erythrocyte glutathione reductase as a template (FIG. 3). We have ignored insertions and deletions, which account for less than 10% of the overall structure and exist mainly in external loops. We have maintained the backbone geometry and have varied the side-chain torsional angles, mutating the necessary residues and preserving as many side-chain dihedral angles as possible (FIG. 4). Where necessary, side chains were extended using the most probable side-chain torsional angle noted in the 25 best-resolution crystal structures in the April 1987 Brookhaven protein data bank,[28] excluding glutathione reductase (FIG. 4). The construction of the model was performed on a μVax 3500 with the FORTRAN program IMPACT[29] and structures generated were analyzed on a

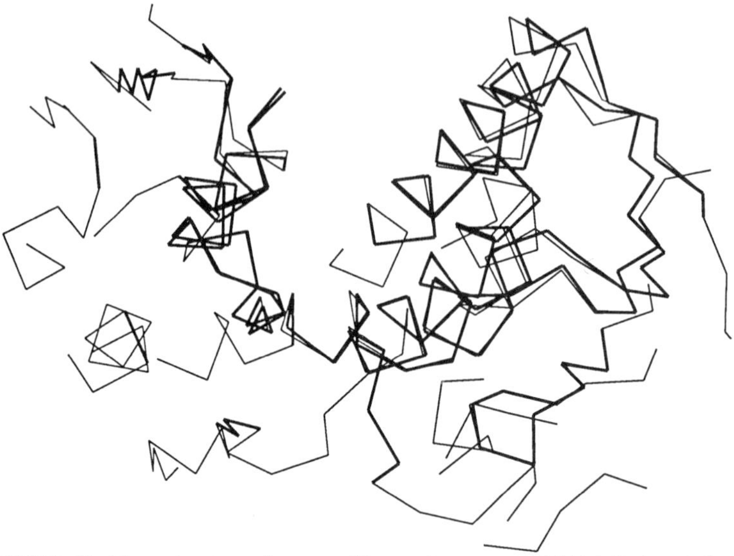

FIGURE 3. Backbone structure of trypanothione reductase model (*thick line*) and glutathione reductase crystal structure (*thin line*).

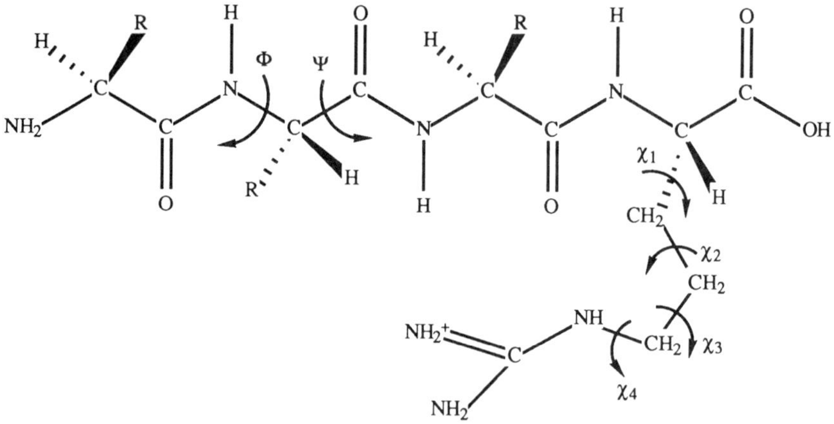

FIGURE 4. Homology model for *Trypanosoma congolense* trypanothione reductase. Backbone geometry was preserved by maintaining Φ,Ψ. Side-chain geometry was preserved as much as possible by maintaining as many side-chain dihedral angles (χ_is) as possible, supplementing with standard geometries.

silicon graphics IRIS 3130 or either an Evans and Sutherland PS 340 or 390 using the commercially available molecular graphics packages INSIGHT, HYDRA, and QUANTA. Obvious large-energy van der Waals contacts resulting from the side-chain mutations were adjusted manually. Side-chain adjustment was necessary only at position 44, which is mutated to a lysine residue and resides in an external beta turn. It was not possible to externalize the side chain of this residue without adjustment of adjacent backbone dihedral angles. We restricted the model to within 21 angstroms of the center of the active site because of the intractability of conformational analysis algorithms to handle such a large structure with current generation supercomputers and because our final intention is the application of molecular dynamics. We wish to apply molecular dynamics to the model to determine those residues in the region of the active site responsible for the substrate specificity in both glutathione reductase and trypanothione reductase.

The resulting homology model of trypanothione reductase, as well as the crystal structure of glutathione reductase, were subject to energy minimization by the molecular mechanics method through use of the X-PLOR version of the CHARMM program[30] on either the IRIS 3130 or a Stellar GS/1000 graphics supercomputer. Minimization of the model structure of trypanothione reductase required the use of constrained minimization, in which residues that were not mutated were allowed to move only at higher cost than those that were mutated. The constrained energy minimization was followed by free minimization in which all atoms were allowed to move. Glutathione was included in the glutathione reductase minimization, and the coordinates were kindly provided by Dr. Georg Schulz. These coordinates are not of the same resolution as the protein crystal structure, and they required constrained minimization. A model of trypanothione was constructed from the glutathione coordinates determined. The use of the molecular mechanics method for minimization required the development of equilibrium geometries and atomic charges for FAD and the spermidine moiety of trypanothione. STO-3G quantum mechanical calculations were performed on the isoalloxazine ring system and spermidine using gaussian 86 on a Cray X-MP 48 supercomputer. The resulting Mulliken populations were used to develop charges. The resulting FAD charges were comparable to those in the literature,[31-33] but this model has the advantage of electric neutrality of the isoalloxazine moiety. The geometry of the isoalloxazine ring system in the crystal structure of glutathione reductase was noted to be in good agreement with the crystal structure of 10-methyliso-alloxazine.[34] Only the isoalloxazine portion of the flavin cofactor was included in these calculations since the adenine moiety and the remainder of the FAD molecule were not within the 21-angstrom sphere. The polar hydrogen force field of CHARMM version 19 was employed, in which hydrogen atoms are considered explicitly only for polar atoms and are included as extended atoms otherwise. A distance-dependent coulombic term was employed, with a dielectric constant of 1. Typical minimizations were 500 steps and required 1 hour of CPU time on the Stellar GS/1000. Resulting structures were examined graphically throughout the minimization calculations. A solvent-accessible surface calculation[35] was performed on the resulting enzyme model structure, and the surface area buried on dimerization was found to be nearly identical, indicating that the active site of trypanothione reductase is not larger than that of glutathione reductase (TABLE 2).

From the determined structures it is apparent that while a great degree of homology is observed in the active-site region of trypanothione reductase, a small region of the active site in one external corner is changed. It is interesting that this region contains three arginine residues in human erythrocyte glutathione reductase (at positions 37, 38, and 347). These arginine residues accommodate the free glycine carboxyls of the

TABLE 2. Solvent-Accesible Surface Area in Human Erythrocyte Glutathione Reductase (GR) vs. *Trypanosoma congolense* Trypanothione Reductase (TR)

Species	Surface Area (Å^2)
GR monomer	18,535.684
GR dimer	31,079.964
TR monomer	19,783.076
TR dimer	33,541.045
Area buried on dimerization:	
(area monomer-0.5 area dimer)	
Area buried GR	2,995.702
Area buried TR	3,012.552

glutathione substrate and are absent in the trypanosomal enzyme. In place of these residues, geometrically, are three acidic residues (at positions 18, 112 and 116) that can accommodate a nitrogen of the spermidine which is amide-bound to the glutathione tripeptide at the glycine carboxyls. Two of these acidic residues (112 and 116) may represent a recognitive site for the spermidine portion of trypanothione. All three of these acidic residues are absent in the human enzyme.

While minimization has proven helpful, it is evident that the exact nature of these interactions will only be understood through use of molecular dynamics. We are currently addressing the importance of these residues and the substrate specificities by molecular dynamics simulations[36,37] in a manner similar to that applied to the apoazurin of *Alcaligenes denitrificans.*[38] We are also undertaking site-directed mutagenesis experiments on the glutathione reductase of *Escherichia coli,* which has been recently cloned and expressed.[39] These experiments provide insight as to the residues important to the substrate specificity of the flavoprotein disulfide reductases.

ACKNOWLEDGMENTS

We wish to acknowledge Dr. Ronald M. Levy, Donna Bassolino, and Dorothea Kominos of the Center of Computational Chemistry at Rutgers University for their help in the preparation of the original homology model; Dr. John Kuriyan and Dr. Klara Osapay of the Laboratory of Biochemistry and Bioorganic Chemistry of the Rockefeller University for their help in the quantum mechanical and molecular mechanics calculations; and Dr. Georg Schulz of the University of Freiburg for providing glutathione coordinates in advance of their submission to the Brookhaven data bank.

REFERENCES

1. WORLD HEALTH ORGANIZATION. 1987. Tropical Disease Research: A Global Partnership. Eighth Programme Report of the United Nations Development Programme(UNDP)/ World Bank/World Health Organization (WHO) Special Programme for Research and Training in Tropical Disease (TDR). WHO. Geneva.

2. DOCAMPO, R. & S. N. J. MORENO. 1984. Free radical metabolites in the mode of action of chemotherapeutic agents and phagocytic cells on *Trypanosoma cruzi*. Rev. Inf. Dis. **6:** 223-228.
3. GODAL, T. 1989. Report of the Eleventh Meeting of the Scientific and Technical Advisory Committee of the UNDP/World Bank/WHO TDR. WHO. Geneva.
4. BOVERIS, A., H. SIES, E. E. MARTINO, R. DOCAMPO, J. F. TURRENS & A. O. M. STOPPANI. 1980. Deficient metabolic utilization of hydrogen peroxide in *Trypanosoma cruzi*. Biochem. J. **188:** 643-648.
5. MESCHNICK, S. R., K. P. CHANG & A. CERAMI. 1977. Heme lysis of the bloodstream forms of *Trypanosoma brucei*. Biochem. Pharmacol. **26:** 1923.
6. MESCHNICK, S. R., S. H. BLOBSTEIN, R. W. GRADY & A. CERAMI. 1978. An Approach to the Development of New Drugs for African Trypanosomiases. J. Exp. Med. **148:** 569-579.
7. MEISTER, A. & M. E. ANDERSON. 1983. Annu. Rev. Biochem. **52:** 711-760.
8. FAIRLAMB, A. H. & A. CERAMI. 1985. Identification of a novel, thiol-containing co-factor essential for glutathione reductase enzyme activity in trypanosomatids. Mol. Biochem. Parasitol. **14:** 187-198.
9. FAIRLAMB, A. H., G. B. HENDERSON & A. CERAMI. 1986. The biosynthesis of trypanothione and N-glutathionyl spermidine in *Crithidia fasiculata*. 1986. Mol. Biochem. Parasitol. **21:** 245-257.
10. FAIRLAMB, A. H., P. BLACKBURN, P. ULRICH, B. T. CHART & A. CERAMI. 1985. Trypanothione: A novel bis-(glutathionyl)spermidine cofactor for glutathione reductase in trypanosomatids. Science **227:** 1486-1487.
11. HENDERSON, G. B., P. ULRICH, A. H. FAIRLAMB & A. CERAMI. 1986. Synthesis of the trypanosomatid metabolites trypanothione, and N^1-mono- and N^8-mono-glutathionylspermidine. J. Chem. Soc., Chem. Commun.: 593-594.
12. HENDERSON, G. B., A. H. FAIRLAMB, P. ULRICH & A. CERAMI. 1987. Substrate specificity of the flavoprotein trypanothione disulfide reductase from *Crithidia fasiculata*. Biochemistry **26:** 3023-3027.
13. SHAMES, S. L., A. H. FAIRLAMB, A. CERAMI & C. T. WALSH. 1986. Purification and characterization of trypanothione reductase from *Crithidia fasiculata*, a newly discovered member of the family of disulfide-containing flavoprotein reductases. Biochemistry **25:** 3519-3526.
14. KRAUTH-SIEGEL, R. L., B. ENDERS, G. B. HENDERSON, A. H. FAIRLAMB & R. H. SCHIRMER. 1987. Trypanothione reductase from *Trypanosoma cruzi*: Purification and characterization of the crystalline enzyme. Eur. J. Biochem. **164:** 123-128.
15. SHAMES, S. L., B. KIMMEL, O. P. PEOPLES, N. AGABIAN & C. T. WALSH. 1988. Trypanothione reductase of *Trypanosoma congolense:* Gene isolation, primary sequence determination and comparison to glutathione reductase. Biochemistry **27:** 5014-5019.
16. BELLOFATTO, V., A. H. FAIRLAMB, G. B. HENDERSON, C. J. BACCHI & G. A. M. CROSS. 1987. Biochemical changes associated with α-difluoromethylornithine uptake and resistance in *Trypanosoma brucei*. Mol. Biochem. Parasitol. **25:** 227-238.
17. FAIRLAMB, A. H., G. B. HENDERSON, C. J. BACCHI & A. CERAMI. 1987. *In vivo* effects of difuoromethylornithine on trypanothione and polyamine levels in bloodstream forms of *Trypanosoma brucei*. Mol. Biochem. Parasitol. **24:** 185-191.
18. FAIRLAMB, A. H., G. B. HENDERSON & A. CERAMI. 1989. Trypanothione is the primary target for arsenical drugs against African trypanosomes. Proc. Natl. Acad. Sci. USA **86:** 2607-2611.
19. HENDERSON, G. B., P. ULRICH, A. H. FAIRLAMB, I. ROSENBERG, M. PEREIRA, M. SELA & A. CERAMI. 1988. "Subversive" substrates for the enzyme trypanothione disulfide reductase: Alternative approach to chemotherapy of Chagas' disease. Proc. Natl. Acad. Sci. USA **85:** 701-729.
20. SEVILLE, M., M. G. VINCENT & K. HAHN. 1988. Modeling the three-dimensional structures of bacterial aminotransferases. Biochemistry **27:** 8344-8349.
21. MURPHY, M. E. P., J. MOULT, R. C. BLEACKLEY, H. GERSHENFIELD, I. L. WEISSMAN & M. N. G. JAMES. 1988. Comparative molecular model building of two serine proteinases from cytotoxic T lymphocytes. Proteins **4:** 190-204.

22. WEBER, I. T., M. MILLER, M. JASKOLSKI, J. LEIS, A. M. SKALKA & A. WLODAWER. 1989. Molecular modeling on the HIV-1 protease and its substrate binding site. Science **243:** 928-931.
23. NAVIA, M. A., P. M. D. FITZGERALD, B. M. MCKEEVER, C. T. LEU, J. C. HEIMBACH, W. K. HERBER, I. S. SIGAL, P. L. DRAKE & J. P. SPRINGER. 1989. Three-dimensional structure of aspartyl protease from human immunodeficiency virus HIV-1. Nature **337:** 615-620.
24. KARPLUS, P. A. & G. E. SCHULZ. 1987. Refined structure of glutathione reductase at 1.54 angstroms resolution. J. Mol. Biol. **195:** 701-729.
25. PAI, E. & G. E. SCHULZ. 1983. The catalytic mechanism of glutathione reductase as derived from X-ray diffraction intermediates. J. Biol. Chem. **258:** 1752-1757.
26. CHOU, P. Y. & G. D. FASMAN. 1974. Conformational parameters for amino acids in helical, beta-sheet, and random coil regions calculated from proteins. Biochemistry **13:** 211-222.
27. RICE, D. W., G. E. SCHULZ & J. R. GUEST. 1984. Structural relationship between glutathione reductase and lipoamide dehydrogenase. J. Mol. Biol. **174:** 483-496.
28. BERNSTEIN, F. C., T. F. KOETZLE, G. J. B. WILLIAMS, E. F. MEYER, M. D. BRICE, J. R. RODGERS, O. KENNARD, T. SHIMANOUCHI & M. TASUMI. 1977. J. Mol. Biol. **112:** 535-542.
29. BASSOLINO, D. A., F. HIRATA, D. KITCHEN, D. KOMINOS, A. PARDI & R. M. LEVY. 1988. Determination of protein structures in solution using NMR data and IMPACT. Int. J. Supercomp. Appl. **12:** 41-61.
30. BROOKS, B. R., R. E. BRUCCOLERI, B. D. OLAFSON, D. J. STATES, S. SWAMINATHAN & M. KARPLUS. 1983. CHARMM: A program for macromolecular energy, minimization, and dynamics calculations. J. Comp. Chem. **4:** 187-217.
31. PLATENKAMP, R. J., M. H. PALMER & A. J. W. G. VISSER. 1987. *Ab initio* molecular orbital studies of closed shell flavins. Eur. Biophys. J. **14:** 393-402.
32. NISHIMOTO, K., H. FUKUNAGA & K. YAGI. 1986. Studies in a model system on the effect of hydrogen bonding at hetero atoms of oxidized flavin on its electron acceptability. J. Biochem. **100:** 1647-1653.
33. NISHIMOTO, K., E. KAI & K. YAGI. 1984. Hydrogen bonding of flavoprotein. II. Effect of hydrogen bonding at hetero atoms of reduced flavin on its activity. Biochim. Biophys. Acta **802:** 321-325.
34. WANG, M. & C. J. FRITCHIE, JR. 1973. Geometry of the unperturbed flavin nucleus. The crystal structure of 10-methylisoalloxazine. Acta Crystallogr. **B29:** 2040-2045.
35. LEE, B. & F. M. RICHARDS. 1971. The interpretation of protein structures: Estimation of static accessibility. J. Mol. Biol. **55:** 379-400.
36. MURGOLO, N. J., G. B. HENDERSON, J. KURIYAN, K. OSAPAY & A. CERAMI. 1989. Modeling of the active site and substrate specificity of trypanothione reductase by homology and molecular dynamics. Abs. Pap. ACS. In press.
37. MURGOLO, N. J., A. CERAMI & G. B. HENDERSON. 1989. Trypanothione. *In* Parasites: Molecular Biology, Drug and Vaccine Design. UCLA Symposia on Molecular and Cellular Biology (New Series, Vol. 131). Alan R. Liss. New York. In press.
38. CHEN, L. X. Q., R. A. ENGH, A. T. BRUNGER, D. T. NGUYEN, M. KARPLUS & G. R. FLEMING. 1988. Dynamics simulation studies of apoazurin of *Alcaligenes denitrificans.* Biochemistry **27:** 6908-6921.
39. GREER, S. & R. N. PERHAM. 1986. Glutathione reductase from *Escherichia coli:* Cloning and sequence analysis of the gene and relationship to other flavoprotein disulfide oxidoreductases. Biochemistry **25:** 2736-2742.

Recent Studies on Thymidylate Synthase

KATHRYN M. IVANETICH AND DANIEL V. SANTI

Departments of Biochemistry and Pharmaceutical Chemistry, and the Biomolecular Resource Center
University of California Medical School
San Francisco, California 94143-0448

TS AND THE dTMP CYCLE

Thymidylate synthase (TS) catalyzes the conversion of dUMP and 5,10-methylenetetrahydrofolate (CH_2-H_4folate) to dTMP and 7,8-dihydrofolate (H_2folate), and is a component of the "dTMP synthesis cycle" (FIG. 1). This cycle refers to the three sequential reactions catalyzed by TS, dihydrofolate reductase (DHFR), and serine transhydroxymethylase (STH) that are required for *de novo* synthesis of dTMP.[1,2] In this cycle, H_4folate serves as a carrier of the one-carbon unit and undergoes obligatory oxidation and reduction during sequential reactions catalyzed by TS and DHFR, respectively. Blockade of this cycle results in depletion of dTMP needed for DNA synthesis and resultant "thymineless death" of cells. Not surprisingly TS and DHFR have been popular targets for chemotherapeutic agents. A number of potent inhibitors of TS are known, the best of which are 5-FdUMP and the 5,8-dideazafolate analog CB3717. Any onc of several DHFR inhibitors (methotrexate, trimethoprim, or pyrimethamine) prevents regeneration of H_4folate from the H_2folate formed with dTMP; when H_4folate pools are depleted, dTMP synthesis ceases and cytotoxicity ensues.

TS Catalysis

The catalytic mechanism of TS (FIG. 2) is well understood.[2] It involves the initial formation of a covalent bond between the 6-position of dUMP and the thiol group of a completely conserved Cys residue of TS. Formation of this covalent adduct serves to activate the 5-position of dUMP for condensation with the one-carbon unit of the cofactor; this gives a covalent ternary complex in which the enzyme is linked to the 6-position of dUMP, and the cofactor to the 5-position. Subsequent proton abstraction, internal redox reaction, and β-elimination provide the methylated pyrimidine nucleotide (dTMP), oxidized cofactor, and catalytically active enzyme. Similar covalent bonds are formed with inhibitors such as FdUMP,[3] resulting in a stable covalent adduct composed of TS, FdUMP and the cofactor that represents an analogue of a steady-state intermediate in the normal reaction. With other 5-substituted dUMPs, covalent addition can result in activation of a latently reactive group at C-5 that can

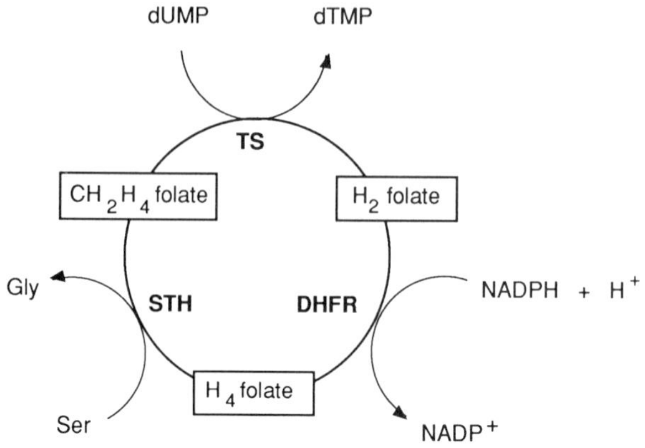

FIGURE 1. TMP cycle showing the metabolic relationships of the enzymes TS, DHFR, and STH.

subsequently inactivate the enzyme. The strategies for development of such "mechanism-based inhibitors" are quite mature, and have been a topic of interest in this laboratory.[2]

TS Structure

TS and DHFR exist as distinct and readily separable proteins in bacteriophage, bacteria, mammalian viruses, yeast, and vertebrates.[1,2] The TS found in the above

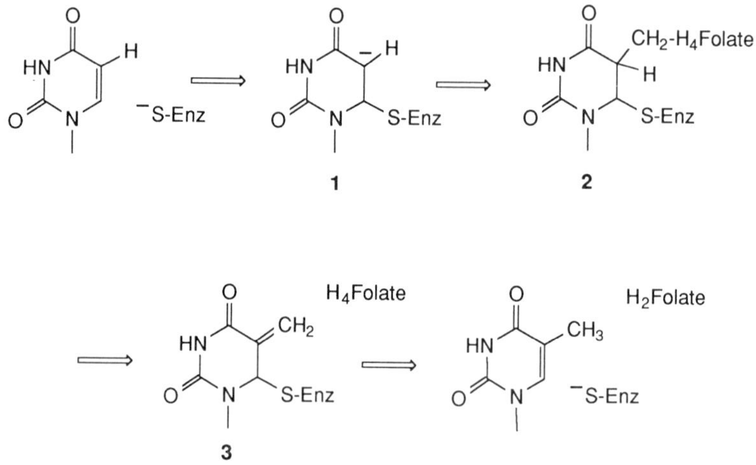

FIGURE 2. The catalytic mechanism of TS showing the formation of covalent steady-state intermediates.

sources is a highly homologous dimer of identical subunits of about 35 kDa; usually, DHFR is a monomer of about 20 kDa.

The TS and DHFR in protozoa exist as a bifunctional protein.[4–6] Depending on species, the apparent sizes usually range from 110 to 140 kDa, with subunit sizes of 55 to 70 kDa. The sequences of the bifunctional TS-DHFR from the protozoans *Leishmania major, Crithidia fasciculata,* and *Plasmodium falciparum* have been predicted from the DNA sequence,[7–10] and the *Leishmania* enzyme has been purified to homogeneity and characterized.[11] Each TS-DHFR subunit consists of two domains, with DHFR at the amino terminus and TS at the carboxy terminus, separated by a junction peptide. The domains are related in size and structure to their monofunctional counterparts in other organisms. It is interesting that in the native protein structural and functional communications exist among domains. We have suggested that the junction peptide may vary in size in certain protozoa.[5]

Primary sequences of TS from some seventeen different sources have revealed that TS is one of the most conserved enzymes (FIG. 3); it has a unit evolutionary period of greater than 22 million years.[12]

In collaboration with Dr. R. Stroud, we have recently reported the X-ray structure of the enzyme from *L. casei,*[12] and now have structures of TS bound to substrates/inhibitors (unpublished data). Also, structures of the *E. coli* and T4 phage TS have been elaborated, and discovery of the structure of the human TS is in progress. Details of the structure of *L. casei* TS are given by Hardy *et al.*,[12] and only a cursory description of features relevant to ligand binding and selectivity is presented here.

L. casei TS crystallizes as a dimer of identical subunits having a two-fold axis of symmetry. All important secondary structural elements of TS are within highly conserved regions; thus, the core structure of *L. casei* TS will undoubtedly be similar to other TSs. The dimer interface is composed of an unusual 6-stranded β-sheet from both monomers. Each monomer comprises a small and large domain, separated by a cleft. The larger domain contains (*a*) the β-strands of the dimer interface; (*b*) a six-turn unusually hydrophobic α-helix, around which the large domain folds; and (*c*) a shallow cavity which contains the active site. The small domain contains the *L. casei* insert (residues 90-139), which is found in no other species.

An interesting, and possibly unique, feature of TS revealed by the crystal structure, is that several side-chain residues of one monomer are shared by the other. This explains why catalytically active monomers of TS have not yet been isolated. Moreover, amino acid residues of one subunit contribute essential components of the active site of the other. For example, Arg 178 and Arg 179 of one monomer provides binding groups for phosphate ion in the active site of the other monomer. The cavity defined as the active site is lined by about 25 residues; 16 of these are conserved among TS of all species, and 8 of these have functional side-chain groups which could play roles in catalysis or binding. Of importance is that they are also nucleophilic targets for potential covalent-bond-forming inhibitors. We anticipate that substrate analogs containing reactive functional groups (potential inhibitors) could be docked into the active site with the reactive moiety precisely juxtaposed to one or more of these groups for covalent bond formation.

HETEROLOGOUS EXPRESSION

Because of source limitations, most of the previous biochemical work on TS has been performed with the enzyme obtained from overproducing strains of methotrexate-

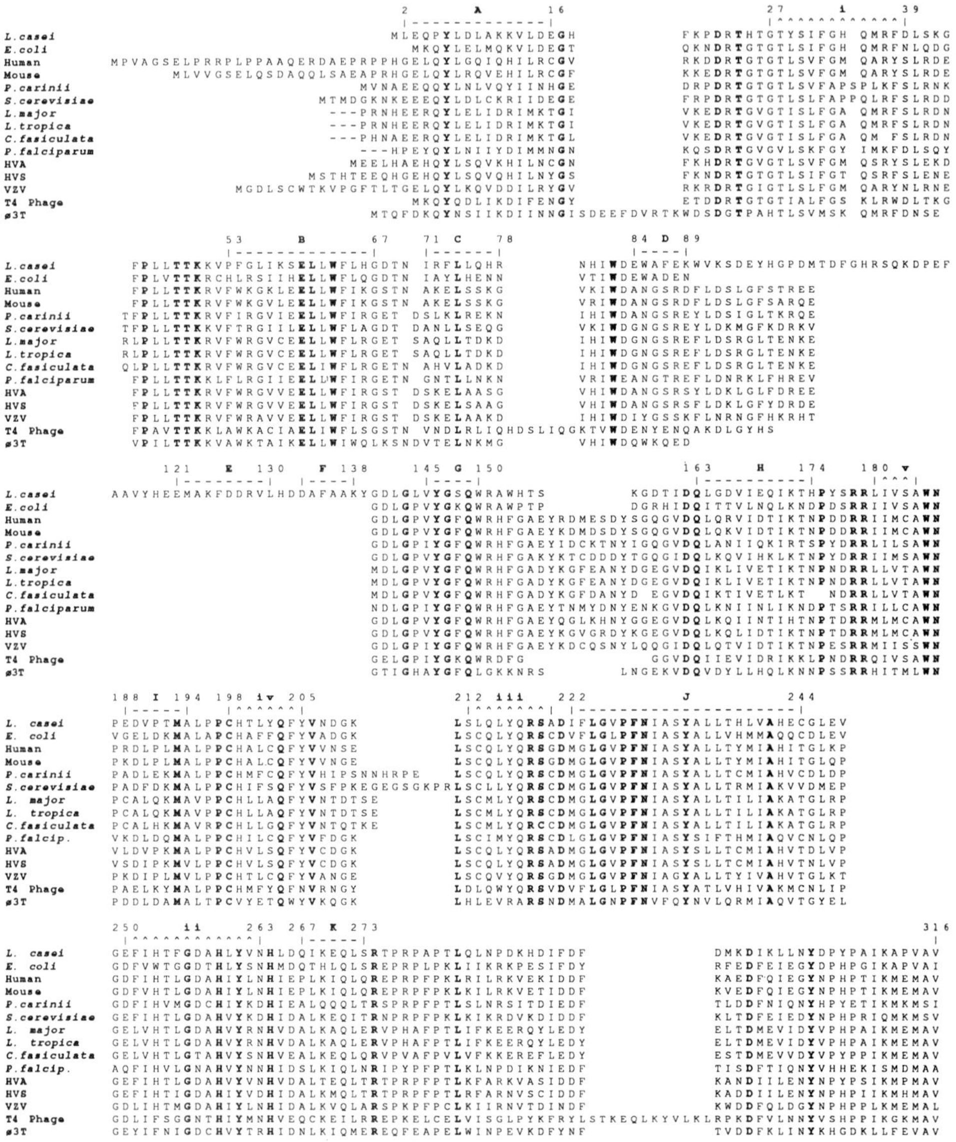

FIGURE 3. Amino acid sequences of TS from different species. The conserved residues are shown in **boldface.**

resistant *L. casei,* in which the enzyme represents about 2% of the total soluble protein.[13,14] Studies of TS structure, function and inhibition are now taking directions that require very large amounts (reagent quantities) of enzyme. In addition, it is an appropriate time to undertake studies of the mutagenesis of TS to uncover more subtle aspects of structure and function. To these ends, several groups have been engaged in cloning the TS gene from various sources, and several high-expression systems have been developed.

We have undertaken a program to express TS from various sources in heterologous systems to provide the large amounts of enzyme necessary for studies in the molecular design of inhibitors. Recently, we reported[15] the expression of *L. casei* TS in *E. coli* in a system where 20% of the total protein is *L. casei* TS. This is some 10-fold higher expression than even the methotrexate-resistant strain of *L. casei,* and provides an unlimited source of this protein. Here, we describe studies that have led to the heterologous expression of TS from the organisms *Leishmania major* and *Pneumocystis carinii;* we also describe the expression of human TS in *E. coli.* With large amounts of the enzymes from both pathogens and host, we can hope to rationally approach the design of new chemotherapeutic agents.

Leishmania *Bifunctional TS-DHFR*

The TS-DHFR from *Leishmania major* is a 120 kDa protein, which consists of two identical subunits.[4,11] Each subunit consists of two domains, with DHFR at the amino terminus and TS at the carboxy terminus, separated by a junction peptide. The complete sequence of the protein is known from DNA sequencing.[7,8] TS-DHFR represents ~ 0.1% of total soluble protein in wild-type *Leishmania* promastigotes. Previously, the major sources of this protein have been antifolate-resistant strains of *L. major,* which produce about 10-fold more TS-DHFR than do wild-type organisms.[4,16] There were two compelling reasons for us to develop expression systems for the *Leishmania* TS-DHFR. First, the low amounts of protein obtainable from protozoan sources place limitations on the type and scope of studies we can consider performing. Second, since transformation systems in *Leishmania* are not available, heterologous expression systems are necessary for any anticipated mutagenesis studies.

The bifunctional TS-DHFR of *Leishmania major* has been cloned and expressed in *E. coli* and *S. cerevisiae.*[17] The strategy involved placing the entire 1560-bp coding sequence, obtained from gDNA, into a parent cloning plasmid which was designed to permit facile introduction of unique restriction sites at the 5′- and 3′-ends. In this manner, the entire coding sequence could be easily subcloned into a variety of expression vectors. High levels of TS-DHFR gene expression were driven by *tac,* pL and T7 RNA *pol* promoters in *E. coli,* and the GAPDH-ADH-2 promoter in *S. cerevisiae* (TABLE 1). In *E. coli,* TS-DHFR accumulated to levels amounting to 7 to 40% of the total cellular protein, but most was present as inactive inclusion bodies. Nevertheless, substantial amounts were soluble in cytoplasmic extracts; up to 2% of the soluble protein was catalytically active TS-DHFR. In the yeast systems, essentially all of the bifunctional protein was soluble and catalytically active, and crude extracts contained about 100-fold more enzyme than did extracts from wild-type *L. major.* The expressed TS-DHFRs from yeast and *E. coli* were purified to homogeneity by methotrexate-Sepharose affinity chromatography. About 10 mg of homogeneous, catalytically active protein was obtained from a 1-liter culture of yeast, whereas 2 mg

TABLE 1. Expression of *Leishmania* TS-DHRF in *E. coli,* Yeast and *Leishmania*[a]

Organism	Plasmid	Vector	Promoter (induction)	% of Total Protein	Specific Activity (U/mg) DHFR	TS
E. coli						
JM105	pE1	pKK223.3	*tac*(IPTG)	7	322	48
X2913(-TS)	pE1	pKK223.3	*tac*(none)	—	195	22
BL21	pE2	pAR3038	T7*pol*(IPTG)	40	247	47
N5151	pE3b	pMG27N-S	pL (heat)	8	136	14
S. cerevisiae						
AB103.1	pE4a	PC1/1	GAPDH-ADH2	7	1885	175
Leishmania						
Wild-type	—	—	—	0.1	20	3

[a] Data from Grumont *et al.*[17]

was obtained from 1 liter of *E. coli* culture. A 200-liter fermentation of the yeast expression system yielded a crude extract containing more than 4 grams of TS-DHFR. The TS-DHFR expressed in yeast was blocked at the N-terminus, as is the enzyme from *Leishmania;* in *E. coli,* the protein was not blocked and showed an N-terminal serine, which corresponds to amino acid 2 of the coding sequence. The enzyme from yeast showed catalytic properties identical to those of the enzyme obtained from *Leishmania.*

Pneumocystis carinii

Pneumocystis carinii, an organism originally thought to be a protozoan but recently reclassified as a fungus,[18] causes disease only in the immunocompromised host.[19] In developed nations, *P. carinii* pneumonia (PCP) is the most common lethal infection of patients with acquired immunodeficiency syndrome (AIDS). Although PCP usually responds to treatment with trimethoprim-sulfamethoxazole or pentamidine, these drugs are often inadequate or cause allergic and toxic side effects when used in AIDS patients. There is a need for new effective therapies for the treatment of PCP.

The development of new therapeutic agents for PCP has been hampered by the lack of an adequate *in vitro* culture system of *P. carinii.* In the absence of continuous *in vitro* cultures there is currently no source of *P. carinii* that can provide sufficient material for biochemical studies. In fact, no protein from this organism has yet been purified. However, DNA libraries have recently been prepared from rat *P. carinii,*[18] allowing the cloning and heterologous expression of genes encoding proteins that are potential targets for drug development. Since TS is the sole *de novo* source of dTMP synthesis, and thymine depletion is cytotoxic to these organisms, TS is an attractive target for the development of chemotherapeutic agents. We have recently isolated the *P. carinii* TS gene and expressed it in *E. coli.*[20]

We tried to isolate the TS gene from *P. carinii* by screening the genomic library with a variety of heterologous hybridization probes, but the attempt failed, presumably because of the unusually high A + T content of *P. carinii.* To obtain a suitable hybridization probe, we used degenerate oligonucleotides as PCR primers to amplify a fragment of the TS gene from *P. carinii* genomic DNA. The strategy was to choose two highly conserved regions of eukaryotic TS, and to prepare a mixture of synthetic oligonucleotide primers that contains all possible sequences of these regions. If the choice of amino acids used to design the degenerate primers was correct, then at least one member of each mixture should anneal to the target TS sequence and serve as a primer in the PCR. Using this approach, we were able to successfully amplify a 403-bp sequence of *P. carinii* TS. The amino acid sequence deduced from this DNA sequence showed significant similarity to residues 145 to 231 of the *L. casei* TS.

Using the PCR product as a hybridization probe, we were able to isolate the *P. carinii* gene from cDNA and gDNA libraries. The cDNA sequence contained a single open reading frame which translated to a protein of 297 amino acids with an M_r of 34,269 Da. The deduced amino acid sequence shows conservation of all of the amino acid residues which are invariant in known TSs (FIG. 3). Overall amino acid identities range from 40% with T4 phage TS, to 60% with human TS, to 65% with the *S. cerevisiae* sequence.

Plasmids were constructed for the expression of *P. carinii* TS in *E. coli.* These contained the TS gene under control of the *lac* or *tac* promoters. These plasmids complemented Thy- *E. coli,* and soluble extracts from cells harboring the plasmids showed TS activity which accounted for about 500 pmol of TS per mg protein, or about 2% of the soluble protein.

As previously described, in protozoa the TS and DHFR exist as a bifunctional protein on the same polypeptide chain, whereas in other organisms the enzymes are clearly distinct and monofunctional. Nucleotide sequence analysis of the flanking sequences of *P. carinii* TS did not reveal proximal open reading frames that could encode DHFR. Further, large DNA electrophoresis demonstrated that TS and DHFR reside on different *P. carinii* chromosomes. Thus, our results support the contention that *P. carinii* is not a protozoan.

P. carinii TS contains all of the conserved amino acid residues contributing to important structural elements identified in the X-ray structure of *L. casei* TS and is therefore likely to have a similar core three-dimensional structure.[12] The amino acid sequence (FIG. 3) shows both of the invariant eukaryote-specific insertions; a 12-amino acid loop at position 90 (between α-D and E helices) and the 8-amino acid loop following residue 157 (between α-G and H helices) of the *L casei* TS. The single amino acid insertion after residue 34 (Ser) has thus far been observed only in the other fungal TS characterized (Pro in *S. cerevisiae*). This insertion is found in the first β-strand of TS, which forms an important interface for subunit contact. Another single amino acid insertion following residue 43 is also present in *S. cerevisiae* and the kinetoplast TSs. The insertion is located on a loop that would connect the first β-strand into the α-helix B. A six-amino acid insertion following residue 210 forms part of an exposed surface loop between β-strands iii and iv. Insertions at this position of TS have thus far only been seen as a nine-amino acid insertion in *S. cerevisiae* TS and a two-amino acid insertion in kinetoplast TSs. Additional differences between human and *P. carinii* TS in nonconserved residues contributing to the active site may provide the basis for molecular design of selective inhibitors of *P. carinii* TS.

Human TS

Although TS has been isolated from human cells,[21,22] the small amounts obtainable are insufficient for intensive investigation. Intensive studies of this enzyme require the amounts only available from recombinant DNA technology. A TS cDNA clone from human fibroblasts has been isolated and expressed in small amounts in a mouse cell line.[23] Nevertheless, this approach has not provided a quantity of human TS that would permit detailed biophysical studies. This laboratory has described the isolation of a full-length cDNA clone of human TS and its expression in *E. coli.*[24] The system provides the large amounts of enzyme needed for studies of protein structure, function and inhibitor design.

We initiated our work by isolating a full-length cDNA clone of TS from a stimulated human T-cell library in pUC9. By screening 1.3×10^5 *E. coli* transformants with synthetic oligonucleotide hybridization probes, thirty-two clones were obtained that contained the full-length coding sequences. One clone, pWHTS-1, which contained a 1.4-kb insert was selected for further study. The coding region was identical to the reported sequence of the TS cDNA from human fibroblasts. The clone pWHTS-1 did not complement TS-deficient *E. coli* c2913 (Thy-), but this was expected, since the 300 bp 5′ flanking sequence does not contain appropriate sequences for transcription or translation in *E. coli.*

In early attempts to express the recombinant human TS gene in *E. coli,* we cloned the coding sequence into vectors that use either the T7 RNA polymerase or *trp-lac* promoters. Human TS of pT7HTS or pJFHTS was not expressed from any of these vectors (TABLE 2). The first successful expression of human TS in *E. coli* utilized a vector based on the constitutive *E. coli* expression system for the *L. casei* TS.[15] The 5′ untranslated region of the TS genomic clone from methotrexate-resistant *L. casei* is 115 bp in length and contains a ribosome binding site at position −7 relative to the initiation codon. The *L. casei* TS expression levels in *E. coli* harboring these plasmids are exceedingly high (10%-20% of the soluble extract), presumably because of unknown regulatory elements in the 5′ untranslated *L. casei* sequence. We therefore constructed a plasmid, pDHTS-BL1, that contained the human TS gene directly fused to the 115 bp 5′ untranslated region of the *L. casei* gene in the phagemid Bluescript.

Constitutive expression of human TS in TS-deficient *E. coli* c2913 (Thy-) harboring pDHTS-BL1 was initially detected by genetic complementation with plasmid pDHTS-B1 on minimal agar lacking thymine. In addition, TS activity was measured directly in soluble extracts of transformed cells grown on LB (TABLE 2). The reason for the enhanced expression imparted by the 115-bp leader sequence from *L. casei* is not known.

In an attempt to increase the level of protein expression, the codon usage in the 5′ coding region of the gene was altered. It was noted that the G + C content in the third position of the first ~80 codons of the coding sequence was 75%, whereas it

TABLE 2. Expression of Human TS in *E. coli*[a]

Plasmid Construct	Vector	Promoter	*E. coli* Host	Specific act[b]	% Soluble[c]
pT7HTS	pAR3040	T7 *pol*	BL21	—[d]	—
			JM107	—[d]	—
pJFHTS	pJF119EH	*trp-lac*	x2913	—[d]	—
			TB-1	—[d]	—
pDHTS-BL1	pDLTS-Nde	*lac*	x2913	0.0024	0.3%
pDHTS-S1	pDLTS-Nde	*lac*	x2913	0.011	1.6%

[a] Data from Davisson *et al.*[24]

[b] Units mg^{-1} at 25°C.

[c] Based on specific activity of pure human enzyme isolated from *E. coli* (0.7 mg ml^{-1}).

[d] Enzyme activity below the limit of detection by assay (<0.0001 units).

was ≈50% in the remaining sequence. While the effect of high G + C sequence on transcription or translation was not established, we altered the codon usage of this region for the purpose of increasing TS expression. A synthetic oligonucleotide containing codons commonly used in highly expressed genes in *E. coli* was used to replace the first 90 bp of the human TS coding sequence. The constitutive level of TS expression from the hybrid construct (pDHTS-S1) was five-fold higher than that directed by the plasmid bearing the native sequence (pDHTS-BL1; see TABLE 2). The observed level of TS expression represents approximately 1.6% of the soluble protein.

Human TS from a 1-liter culture of *E. coli* c2913 containing plasmid pDHTS-S1 was purified to near homogeneity by phenyl-Sepharose and N^{10}-formyl-5,8-dideazafolate-Sepharose affinity chromatography. On 12% SDS-PAGE, the purified preparation shows a single major component with a molecular mass of 35.8 kDa. The yield of purified human TS from 1 liter of *E. coli* culture, or about 7 g of wet cells, was 3.7 mg, which surpasses any reported isolation of the enzyme. For comparison, a yield of 66 μg of pure TS was obtained from 25 g of human leukemic cells grown in culture.[21]

Human TS expressed in Thy- *E. coli* has properties similar to the authentic enzyme isolated from human cells. One difference between the human thymidylate synthase expressed in *E. coli* and that from transfected mouse cells[23] appears at the N-terminus. The expressed human TS has the N-terminal methionine residue blocked, presumably as a formyl-Met residue. We do not know the sequence of authentic human TS.

The heterologous expression system and purification procedure described herein provides a plentiful source of human TS. Although the N-terminal Met is blocked, the enzyme is fully active and has properties similar to those reported for preparations of the enzyme from human leukemic cells.

PERSPECTIVES

We now have generic approaches for obtaining large amounts of TS from almost any organism. Here we described the heterologous expression systems used to obtain reagent quantities of TS from the protozoan *Leishmania,* the fungus *Pneumocystis,* and from the human. The availability of this important enzyme from pathogens as well as host, together with increasing knowledge of structure-function relationships of TS, makes us believe that rational structure-based approaches to the development of species-selective inhibitors are now possible. If put to use, TS would become an important drug target for a variety of infectious diseases.

REFERENCES

1. BLAKELY, R. L. 1984. *In* Folates and Pteridines. R. L. Blakely & S. J. Benkovic, Eds. Vol. **1:** 191-253. Wiley. New York.
2. SANTI, D. V. & P. V. DANENBERG. 1984. *In* Folates and Pteridines. R. L. Blakely & S. J. Benkovic, Eds. Vol. **1:** 343-396. Wiley. New York.
3. SANTI, D. V., C. MCHENRY, R. T. RAINES & K. IVANETICH. 1987. Biochemistry **26:** 8606-8613.

4. CODERRE, J. A., S. M. BEVERLEY, R. T. SCHIMKE & D. V. SANTI. 1983. Proc. Natl. Acad. Sci. USA **80:** 2132-2136.
5. GARRETT, C. E., J. A. CODERRE, T. D. MEEK, E. P. GARVEY, D. M. CLAMAN, S. M. BEVERLEY & D. V. SANTI. 1984. Molec. Biochem. Parasitol. **11:** 257-265.
6. FERONE, R. & S. ROLAND. 1980. Proc. Natl. Acad. Sci. USA **77:** 5802-5806.
7. GRUMONT, R., W. L. WASHTIEN, D. CAPUT & D. V. SANTI. 1986. Proc. Natl. Acad. Sci. USA **83:** 5387-5391.
8. BEVERLEY, S. M., T. E. ELLENBERGER & J. S. CORDINGLEY. 1986. Proc. Natl. Acad. Sci. USA **83:** 2584-2588.
9. BZIK, D. J., W. B. LI, T. HORII & J. INSELBURG. 1987. Proc. Natl. Acad. Sci. USA **84:** 8360-8364.
10. HUGHES, D. E., O. A. SHONEKAN & L. SIMPSON. 1989. Mol. Biochem. Parasitol. **34:** 155-166.
11. MEEK, T. D., E. P. GARVEY & D. V. SANTI. 1985. Biochemistry **24:** 678-686.
12. HARDY, L. W., J. S. FINER-MOORE, W. R. MONTFORT, M. O. JONES, D. V. SANTI & R. M. STROUD. 1987. Science **235:** 448-455.
13. CRUSBERG, T. C., R. LEARY & R. L. KISLIUK. 1970. J. Biol. Chem. **245:** 5292-5296.
14. DUNLAP, R. B., N. G. L. HARDING & F. M. HUENNEKENS. 1971. Biochemistry **10:** 88-97.
15. PINTER, K., V. J. DAVISSON & D. V. SANTI. 1988. DNA **7:** 235-241.
16. GARVEY, E. P., J. A. CODERRE & D. V. SANTI 1985. Mol. & Biochem. Parasitol. **17:** 79-91.
17. GRUMONT, R., W. SIRAWARAPORN & D. V. SANTI. 1988. Biochemistry **27:** 3776-3784.
18. EDMAN, J. C., J. A. KOVACS, H. MASUR, D. V. SANTI, H. J. ELWOOD & M. L. SOGIN. 1988. Nature **334:** 519-522.
19. MILLS, J. 1986. Rev. Infect. Dis. **8:** 1001-1011.
20. EDMAN, U., J. C. EDMAN, B. LUNDGREN & D. V. SANTI. 1989. Proc. Natl. Acad. Sci. USA. **86:** 6503-6507.
21. LOCKSHIN, A., R. G. MORAN & P. V. DANENBERG. 1979. Proc. Natl. Acad. Sci. USA **76:** 750-754.
22. DOLNICK, B. J. & Y. CHENG. 1977. J. Biol. Chem. **252:** 7697-7703.
23. SHIMIZU, K., D. AYUSAWA, K. TAKEISHI & T. SENO. 1985. J. Biochem. **97:** 845-850.
24. DAVISSON, V. J., W. SIRAWARAPORN & D. V. SANTI. 1989. J. Biol. Chem. **264:** 9145-9148.

Studies of Cachexia in Parasitic Infection

KEVIN J. TRACEY[a,b] AND ANTHONY CERAMI[b]

[a] *Division of Neurosurgery*
New York Hospital-Cornell University Medical Center
New York, New York 10021

[b] *Laboratory of Medical Biochemistry*
The Rockefeller University
New York, New York 10021

Chronic illness caused by infection with parasites, viruses, or bacteria is frequently associated with a potentially fatal syndrome termed "cachexia." The stricken host dies from progressive weight loss, anemia, immune suppression, and terminal organ injury, even when the invasive burden may be relatively small. Until recently the biochemical basis of these harmful effects of infection-associated cachexia was not understood. They are now known to be mediated primarily by endogenous factors released in response to invasive infection. The search for these mediators led to the identification, isolation, and cloning of the cytokine known as cachectin/TNF (tumor necrosis factor).

Investigation of the biological effects of cachectin/TNF subsequently confirmed its role as a mediator of cachexia. Further studies revealed that cachectin is also an important mediator of septic shock, another syndrome of injurious host responses elicited by acute bacterial infection. The realization that endogenous factors, produced acutely or chronically during infection and inflammation, may mediate lethal syndromes in the host has advanced our understanding of the pathophysiology of infectious illnesses, and led to the investigation of novel treatment modalities. In this paper we will briefly review the history of cachectin/TNF, and discuss its role as an endogenous mediator of the hosts' responses to infection.

HISTORY OF CACHECTIN/TNF

Severe cachexia develops in rabbits infected with *Trypanosoma brucei;* with advancing infection they lose up to 50% of lean body weight, become moribund, and die.[1] In this depleted state, a paradoxical increase of serum triglycerides occurs because of a suppression of lipoprotein lipase (LPL), a membrane-bound enzyme necessary in the clearance of serum lipids. During their search for humoral mediators of cachexia, Kawakami and Cerami reasoned that a host factor, released in response to infection, acted to suppress LPL, and participated as a mediator of the resultant catabolic changes and cachexia.[2] These investigators used endotoxin-sensitive (C3H/HeN) and

-resistant (C3H/HeJ) mice and identified the presence of a humoral factor, released during endotoxemia in the endotoxin-sensitive strain, that suppressed LPL in the resistant mice.[2] Beutler *et al.*,[3] using the inhibition of LPL in the adipocyte cell line 3T3-L1[4] as a bioassay, isolated the active factor from the incubation medium of an endotoxin-treated murine macrophage cell line (RAW 264.7), and named it ***cachectin*** for its presumed role in cachexia. The N-terminal amino acid sequence of murine cachectin[5] was found to be strongly homologous to human tumor necrosis factor (TNF),[6] a molecule studied by independent scientists for its ability to kill some tumor cells. Subsequent cloning of the cDNA for the gene encoding cachectin[7] later showed that it was identical to TNF.

Macrophages and other immunocompetent cells release relatively large amounts of cachectin/TNF when exposed to a variety of bacterial, viral, or parasitic factors. During endotoxemia in rabbits,[8] baboons,[9] or man,[10] very high serum cachectin/TNF levels are achieved within hours. Cachectin/TNF rapidly leaves the circulation, binds to high-affinity receptors,[8,11] and induces a broad range of biological responses.[12–14] Some of these systemic effects are listed in TABLE 1. Recent investigations have revealed that acutely elevated serum cachectin/TNF levels, as occur during endotoxemia, bacteremia, or the administration of cachectin/TNF, triggers the lethal effects of septic shock and multiple organ system failure (MOSF). Moreover, chronic cachectin/TNF production or administration will induce the deleterious responses that are characteristic of cachexia.

CACHECTIN/TNF INDUCES CACHEXIA

The first evidence of cachectin/TNF's role in cachexia was provided by studies of mice given injections of a dialyzed conditioned medium from LPS-induced peritoneal macrophages.[15] The treated mice developed weight loss and anorexia, which was attributed to cachectin/TNF present in the medium. The subsequent availability of human recombinant cachectin/TNF led to detailed investigations of the molecular basis of cachexia.

TABLE 1. The Systemic Effects of the Administration of Cachectin/TNF

Dosage Schedule	
Acute, high-dose	Chronic, low-dose
Shock	Anorexia
Fever	Weight loss
Hypotension	Anemia
Decreased cardiac output	Net protein catabolism
Pulmonary edema	Net lipid catabolism
MOSF	Acute-phase protein synthesis
Intravascular dehydration	Neutrophilia
Catabolic hormone release	Death
Hyperglycemia followed by hypoglycemia	
Neutropenia followed by neutrophilia	
Acute-phase protein synthesis	
Death	

Recombinant cachectin/TNF induces a catabolic state in adipocytes *in vitro* by causing a suppression of the transcription and translation of several key lipogenic enzymes.[16] Because lipolysis is enhanced and lipogenesis suppressed,[17] cachectin/TNF-exposed lipid-laden adipogenic TA1 cells become depleted of intracellular lipid and revert to the morphologic configuration of normal fibroblasts. This model of *in vitro* cachexia is reversed if cachectin/TNF is removed from the medium. The similarity of these catabolic cellular effects to *in vivo* cachexia led to the suggestion that one important biologic role of cachectin/TNF is to mobilize energy stores during infection.

A similar state of enhanced catabolism and energy mobilization is observed in skeletal muscle cells treated with cachectin/TNF. Within minutes after the addition of cachectin to the medium, glycogenolysis is stimulated in L6 myocytes, which become depleted of glycogen stores.[18] Large quantities of lactate are released by the catabolic muscle cells. The appearance of cachectin/TNF during infection can therefore trigger the mobilization of endogenous energy stores from both peripheral adipose and muscle tissues.

The liver of cachectic animals is often metabolically active because of increases in rates of gluconeogenesis, acute-phase protein synthesis, and ureagenesis. Studies of hepatocytes *in vitro* indicate that cachectin/TNF mediates increased transcription rates for several of the acute-phase protein genes[19] and enhanced glucagon-dependent amino acid uptake.[20] This suggests that during infection, secreted cachectin/TNF both stimulates essential hepatic protein synthesis, and induces the release of the necessary substrates from peripheral tissue stores.

The net effects of the persistence of these cellular responses to cachectin/TNF *in vivo* is the development of cachexia. This was demonstrated by Oliff *et al.*,[21] who implanted a genetically engineered cachectin-secreting cell line into the hindlimbs of nude mice. The growth of cachectin/TNF-secreting tumors produced severe cachexia, but control animals bearing tumors not secreting cachectin/TNF did not become cachectic. The presence of a single gene product, cachectin/TNF, induced weight loss, weakness, and anorexia associated with significantly increased mortality rates. Cachexia is also induced in Sprague-Dawley rats injected twice daily with recombinant human cachectin/TNF.[22] Body composition analysis indicated that lipid and protein depletion occurred in a manner that was similar to the cachexia of infection. Partially starved, pair-fed animals not given cachectin/TNF tended to preferentially retain endogenous protein and utilize lipid, suggesting that cachectin-induced catabolism of peripheral tissue energy stores overrides the protein-sparing mechanisms normally observed in unstressed starvation. Anemia due to decreased red blood cell mass, another hallmark of the cachectic state, was also observed in these animals.

Other studies indicate that cachectin/TNF induces significant alterations in lipid metabolism that contribute to the paradoxical lipemia of cachexia. Hepatic lipid biosynthesis is increased[23] and peripheral lipid clearance is reduced secondary to suppression of LPL.[24] Similar effects are seen in humans given cachectin/TNF: hyperlipidemia, increased rates of whole-body glycerol and free fatty acid turnover, and accelerated rates of whole-body lipolysis are observed within hours.[25] These biological responses to cachectin/TNF are quite similar to the altered lipid metabolism associated with human cachexia.

Tolerance to the biological effects of cachectin/TNF may occur within 7 days of repeated intraperitoneal injections of recombinant human cachectin, but the mechanism of this tachyphylaxis is unknown.[22] Recent studies suggest that it is not due to a humoral immune response or to altered metabolism of cachectin/TNF during repeated episodic administration.[26] The role of uncharacterized inhibitory or carrier molecules in the regulation of the deleterious effects of cachectin/TNF has been suggested,[27] but remains unproved. Inter-species differences may be important when assessing the degrees of biological responsiveness to heterologous protein preparations, as is illustrated by studies showing that recombinant murine cachectin/TNF induces the proliferation of murine thymocytes in the presence of a comitogenic stimulus, but recombinant human cachectin does not.[28] A better understanding of the molecular basis of tolerance to cachectin/TNF may lead to future advances in the therapy of cachexia.

The multiplicity of biological effects induced by cachectin/TNF is in part dependent upon the biosynthesis of other endogenous secondary mediators (TABLE 2). These factors act systemically, and in a local or paracrine manner, to amplify and synergistically enhance the pathophysiological derangements induced by cachectin/TNF. One of these is a pluripotent cytokine, interleukin-1, which is induced by cachectin,[29] and has been implicated in a variety of inflammatory responses.[30] In addition to inducing anorexia, fever, and cortisol release, IL-1 synergistically increases the toxicity of cachectin/TNF.[31] Other hormones known to participate in catabolic hypermetabolism (including epinephrine, norepinephrine, glucagon, and cortisol) are also induced by cachectin/TNF.[20,32] Endotoxin/LPS, which may be present by association with the infectious agent or via altered gut absorption during cachexia, is also capable of synergistically enhancing the toxicity of cachectin/TNF.[33] The complex relationship between these other secondary mediators of cachectin/TNF-induced cachexia is an important area for additional study.

The use of antagonists to cachectin/TNF in the treatment of cachexia has been proposed,[21,22] but the role of cachectin/TNF in human cachexia remains uncertain. Several investigators have identified cachectin/TNF in the serum of patients with a variety of diseases known to be associated with cachexia, including parasitic infection,[34] cancer,[35] and acquired immunodeficiency syndrome (AIDS).[36] Others have not detected increased levels in patients afflicted with the cachexia of cancer[37]; the authors of the latter report indicate, however, that cachectin/TNF is known to be biologically active at concentrations below the limits of detection of their assay, and it may circulate

TABLE 2. Endogenous Factors Induced by the Cytokine Cachectin/TNF

Cytokines	Cachectin/TNF IL-1 IL-6 CSF GM-CSF
Growth Factors	PDGF TGF-β
Eicosanoids	Prostaglandins Leukotrienes Platelet-activating factor
Hormones	Epinephrine Norepinephrine Glucagon Cortisol
Acute-phase Proteins	C-reactive protein α_1-acid glycoprotein α_2-macroglobulin Complement proteins factor B and C3 α_1-antichymotrypsin

only periodically in cancer patients. Our own studies indicate that the administration of monoclonal anti-cachectin/TNF antibodies protects to a degree against the cachectin/TNF-induced cachexia in animals.[22]

CACHECTIN/TNF IN SEPTIC SHOCK

Acute bacterial infection in mammals frequently leads to a syndrome of hypotension, lethal tissue injury in the lungs and other organs, and death within hours. Termed "septic shock," the mortality of this syndrome in man exceeds 50%, and accounts for more than 50,000 deaths per year nationwide. Early evidence of cachectin/TNF's role in septic shock was at first surprising. When laboratory animals were infused with highly purified human recombinant cachectin/TNF they developed falling blood pressure, increased respiratory rate, lactic acidosis, and shock.[32,38] Hemoconcentration and wide variations in serum glucose levels developed prior to abrupt death by respiratory arrest. Postmortem examination revealed inflammation and extensive tissue injury in critical organs; pulmonary edema, adrenal hemorrhage, acute renal tubular necrosis, and gastrointestinal hemorrhagic necrosis were invariably present. This constellation of pathophysiological changes closely mimics endotoxemia or septic shock in both animals and man.

The mechanisms of cachectin-induced shock and multiple organ system injury have since been widely investigated. As described above, cachectin/TNF induces many endogenous secondary mediators that propagate systemic toxicity and tissue injury (TABLE 2). Both IL-1 and LPS, which are ubiquitous during Gram-negative infections when cachectin is also released, synergistically increase the lethality of cachectin.[31,33] Interferon-γ and IL-1 also potentiate cachectin's toxicity and ability to cause shock. Platelet-activating factor is a potent, vasoactive eicosanoid induced by cachectin/TNF[39] that in part mediates hypotension and shock.

Although the deleterious sequelae of septic shock appear to be mediated by a cascade of humoral responses, the importance of cachectin's role is underscored by studies showing that lethal septic shock can be prevented by neutralizing cachectin/TNF. We have utilized a clinically relevant model of overwhelming sepsis in baboons given intravenously a lethal dose of live *E. coli* (1.2×10^{11} organisms/kg).[9] Neutralizing monoclonal anti-cachectin/TNF antibody fragments ($F(ab')_2$) prevented the characteristic increase of serum cachectin/TNF levels after bacterial infusion, and protected baboons from shock, pulmonary failure, and death.[9] Although an antibiotic was not given until after 8 hours, dramatic protection resulted from inhibiting the cachectin/TNF normally released in response to infection. Whereas nonimmunized control animals succumbed to septic shock and critical organ injury in 13.3 ± 3.5 hours (mean $\pm$ SE, $n = 6$), none of the animals that received anti-cachectin mAb 2 hours before bacteremia succumbed.[9] Thus, although the magnitude of the bacteremia was similar between controls and the antibody-treated baboons, septic shock and lethal tissue injury did not develop when cachectin/TNF was neutralized.

Similar results using anti-cachectin/TNF antibodies have shown improved survival in endotoxemic mice[40] and rabbits[41] and support the concept that cachectin/TNF is an essential primary mediator of shock and tissue injury. At the present time, cachectin/TNF is the only endogenous mediator that has been found to induce a syndrome of septic shock after systemic administration, which when inhibited during bacteremia prevents septic shock. These animal studies suggest that cachectin/TNF antagonists may be useful in the treatment of human sepsis. In man, increased mortality correlates with increased serum cachectin/TNF levels in meningococcal infection[42] and purpura fulminans caused by Gram-negative septicemia.[43] Cachectin/TNF is also detected more frequently in the serum of burned patients who become septicemic or who eventually succumb to their burn injury.[44] Intermittent release of cachectin/TNF occurred during the prolonged post-burn hospitalization period,[44] indicating that episodic cachectin/TNF appearance may propagate MOSF in protracted critical illness.

The data available to us suggest that the administration of cachectin/TNF antagonists may abrogate the deleterious effects of cachectin/TNF released either in large amounts during acute infection, or intermittently during prolonged critical illness and MOSF. Inhibiting the toxicity of cachectin/TNF may minimize the stimulus to persistent tissue injury and improve survival. In the absence of an appropriate animal model for prolonged human critical illness and organ failure, further studies are needed to determine the effects of such therapies both in acute septic shock and as prophylaxis in patients known to be at high risk for the development of acute septicemia.

SUMMARY

Cachexia and septic shock, syndromes associated with chronic and acute infection, respectively, are mediated by endogenous factors. The search for humoral mediators of cachexia led to the isolation of the cytokine known as cachectin/TNF. A biologic role for cachectin/TNF in cachexia has been identified: it induces a catabolic state in adipose and skeletal muscle cells *in vitro,* and animals persistently exposed to it *in vivo* become cachectic. Cachectin/TNF was also discovered to be a primary, essential mediator of septic shock. The acute administration of the recombinant protein causes shock, tissue injury, and derangements of metabolic homeostasis that mimic endotoxemia and septic shock syndrome. Anti-cachectin antibodies protect against the lethal effects of septic shock and cachexia, suggesting that this mediator has a central role as a trigger to the inflammatory and deleterious host responses to infection. Future investigations will undoubtedly be directed towards the effects of inhibiting cachectin/TNF in the treatment of the complications of infectious disease.

[**Note added in proof:** Neutralizing endogenous cachectin/TNF with specific antibodies has been shown to abrogate anorexia and changes in body lipid and protein metabolism in tumor-bearing mice.[45] These data support the suggestion that this cytokine participates as a mediator of cachexia in some paraneoplastic syndromes, and provides another model for studying the pathogenesis of cancer cachexia.]

REFERENCES

1. ROUZER, C. A. & A. CERAMI. 1980. Mol. Biochem. Parasitol. **2:** 31-38.
2. KAWAKAMI, M. & A. CERAMI. 1981. J. Exp. Med. **154:** 631-639.
3. BEUTLER, B., J. MAHONEY, N. LETRANG, P. PEKALA & A. CERAMI. 1985. J. Exp. Med. **161:** 984-995.
4. KAWAKAMI, M., P. H. PEKALA, M. D. LANE & A. CERAMI. 1982. Proc. Natl. Acad. Sci. USA **79:** 912-916.

5. BEUTLER, B., D. GREENWALD, J. D. HULMES, M. CHANG, Y. C. PAN, J. MATHISON, R. ULEVITCH & A. CERAMI. 1985. Nature **316:** 552-554.
6. CARSWELL, E. A., L. J. OLD, R. L. KASSEL, S. GREEN, N. FIORE & B. WILLIAMSON. 1975. Proc. Natl. Acad. Sci. USA **72:** 3666-3670.
7. CAPUT, D., B. BEUTLER, K. HARTOG, R. THAYER, S. BROWN SHIMER & A. CERAMI. 1986. Proc. Natl. Acad. Sci. USA **83:** 1670-1674.
8. BEUTLER, B. A., I. W. MILSARK & A. CERAMI. 1985. J. Immunol. **135:** 3972-3977.
9. TRACEY, K. J., Y. FONG, D. G. HESSE, K. R. MANOGUE, A. T. LEE, G. C. KUO, S. F. LOWRY & A. CERAMI. 1987. Nature **330:** 662-664.
10. HESSE, D. G., K. J. TRACEY, Y. FONG, K. R. MANOGUE, M. A. PALLADINO, JR., A. CERAMI, G. T. SHIRES & S. F. LOWRY. 1988. Surg. Gynecol. & Obstet. **166:** 147-153.
11. PALLADINO, M. A., JR., M. R. SHALABY, S. M. KRAMER, B. L. FERRAIOLO, R. A. BAUGHMAN, A. B. DELEO, D. CRASE, B. MARAFINO, B. B. AGGARWAL, I. S. FIGARI, D. LIGGIT & J. S. PATTON. 1987. J. Immunol. **138:** 4023-4032.
12. TRACEY, K. J., S. F. LOWRY & A. CERAMI. 1987. Ciba Foundation Symposia **131:** 88-108.
13. TRACEY, K. J., S. F. LOWRY & A. CERAMI. 1988. J. Infect. Dis. **157:** 413-420.
14. CERAMI, A., K. J. TRACEY, S. F. LOWRY & B. BEUTLER. 1987. Recent Prog. Horm. Res. **43:** 99-112.
15. CERAMI, A., Y. IKEDA, N. LETRANG, P. J. HOTEZ & B. BEUTLER. 1985. Immunol. Lett. **11:** 173-177.
16. TORTI, F. M., B. DIECKMANN, B. BEUTLER, A. CERAMI & G. M. RINGOLD. 1985. Science **229:** 867-869.
17. PEKALA, P. H., M. KAWAKAMI, C. W. ANGUS, M. D. LANE & A. CERAMI. 1983. Proc. Natl. Acad. Sci. USA **80:** 2743-2747.
18. LEE, M. D., A. ZENTELLA, P. H. PEKALA & A. CERAMI. 1987. Proc. Natl. Acad. Sci. USA **84:** 2590-2594.
19. PERLMUTTER, D. H., C. A. DINARELLO, P. I. PUNSAL & H. R. COLTEN. 1986. J. Clin. Invest. **78:** 1349-1354.
20. WARREN, R. S., D. B. DONNER, H. F. STARNES, JR. & M. F. BRENNAN. 1987. Proc. Natl. Acad. Sci. USA **84:** 8619-8622.
21. OLIFF, A., D. DEFEO JONES, M. BOYER, D. MARTINEZ, D. KIEFER, G. VUOCOLO, A. WOLFE & S. H. SOCHER. 1987. Cell **50:** 555-563.
22. TRACEY, K. J., H. WEI, K. R. MANOGUE, Y. FONG, D. G. HESSE, H. T. NGUYEN, G. C. KUO, B. BEUTLER, R. S. COTRAN, A. CERAMI & S. F. LOWRY. 1988. J. Exp. Med. **167:** 1211-1227.
23. FEINGOLD, K. R. & C. GRUNFELD. 1987. J. Clin. Invest. **80:** 184-190.
24. ZECHNER, R., T. C. NEWMAN, B. SHERRY, A. CERAMI & J. L. BRESLOW. 1988. Mol. Cell. Biol. **8:** 2394-2401.
25. STARNES, H. F., JR., R. S. WARREN, M. JEEVANANDAM, J. L. GABRILOVE, W. LARCHIAN, H. F. OETTGEN & M. F. BRENNAN. 1988. J. Clin. Invest. **82:** 1321-1325.
26. FRAKER, D. L., M. C. STOVROFF, M. J. MERINO & J. A. NORTON. 1988. J. Exp. Med. **168:** 95-105.
27. SECKINGER, P., S. ISAAZ & J.-M. DAYER. 1988. J. Exp. Med. **167:** 1511-1516.
28. RANGES, G. E., A. ZLOTNIK, T. ESPEVIK, C. A. DINARELLO, A. CERAMI & M. A. PALLADINO, JR. 1988. J. Exp. Med. **167:** 1472-1478.
29. DINARELLO, C. A., J. G. CANNON, S. M. WOLFF, H. A. BERNHEIM, B. BEUTLER, A. CERAMI, I. S. FIGARI, M. A. PALLADINO, JR. & J. V. O'CONNOR. 1986. J. Exp. Med. **163:** 1433-1450.
30. DINARELLO, C. A. 1988. FASEB.J **2:** 108-115.
31. WAAGE, A. & T. ESPEVIK. 1988. J. Exp. Med. **167:** 1987-1992.
32. TRACEY, K. J., S. F. LOWRY, T. J. FAHEY, 3RD, J. D. ALBERT, Y. FONG, D. HESSE, B. BEUTLER, K. R. MANOGUE, S. CALVANO, H. WEI, A. CERAMI & G. T. SHIRES. 1987. Surg. Gynecol. Obstet. **164:** 415-422.
33. ROTHSTEIN, J. L. & H. SCHREIBER. 1987. Ciba Foundation Symposia **131:** 124-139.
34. SCUDERI, P., K. E. STERLING, K. S. LAM, P. R. FINLEY, K. J. RYAN, C. G. RAY, E. PETERSEN, D. J. SLYMEN & S. E. SALMON. 1986. Lancet **2:** 1364-1365.
35. BALKWILL, F., R. OSBORNE, F. BURKE, S. NAYLOR, D. TALBOT, H. DURBIN, J. TAVERNIER & W. FIERS. 1987. Lancet **2:** 1229-1232.

36. Lahdevirta, J., C. P. J. Maury, A.-M. Teppo & H. Repo. 1988. Am. J. Med. **85:** 289-291.
37. Socher, S. H., D. M. Martinez, J. B. Craig, J. G. Kuhn & A. Oliff. 1988. J. Natl. Cancer Inst. **80:** 595-598.
38. Tracey, K. J., B. Beutler, S. F. Lowry, J. Merryweather, S. Wolpe, I. W. Milsark, R. J. Hariri, T. J. Fahey, 3rd, A. Zentella, J. D. Albert, G. T. Shires & A. Cerami. 1986. Science **234:** 470-474.
39. Camussi, G., F. Bussolino, G. Salvidio & C. Baglioni. 1987. J. Exp. Med. **166:** 1390-1404.
40. Beutler, B., I. W. Milsark & A. C. Cerami. 1985. Science **229:** 869-871.
41. Mathison, J. C., E. Wolfson & R. J. Ulevitch. 1988. J. Clin. Invest. **81:** 1925-1937.
42. Waage, A., A. Halstensen & T. Espevik. 1987. Lancet **1:** 355-357.
43. Girardin, E., G. E. Grau, J.-M. Dayer, P. Roux-Lombard, the J5 Study Group & P.-H. Lambert. 1988. N. Engl. J. Med. **319:** 397-400.
44. Marano, M. A., Y. Fong, L. L. Moldawer, S. E. Calvano, K. J. Tracey, P. S. Barie, K. R. Manogue, A. Cerami, G. T. Shires & S. F. Lowry. 1988. Surg. Gynecol. & Obstet. In press.
45. Sherry, B. A., J. Gelin, Y. Fong, M. Marano, H. Wei, A. Cerami, S. F. Lowry, K. G. Lundholm & L. L. Moldawer. 1989. Anticachectin/tumor necrosis factor-alpha antibodies attenuate development of cachexia in tumor models. FASEB J. **3:** 1956-1962.

Epidemiologic Problems and Prospects

P. G. SMITH

Tropical Epidemiology Unit
London School of Hygiene and Tropical Medicine
London WC1E 7HT, England

INTRODUCTION

Remarkable advances have taken place in the biomedical sciences over the last decade or so and it was with great foresight that decisions were taken for increased investment in tropical disease research over the same period. Many laboratory scientists have been attracted to work to increase understanding of tropical diseases, especially at the cellular and molecular level, with the objective of developing new and improved tools for disease control. Much of this work has been done in laboratories in developed countries, but not all of it, and there has been some progress in the transfer of technical skills and knowledge to groups in the areas where tropical diseases are endemic. From this blossoming of research new tools are being developed that hold great potential for the control of some of the major disease problems in the Third World. For example, in its most recent report, the WHO Tropical Disease Research Programme (TDR) lists more than 50 such products of research in which scientists supported by the TDR Programme have participated.[1] Significant problems have arisen, however, in obtaining rigorous evaluations of these new tools in field situations. While promising results have been obtained in laboratory investigations or in small trials in clinical settings, it has been difficult to develop the necessary field research studies to evaluate tools in situations in which they may be useful for disease control. This is due, largely, to the dearth of persons with appropriate training in epidemiology and other field-related disciplines in tropical disease endemic areas, and even those with the appropriate skills often find that the local logistic obstacles to such research are overwhelming.

An expanded program of field research is essential to evaluate and monitor the effectiveness of both new and existing disease control tools if such tools are to be deployed rationally. The development of such a program should be, and has become, an important priority for many of the agencies supporting research on tropical diseases. In this paper I discuss the kinds of field research that are required and the different possible approaches to the epidemiologic evaluation of various forms of intervention. I also put forward some ideas that have been developed within the TDR Programme that are aimed at strengthening field research in the tropical disease endemic areas.

WHAT KINDS OF FIELD RESEARCH ARE REQUIRED?

When a new tool or means of intervention shows promise in laboratory studies or in initial clinical trials it is important that, at an early stage, field trials are undertaken with the objective of determining the usefulness of the tool in situations close to those in which it might be used for eventual disease control, and also to find out whether there are any adverse effects that may have gone undetected in small studies. Often these initial field studies will be in the form of randomized controlled trials. It is vital that such studies are conducted at a relatively early stage in the evaluation of a new tool, especially if it is a preventive or curative intervention, and that the studies are of sufficient size to be expected to yield unequivocal results. If the studies are too long delayed or are poorly designed or conducted or are too small, proper evaluation may be compromised. If field trials are delayed, at some point the weight of evidence suggesting that an intervention is effective may become such that ethical considerations may rule out a properly controlled trial. A recent example, illustrating the kinds of problems that may arise, was the trials of the mass application of ivermectin in areas where onchocerciasis is endemic. Studies predominantly in clinical settings, each involving at most a few hundred patients, had indicated that ivermectin was effective in clearing microfilariae from the skin of onchocerciasis patients. When large-scale field trials were being planned some investigators had reservations about the ethical acceptability of including untreated groups in these studies because of the accumulating evidence of good results from clinical studies. My purpose here is not to reopen that particular debate but to use the example to illustrate that the longer field evaluation is delayed, the more difficult it may be to undertake properly controlled studies.

After the initial demonstration of efficacy in field trials there is a need, for some interventions, to conduct further research on the best strategy with which to use the intervention for disease control. This might include consideration of issues such as whether all in a community should be treated or just those with evidence of current infection or those with an intensity of infection above a certain level, and what is the appropriate dose and frequency of application. Determining the desirable frequency of application is likely to be of special importance for interventions against parasitic diseases. For many of these diseases reinfection is common and repeated application of curative therapy, or even repeated vaccination, may be necessary for the purposes of disease control. An example where studies of this kind may be required is with respect to drug treatment of schistosomiasis. Drugs have been available for some time that after a single dose will reduce egg loads to a low level. However, in most endemic areas reinfection is common and egg counts rise again after treatment. The speed of this rise is dependent on the pressure of infection in the community and thus different re-treatment strategies, to keep egg counts at a low level, are likely to be necessary in different communities. It seems that additional studies are needed, however, to experiment with different re-treatment strategies for the prevention of *morbidity.* Treating every year, for example, may be required to maintain low egg counts, but it may be necessary to treat less frequently, say every 2 or 3 years, to prevent significant schistosomiasis-related morbidity. Such questions are of great importance in situations where health budgets are very small, but to date few, if any, studies seem to have been conducted to evaluate the impact of different re-treatment strategies on morbidity, rather than on egg counts. Very similar issues are likely to arise with the use of ivermectin for the treatment of onchocerciasis.

In addition to initial field studies of efficacy and studies to evaluate plans for different disease control strategies, there is a need for operational research studies to devise control schemes so as to maximize the coverage of the at-risk population with the intervention under study for a given cost. This is now the most pressing area for the development of field research strategies. Such research is likely to be multidisciplinary in nature, requiring, for example, the interaction of epidemiologists, social scientists, and economists. Initially it is likely to be descriptive research aimed at developing hypotheses as to why coverage is low or variable, but it should lead to studies in which the effectiveness of different delivery strategies is compared. This area of research is of great importance even in the absence of new biomedical interventions since, as has been argued previously, an enormous impact could be made on disease burdens if only we could effectively apply the interventions we already have. Operational research of this kind is usually not easy and it is not surprising that it has been relatively neglected, given the shortage of field research personnel in the tropical disease endemic areas. In developing capacity for field research the ultimate challenge is in this area.

TOOLS FOR RESEARCH OR FOR CONTROL?

One of the dangers in the rapid advance of biomedical science is that it may produce tools that look exciting in the laboratory, but that have little value for disease control. To the extent possible, research directions should be demand-based, steered by the needs of disease control programs. It is important to distinguish clearly between those tools that may be of value for research purposes and those that may be useful in disease control programs. Some, of course, are useful for both, but problems may arise if tools developed for research are uncritically advocated for use in control at too early a stage. A current example of a development of this kind is that of serologic tests for the early diagnosis of leprosy. It is argued that if there was a sensitive and specific test for the early diagnosis of leprosy, at say a pre-clinical stage, it may be possible to implement treatment before there had been much transmission of the infection to others, and thus through a vigorous program of screening and treatment to reduce rapidly the incidence of new disease in a community. Those experienced in leprosy control point out that even with existing diagnostic methods, through clinical screening, such potential exists, but is not fulfilled. In many endemic areas only a small proportion of patients have their disease detected and treated because of failings in the control program due to financial, organizational and other constraints. Nonetheless, much research has been done on serodiagnostic tests for early detection of leprosy and some have advocated the use of such tests in control programs. Some data collected recently by Convit and his colleagues in Venezuela on one of these tests illustrates why there has been excitement about such tests, but also why at present they are a research rather than a control tool. Full details of these results are to be published elsewhere and I am grateful to Dr. Convit and his colleagues for allowing me to summarize some of the findings here.

A randomized controlled trial of an armadillo-derived *M. leprae* vaccine is being conducted in Venezuela. The participants are the household members and other close contacts of leprosy patients. Before vaccination, each trial entrant had a serum sample taken which was analyzed using the ELISA test for antibodies to phenolic glycolipid 1 (PGL1). For each individual, antibody level, as assessed by optical density in the ELISA test, was expressed as a ratio relative to that of sera taken from a pool of "positive" controls, who were known to give a strongly positive test result (mostly

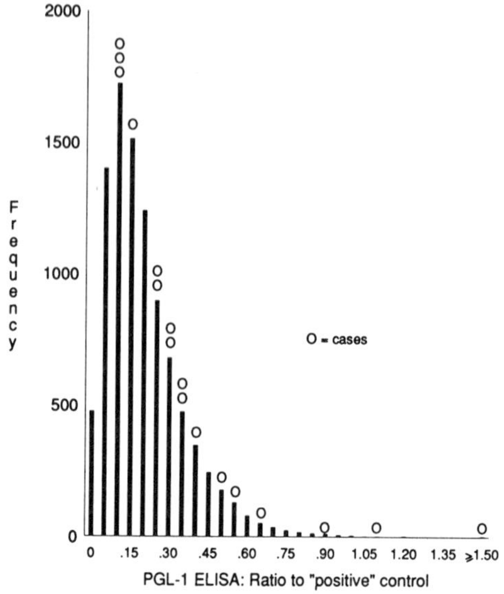

FIGURE 1. Venezuela leprosy vaccine trial. Distribution of antibody assays for phenolic glycolipid 1 among 9,542 contacts of leprosy patients at entry to the trial. Shown separately are the results for the 17 contacts who developed leprosy in the 3 years after entry to the trial. The antibody assays are expressed as the optical densities in the ELISA tests relative to the values for "positive" control sera.

patients with lepromatous leprosy). FIGURE 1 shows the distribution of these ratios in about 9,500 contacts, a sample of those entered into the trial. Shown separately are the ratios for 17 contacts who were diagnosed as having clinical leprosy within 3 years of entry to the trial. The results are summarized in TABLE 1. There is a highly significant association between the assayed PGL1 antibody level and the risk of

TABLE 1. Assays for Antibodies to Phenolic Glycolipid 1 in the Venezuelan Leprosy Vaccine Trial

Ratio to Positive Control	No. of Contacts Tested	Cases of Leprosy in 3 Years	Rate per 1000	Relative Risk	
<.25	6346	4	0.6	1.0	
0.25–	2642	7	2.6	4.2	
0.50–	474	3	6.3	10.0	
0.75–	70	1[a]	14.3	22.7	19.8[b]
1.00+	10	2[a]	200.0	317.5	
Total	9542	17	1.8		

NOTE: ELISA antibody assays for phenolic glycolipid 1 among 9542 contacts of leprosy patients at entry to the trial are shown, related to leprosy incidence in the following three years. The antibody assays are expressed as the optical densities in the ELISA tests relative to "positive" control sera.

[a] Two cases were detected through special survey of those with high antibody levels.

[b] Relative risk if two cases detected through special survey are ignored.

developing clinical leprosy in the three years after the test, such that those with levels above 75% of that of the positive control sera are more than twenty times more likely to be diagnosed with leprosy than those with antibody level of less than 25% of the positive control. There is also a gradient in risk—the higher the antibody level, the higher the risk. These results also suggest, however, that the test is likely to be of very little value as a screening test to pick up those at high risk of leprosy. For example, 80 of 9,542 contacts had a level of above 75% of the positive control, but only 3 of 17 cases of leprosy occurred in this group. Eleven of the 17 cases occurred in 8,988 contacts with antibody levels of below 50% that of the positive control sera. Thus, by screening a large number of sera, the test might be used to identify a small number of individuals at relatively high risk of leprosy, but most cases would be missed, unless the cut-off level for the at-risk group was set at such a level that most of those tested would fall into the category! The test may have value for epidemiologic assessment, but at present it seems unlikely that it will be a useful screening tool in control programs.

EPIDEMIOLOGIC METHODS TO EVALUATE NEW INTERVENTIONS

Randomized Controlled Trials

Randomized controlled trials, preferably double-blind and often placebo-controlled, should play a central role in the evaluation of new forms of intervention against disease. In many instances they are the method of first choice for the evaluation of new medical procedures and vaccines and for the objective assessment of side effects. The superiority of this study design over other methods is well recognized, and guidelines for the design and conduct of such trials have been extensively documented. Some special issues arise in the conduct of trials on infectious diseases when one of the outcomes of interest is a reduction in disease transmission. Sometimes this is the major objective of an intervention (for example, improvements in environmental sanitation and water supply to reduce diarrhea morbidity or the use of insecticide spraying for malaria control). In other circumstances, this may be a desirable side effect of treating individuals (for example, mass treatment with ivermectin against onchocerciasis). To assess the impact of such interventions it is either impossible or inappropriate to randomize the intervention by individual since, for proper evaluation, the measure should be applied to a "transmission unit." This may be a village, or in the case of vector-borne diseases, an area corresponding to the movements of both individuals and vectors. Thus, if different intervention strategies are to be compared, the appropriate randomization is by transmission unit. This poses two potential problems. First, for many infections the transmission unit may be difficult to define geographically because of incomplete knowledge of the local transmission cycle and, second, the number of transmission units required for a statistically valid study may be large. It is not uncommon in such situations for a "treated" village to be compared with a "control" village without proper consideration of the likely "natural" variations between villages, making these studies difficult or impossible to interpret. It has become apparent that for many, and indeed probably most, parasitic and infectious diseases the rates of infection and intensity of infection are substantially different over quite small areas and even in the same area at different times. This implies that studies in which villages or similar areas are the units of randomization must be large enough to take account of "natural" variation between villages when attempting to distinguish effects due to the intervention from those due to other causes.

Phased Introduction

There are circumstances in which randomized controlled trials, with individual or group randomization, may be ruled out but, nonetheless, an estimate is required of the efficacy of an intervention.[2] One such situation arises when substantial evidence already exists that an intervention is likely to be effective. For example, a sequence of studies has been planned for the evaluation of potential malaria vaccines. After the safety and acceptability of a vaccine has been assessed in nonimmune volunteers, small controlled trials will be conducted in areas not endemic for malaria; these trials will use artificial challenge with malaria parasites. Such trials will be extended in malaria-endemic areas to nonimmune immigrants and then to the indigenous population. The outcome measured in these studies will be the development of parasitemia and possibly mild symptoms of malaria. It is unlikely that many in the trials will develop severe malaria since the participants will be carefully monitored and will be treated as soon as evidence of malaria is detected, since it would be unethical to do otherwise. At the end of this sequence of studies a moderate or high efficacy may have been demonstrated for a vaccine, but against endpoints that are not those of greatest public health importance. Death is the most important consequence of malaria, but it is arguable whether this is an allowable endpoint in a trial when effective treatments for malaria are available. It is unlikely that any vaccine will completely prevent parasitemia and it is conceivable that those who do not respond to the vaccine are those who would respond abnormally to malaria in the absence of vaccination and die rather than develop immunity. This may be unlikely, but since it is not known why some children die of malaria and others do not we cannot be certain. Trials with death as the endpoint may be opposed on ethical grounds, but if such trials are vetoed some other method of evaluation of the effect on mortality will have to be found.

In some ways an analogous situation has arisen with respect to hepatitis B vaccination and liver cancer. Numerous epidemiologic studies have shown that the hepatitis B carrier state is so strongly associated with the development of liver cancer that it seems very likely that the association is causal. Hepatitis B vaccines have been developed that give good protection against the carrier state and, therefore, it is believed that such vaccination will also protect against the development of liver cancer and other hepatitis B-associated liver diseases. Some argue that this indirect evidence is so strong that controlled trials to assess the protective effect of the vaccine against liver cancer are unacceptable. Not all share this view, but if controlled trials are not to be conducted it would seem prudent to undertake some other form of assessment.

One approach is that being employed in The Gambia to evaluate hepatitis B vaccine against this endpoint.[3] The regular vaccination program in The Gambia is carried out by mobile teams, each team being responsible for a different part of the country. Hepatitis B vaccine (which must be given shortly after birth) was introduced initially into the regimen of one team, selected at random. Once established into the routine activities of that team it was introduced into a second team, chosen at random, and a few months later into a third team, and this expansion will continue until national coverage is achieved (FIG. 2). During this phased introduction of the vaccine,

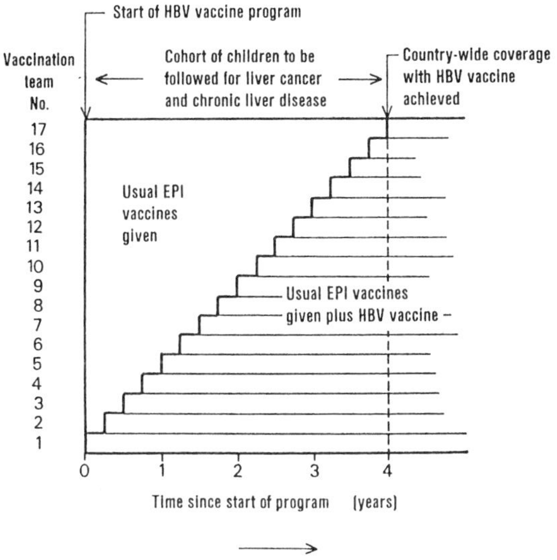

FIGURE 2. Phased introduction of hepatitis B vaccination in The Gambia. (From The Gambia Hepatitis Study Group.[3] Reproduced by permission of the American Association for Cancer Research, Inc.)

records are being kept of attenders at all vaccination clinics regardless of whether or not hepatitis vaccine has yet entered the team's schedule of vaccinations. In this way vaccinated and unvaccinated cohorts will be defined whose members may be followed for the subsequent development of liver diseases.

The proposed design is not as efficient statistically as randomizing at the individual level, but it does have some advantages. Many forms of health intervention are introduced in a progressive fashion, but usually are not planned with evaluation in mind. With the addition of the element of randomization of areas, and possibly also the institution of registration systems to identify those who receive or do not receive the intervention (although this may be unnecessary for interventions whose impact occurs soon after administration), many forms of interventions might be evaluated using a scheme of this kind. For example, the protective efficacy of malaria vaccines against death might be evaluated in this way if and when vaccination is introduced on a large scale, with infant and child mortality being measured in areas before and after the implementation of vaccination.

Case-Control Studies

The case-control approach has been much used to study the etiology of chronic diseases in developed countries, but has been employed relatively rarely for the study of tropical diseases. One reason for this has been the great shortage of trained epidemiologists in the developing world, and, in part, to the bias against such designs for the evaluation of interventions. In principle, the approach is simple: we take a group of cases with the disease of interest and a group of controls, who do not have the disease, and we compare the histories of exposure to the factor under study in the two groups. If the exposure is a supposedly protective intervention we expect fewer "cases" than "controls" to have a history of exposure and a direct estimate of the protective effect may be made from the difference.[4]

Clearly case-control methods can only be used once an intervention has been employed on a widespread basis for some time and a reliable history of exposure to the intervention can be obtained, but in these circumstances it may be a useful approach. A recent example of the use of this method has been in studies to evaluate the efficacy of BCG vaccination.

Randomized controlled trials of BCG vaccination have given conflicting results. In some trials the vaccine appeared to offer good protection against tuberculosis, but some trials in the United States and, most recently, the large trial in South India have indicated little effect. Many millions of doses of BCG have been given to children in Africa, but until recently there had never been any evaluation of whether this has had any effect on the incidence of tuberculosis in any African country. Furthermore, few of the controlled trials have involved vaccination of neonates, but this is when BCG is given in most routine programs. Tuberculosis is a major health problem in much of the Third World, but it is beyond the resources of most developing countries to set up randomized trials to assess the effect of BCG vaccination. The case-control approach seemed particularly appropriate to obtain a retrospective assessment of past vaccination policies.

Some such studies have either been completed or are well advanced and FIGURE 3 summarizes preliminary findings from ten of them.[5] These results have been discussed

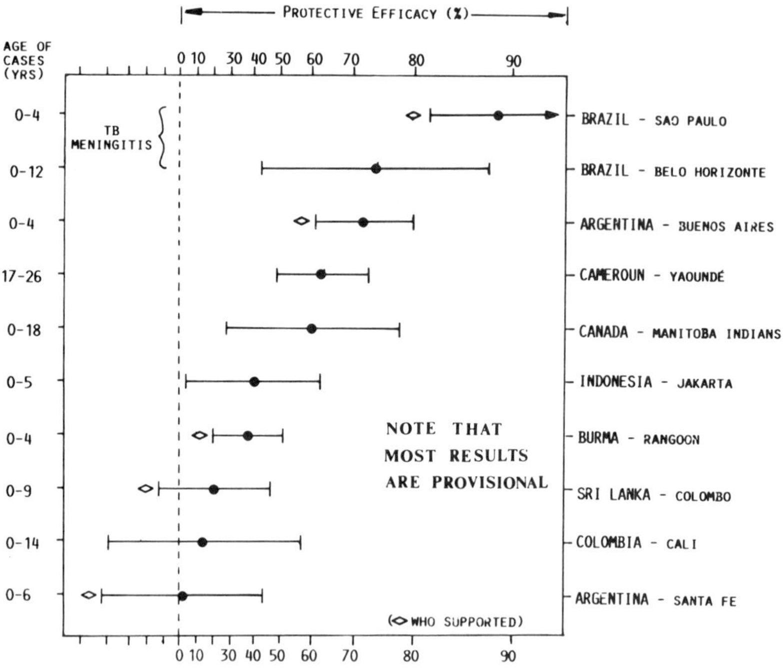

FIGURE 3. Protective efficacy of the BCG vaccine against tuberculosis as measured in ten case-control studies (the *bars* show the 95% confidence limits on the estimate of protective efficacy). (From Smith *et al.*[5] Reproduced by permission.)

in more detail elsewhere,[5,6] and I wish to stress only a few points. First, unlike the controlled trials, most of these studies were conducted in developing countries. Second, whereas the ten or so controlled trials have been done over a 40- to 50-year period, all of the case-control studies were completed in about 5 years. Third, the cost of these studies has been a small fraction of that of the controlled trials. It would be unwise to suggest that case-control studies do not present problems of interpretation, and some of the difficulties of this study design are magnified when they are conducted in developing countries. However, the technique has been used increasingly in recent years for studies on tropical diseases and, while not a substitute for randomized controlled trials, may be a valuable approach when such trials are ruled out for whatever reason.

HOW TO INCREASE THE CAPACITY FOR FIELD RESEARCH

Increasing the capacity for scientists in areas where tropical diseases are endemic to undertake field research studies is an important public health priority and is of special concern to those programs developing new methods of intervention against tropical diseases. The WHO Tropical Diseases Research Programme (TDR) has given this objective high priority and the initiatives I will describe have been recently taken in the Programme. Because I have worked on these aspects with the TDR for the past year, my perspective is a little biased, and I would mention that other groups are active in this area also.

Fellowships for Advanced Epidemiological Field Research Training

In the laboratory sciences practical skills are learned only in small part in postgraduate courses, but are mostly acquired working in laboratories as junior researchers under the supervision of experienced scientists. The same has been true for epidemiologists working in developed countries.

Many of the skills needed for successful field research on tropical diseases are not taught in courses, especially in developed countries, where the opportunities for relevant fieldwork experience may be, at best, limited. Unfortunately, opportunities for "apprenticeship" training in the developing countries are very limited since, in many countries, there are no established traditions of field research and experienced field epidemiologists are few.

In an attempt to exploit ongoing training opportunities in field studies in tropical disease endemic areas TDR is providing fellowships to attach junior researchers to successful field projects, often in countries other than their own, for a period of two or three years to develop their skills in the design, conduct, and analysis of epidemiologic investigations. The fellowships are intended for those who have a basic grounding in epidemiology, but who lack supervised field experience.

Outline Protocols for Priority Field Studies

The "investigator-initiated" method of allocating funds for research does not work well for field research on tropical diseases. The experience within TDR has been that the quality of submitted proposals has been generally poor and often the objectives of the research proposed are not those accorded highest priority for funding. To improve this situation it is planned that the proposal review committees will play a more active role in stimulating field research. The committees themselves or field studies subcommittees will be charged with the responsibility to list priorities for field research and, further, to outline protocols for this research. Where possible, scientists from the tropical disease endemic areas, who might be able to undertake research of the kind likely to be proposed, will be included in the committees so that they can take an active part in the drafting process.

To convert outline protocols into specific proposals for funding, adapted to local circumstances, is in itself a substantial undertaking. There are several ways in which this process may be facilitated. First, the assistance of a consultant might be sought, ideally from the endemic area. Such consultants would be charged not only to give assistance with the design of the study, but also to advise, on an ongoing basis, on its conduct and analysis. Second, potential investigators might be brought together for a special protocol development workshop at which the participants, together with consultants, would work together to expand outline protocols into detailed and costed study designs adapted to their own geographic areas and circumstances. Such consultants and workshops could be organized as part of the activities of field research networks.

Field Research Networks

In developed countries recently trained epidemiologists have easy access to others working on similar problems to whom they can turn for advice and support. Such a mechanism is usually not available in developing countries, where the scarcity of trained manpower is such that an epidemiologist or social scientist may be in a position of considerable isolation. The schools of public health and other institutions that are responsible for training such individuals are usually unable to provide much supervision or guidance to students once courses have finished.

The Tropical Disease Research Programme has launched a major new initiative aimed at strengthening capacity for field research in the endemic areas through the creation and promotion of regional networks of field researchers and centers. It has proposed to build up links between field researchers in the endemic areas by the organization of regular regional workshops bringing together those conducting TDR-related field studies. At these workshops investigators will be able (1) to exchange ideas and information on methods developed in the context of their own field studies; (2) to design protocols for new studies; (3) to be briefed by "experts" on new developments (e.g., priority issues for research or new field tools); and (4) to present preliminary results from field studies for critical review. Short instructional courses on particular methods or techniques might be run in conjunction with such workshops. Workers in developed countries will contribute to the networks, and emphasis will be placed on the transfer of skills to those in the tropical disease endemic areas.

The functions of the proposed networks are summarized in TABLE 2.

Initially these networks will be focused on those doing field research on diseases included in the TDR Programme. Once the networks are well established, it is likely that those with other disease interests will be added.

The development of field research in close liaison with national disease control programs is viewed as especially important since it is through such links that newly

TABLE 2. Functions of Field Research Networks

1. To facilitate communication between field researchers in the endemic areas in order to strengthen their capacity to conduct multidisciplinary field studies.
2. To facilitate continuing training in field research, through regular workshops and short training courses organized at regional centers.
3. To serve as a focus for collaborative research studies and to provide a mechanism by which protocols would be developed for high-priority field studies.
4. To foster the links between field researchers and national disease control programs.
5. To disseminate information through the network on new advances in field research methods and tools.
6. To provide a focus for the strengthening of regional resource centers so that they could provide assistance or advice for individual researchers on special aspects of field studies.
7. To promote further field research studies by appropriate expansion of the network to include additional researchers and institutions.
8. To link field researchers in the endemic areas with those in developed countries, with the objective of transfer of skills.

developed disease control tools may be introduced into widespread use and subjected to ongoing evaluation. Thus, there will be a preference to include in the networks those research groups that are either national control programs or that have established close links with such programs.

The importance of integrating those with social science skills and experience into the research networks should be stressed. The social component is likely to be critically important in evaluating the performance of new means of intervention in disease control programs, as also will be the contribution of health economists.

SUMMARY

Rapid advances in the biomedical sciences are producing new means of intervention against many of the major tropical diseases. The discovery of new drugs, vaccines and diagnostic tests, however, is only the first, though important, step down an often long and difficult road to their effective deployment in disease control programs. The blossoming of interest in tropical diseases among those in the laboratory sciences has not been paralleled by the required expansion in the number of scientists undertaking field research in the areas where such diseases are endemic. In consequence, it may be difficult to ensure the proper evaluation of new interventions in realistic disease control situations. There is also a danger that some tools developed for research purposes may be uncritically introduced into control programs without adequate consideration of their true utility.

Developing field research capacity in the tropical disease endemic areas is an urgent priority if the new tools and interventions are to be employed optimally. Some methods for achieving this are discussed and possible epidemiologic approaches to the evaluation of interventions against tropical diseases are outlined.

REFERENCES

1. WORLD HEATH ORGANIZATION. 1987. Tropical Disease Research: A Global Partnership: Eighth Programme Report. WHO. Geneva.
2. SMITH, P. G. 1987. Evaluating intervention against tropical diseases. Int. J. Epidemiol. **16:** 159-166.
3. THE GAMBIA HEPATITIS STUDY GROUP. 1987. The Gambia Hepatitis Intervention Study. Cancer Res. **47:** 5782-5787.
4. SMITH, P. G. 1982. Retrospective assessment of the effectiveness of BCG vaccination against tuberculosis using the case-control method. Tubercle **62:** 23-35.
5. SMITH, P. G. 1987. Case-control studies of the efficacy of BCG against tuberculosis. *In* Proceedings of the 26th World Congress of the International Union against Tuberculosis, Singapore 4-7 November 1986: 73-79. Professional Postgraduate Services International. Japan.
6. FINE, P. E. M. 1988. BCG vaccination against tuberculosis and leprosy. Brit. Med. Bull. **44:** 691-703.

Recent Occurrences in the Discovery and Development of Drugs to Treat HIV Infections

JOHN J. McGOWAN

Developmental Therapeutics Branch, AIDS Program
National Institute of Allergy and Infectious Diseases
National Institutes of Health
Bethesda, Maryland 20892

INTRODUCTION

The identification of HIV as the cause of AIDS has allowed researchers to explore methods to treat, prevent, and potentially cure the disease. Early successes have allowed for testing programs to identify potential therapies that have proved successful in treating those infected with HIV. However, the ability to safely administer these drugs around the world for all infected with HIV is still subject to question. Drug toxicities, costs and the requirements for other support systems needed to administer the current therapies make it unlikely that existing Western treatments will be widely used in developing countries. Traditional healers in Africa, the Americas, and in Asia continue to provide methods of treatment for the general population.[19] The traditional healer is now using herbs and other extracts from plants to potentially treat HIV infections. The evaluation of these traditional medicines as therapies for those infected with HIV is a new challenge confronting the world today. Western medical science derives from principles different from those of traditional healing. Communication between the cultures that support these traditional clinical efforts and Western cultures could be improved upon. A concerted effort to improve communication between the botanist, chemist, biologist, pharmacologist, ethnobotanist and traditional healer must be accomplished to ensure that the best treatments for HIV are made available in both developing and developed countries.

The current effort to discover new treatments for HIV is massive. Academic, public, private and government sectors around the world have responded with an unprecedented search for antiviral drugs to treat HIV. The Medical Research Council in England, the Institut Pasteur in France, and the National Institutes of Health in the United States all serve as examples of Western government-sponsored research programs. In addition, the private sector around the world has responded to the challenge to find therapies to treat HIV infections.

In this communication, an example of the NIH's program on drug discovery is given. The series of bioassays utilized in these efforts are presented and it is seen that traditional medicines could be tested for potential anti-HIV activities in these assays.

NIH PROGRAMS FOR DRUG DISCOVERY AND DEVELOPMENT

The NIH has launched a coordinated and comprehensive effort to facilitate all steps of research and development leading to possible therapies for AIDS (FIG. 1). The emphasis of the NIH is to stimulate discovery through basic and applied research in the public and private sector and to encourage the development of newly discovered drugs by the private sector.

Two fundamental approaches are taken to identify new drugs for development: random drug screening and rational drug design (FIG. 2).

The National Institute of Allergy and Infectious Diseases (NIAID) has the lead responsibility to support basic research that relates to drug discovery and development and animal models that can be used for drug evaluation. The NIAID also assumes the lead in multidisciplinary research on rational approaches leading to targeted drug discovery and development through the National Cooperative Drug Discovery Group Program for the Treatment of AIDS (NCDDG-AIDS). The NIAID discovery effort is coordinated with a program on X-ray crystallography sponsored by the National Institute of General Medical Science.

The National Cancer Institute (NCI) has assumed responsibility for random drug screening. The NCI has established a program for the acquisition and testing of novel compounds in a centralized screening facility at the Frederick Cancer Research Facility in Frederick, Maryland. Included in the acquisition effort is the random selection of

---

Office of the Director, NIH

- Intramural Program on AIDS Therapies
- NIGMS Targeted Antiviral Program

Developmental Therapeutics Program, DCT, NCI

- Contract Resources for Preclinical Drug Development

Developmental Therapeutics Branch, AIDSP, NIAID

- National Cooperative Drug Discovery Group Program for AIDS
- Animal Models for Testing Efficacy of Drugs
- Animal Models to Examine Combination Therapies
- NIH Research and Reference Reagent Program
- All Grants Relating to AIDS Drug Development

FIGURE 1. NIH Programs in AIDS drug discovery and preclinical development. Three organizations are primarily involved in the discovery of new drugs for AIDS. The Office of the Director, NIH, supports 35 intramural grants on targeted AIDS research for a total of 4.6 million dollars and eight grants awarded by the National Institute of General Medical Sciences, primarily to analyze the three-dimensional structure of the viral proteins, for a total of 5.9 million dollars. The National Cancer Institute supports contracts for natural product isolation, large-scale random drug screening, formulation, scale-up drug synthesis, pharmacology, and toxicology leading to the filing of the IND by the NIAID with the FDA. The cost of the NCI contract program is approximately 45 million dollars. The focus of the National Institute of Allergy and Infectious Diseases has been the National Cooperative Drug Discovery Group Program for AIDS, which has a total budget of 20 million dollars. In addition, the NIAID funds grants relating to drug research for 5 million dollars and development and centralized testing facilities to analyze drugs in animal retroviral vectors for a total of million dollars.

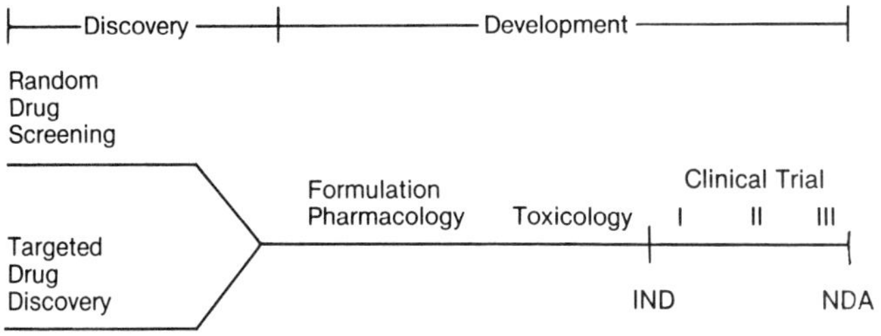

FIGURE 2. Typical steps necessary for entering a Phase I clinical trial of a drug in the United States. Drugs are initially discovered through random drug screening and rational drug design. Scale-up synthesis of the drug from mg per kilogram quantities is required, with concurrent formulation of the drug for intravenous or oral delivery, followed by the pharmacokinetic and toxicology studies needed to support the rationale of the clinical trial study design, filing of the investigational new drug application (IND) with the FDA, and approval of the new drug application (NDA) by the FDA.

plant and marine organisms. Extracts or active principles prepared from these acquired organisms will be tested for potential activity against HIV. In a standardized assay, different extracts and structural entities are tested to determine whether they can inhibit HIV replication *in vitro*. The screening facility has been fully operational for more than a year and will test at least 10,000 compounds a year. Compounds from any source are considered for screening, but an emphasis is placed on those compounds with unique structural features or evidence of biological activity.

Traditional preparations could be examined in a series of biological assays, through either program at the NIH, to verify the claim(s) made for their potential use to treat HIV infections. As reported by Farnsworth *et. al.*,[19] 88 chemical compounds purified from 119 plant extracts were examined and found to be active therapeutically for disease or symptoms being treated by traditional medicine. This supports the rationale to examine traditional medicines and the isolated natural products in bioassays which are available (TABLE 1).

Any cell culture or biochemically based assays could be used to evaluate a traditional medicine. The western-based model given (TABLE 2) recognizes the differences between western and traditional healers and provides a framework to guide scientific evaluation of a therapeutic agent which might be used in the treatment of HIV infections.

Any purified principles provided from traditional medicine could enter the programs described within the NIH. After consultation with the supplier, an active compound may enter preclinical development within the NCI, NIAID, or the private sector and lead to an INDA from the FDA (FIG. 2). The NIAID may also provide confirmatory evaluation of the compound and testing for potential efficacy in animal models (TABLE 2 and FIG. 3).

A number of drugs have been discovered through these programs that will not be discussed. However, two deserve comment: The first is castanospermine,[10,11] a natural product isolated from the Australian chestnut tree and identified as active against HIV by the Haseltine NCDDG-AIDS Group at the Dana-Farber Center in Boston. Castanospermine represents a new class of compounds which block glycosylation of the viral glycoprotein. The drug has shown some efficacy in a murine retrovirus model.[12] However, the toxicities associated with the concentration required for effective

TABLE 1. Examples of Biochemical and Cell-Culture-Based Assays Now Being Used to Determine Anti-HIV Activity

Biochemical/Cell Culture Assay	Viral Function Being Measured
Polymerization/viral replication	Reverse transcriptase
Ribonuclease/viral replication	Ribonuclease H
Proteolysis/viral replication	Protease
CD4 binding/cell fusion	GP120; viral-envelope-mediated fusion
Protein aggregation/viral replication or virion assembly	p24 protein interaction
GTPase/viral replication	nef
Phosphorylation/viral replication	nef

treatment cause doubt as to whether this compound is a viable clinical candidate. However, several pharmaceutical companies are developing analogues of castanospermine which are more active and appear less toxic than castanospermine.[3]

The second compound is the receptor for HIV-recombinant soluble T4 (rsCD4).[1,2] Through genetic engineering several of the NCDDG-AIDS groups have made recombinant soluble CD4 receptor to HIV (rsCD4).[1] Clinical evaluations of the drug have been initiated by Biogen and Genentech. Variations of this therapeutic protein are under development at several companies including Biogen, Smith, Kline and French, Genelabs, and Upjohn.

TABLE 2. Generalized Scheme Recommended for Evaluation of Extracts from Traditional Therapies for Potential Activity against HIV

Action
1. Authenticated extract provided for analysis
2. Single assay to detect potential activity and toxicity of a traditional medicine
3. Analyze data and determine future priorities High-priority extracts with antiviral effect > toxic effect to cells Lower priority if toxicity = or > than anti-HIV effect; then stop analysis
3. Crude (partial) purification of extract by chemical or physical methods
4. Confirmation of antiviral activity and toxicity data of extract and fractions of the extract in a variety of assays
5. If active fraction(s) identified, then carry out: *A.* Chemical identification of active compound(s) *B.* Biochemical assays of active fraction *C.* *In vivo* efficacy and toxicity studies in appropriate animal model system
6. Depending upon information provided in Step 5, prioritize compounds for potential clinical evaluation

NOTE: No one assay is ideal, but a number are currently being utilized. The scheme provided attempts to show the cost and benefit of a single cell assay followed by more detailed confirmatory assays should an active compound(s) be identified. The key for success of any therapeutic agent is that it not be cytotoxic. Therefore, careful analysis of cytotoxicity should be made. Tests should examine how long the cells will survive and how actively they will replicate in the presence of the drug. Systems that are simple, reproducible, and affordable should be chosen to determine the antiviral effect. The endpoint could vary from amount of cell survival, syncytium formation, p24 expression, reverse transcriptase levels in the supernatant, or fluorescence of viral antigens. All these work, but trade-offs in detection are realized.

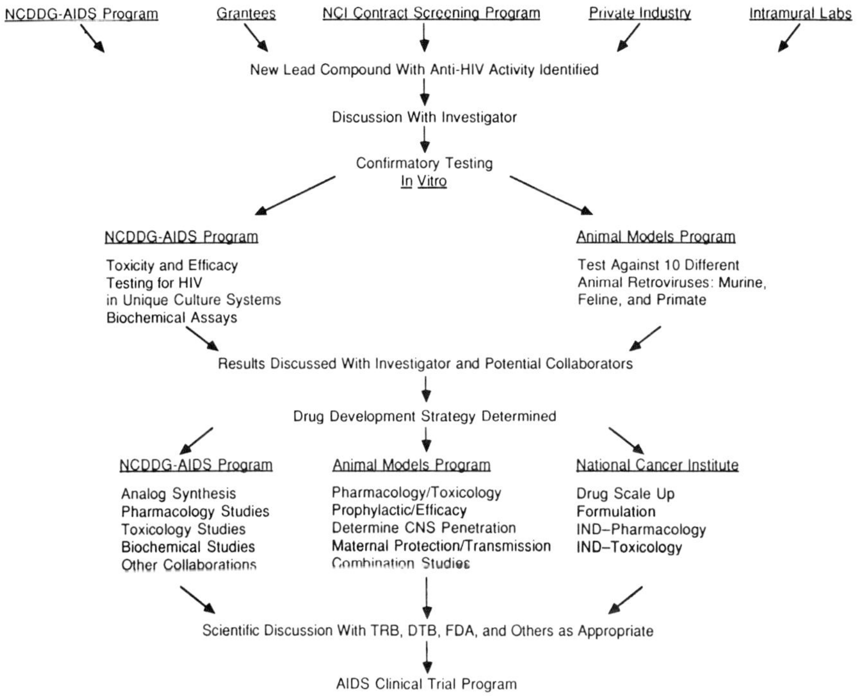

FIGURE 3. Schematic diagram of how the NIH functions in drug development. Any compound can be submitted to the National Cancer Institute Screening Program to obtain initial information about the potential activity of drug.

The flow chart shown here describes what happens if a sponsor already has some initial data and would like to have confirmatory testing. Compound with data relating to its anti-HIV activity and solubility is provided by any source. This is a key point, because at present, an ideal screen for drugs for AIDS does not exist. Each cell line and each biochemical assay has its pitfalls. Therefore, before a costly decision is made to develop a drug the NIAID assists by testing the compound blinded *in vitro* in different cell lines (macrophage, T cell and others) infected with HIV, SIV, FELV, MulV and other related retroviruses. Many investigators desire as much information about the potential efficacy of a compound as can be obtained.

Confirmatory test results are obtained. Meetings occur between branch staff and supplier to discuss results and potential collaborations, either in the animal models program, the NCI program, the NCDDG-AIDS program, or in studies by other grantees.

An outline of drug development strategy is made and initial animal testing begins (both for efficacy and pharmacology). As data are collected, the meetings increase in frequency and the number of persons involved increases as well. AIDS Program staff then facilitate the further development of compounds to clinical trials by bringing together sponsors, scientists from the Food and Drug Administration, and clinical scientists within the AIDS Program Treatment Research Branch to design protocols for Phase I studies in patients.

The success of the NCI-managed NIH drug development, especially the pioneering efforts of Broder, led to the discovery and entry of azidothymidine or zidovudine (AZT),[15] dideoxycytidine (ddC),[13] and dideoxyadenosine and dideoxyinosine (ddA/ddI)[14] into clinical trials.

Two additional anti-retroviral drugs discovered through NIH programs have recently entered clinical trials in 1989. These drugs are AZdU and d4T.

NUCLEOSIDE ANALOGUES PREDICTED TO ENTER CLINICAL TRIALS IN 1989

At present, AZT (zidovudine) has been licensed to treat those infected with HIV. Other drugs are being studied clinically, including ampligen, ddC, ddI, rsCD4, and dextran sulfate. The success of AZT and the early promise of other compounds now in clinical trials provide hope that effective treatments will be achieved that prevent the progression of disease.

No single therapeutic agent is likely to fulfill all the objectives in a treatment strategy, however. Combinations of drugs targeted against HIV are likely to be used. Differences in drug metabolism and toxicity will be key in selecting alternating regimens of drugs to stop disease progression and restore the immune system. Thus, in HIV therapy multiple drugs that work at different metabolic steps or have different toxicities need to be identified. The drugs to be used should have the following characteristics: they should require infrequent dosing, have few, if any, side effects, and be orally bioavailable.

Because of the success of the nucleoside analogue AZT, a series of other nucleoside analogues have been evaluated preclinically and soon will enter clinical trial. The target for all these particular drugs is the HIV reverse transcriptase, which presumably incorporates them into viral DNA and stops the elongation of the viral DNA.[15] These drugs potentially may be safer, more effective, and cheaper than AZT. However, these drugs will still be of great value if they are effective and do not cause hematopoietic damage, but carry somewhat more acceptable toxicity. So with respect to AZT the following questions are raised and discussed for each drug. Is it active against HIV? Is it orally bioavailable? Is it less toxic than AZT?

D4T, AZdU, and AZT are similar in structure (FIG. 4). D4T and AZdU are active against HIV in several cell lines.[5,6] The therapeutic index varies according to the assay conditions and cell lines (TABLE 3). Like AZT, AzdU and D4T are orally bioavailable. AZdU and D4T are both less toxic when compared to AZT in the granulocyte-macrophage colony-forming assay.[4-6,18] The triphosphate form of D4T or AZdU is comparable to AZT in competing as substrate with the HIV reverse transcriptase. At present, a base of information to determine significance of these preclinical tests has not been established. Making an accurate prediction of clinical efficacy or safety of these compounds is not yet possible. Yet these tests present a method to "prioritize" candidate compounds and allocate resources for future development. Only through further controlled clinical trials can insight be gained about the merit of these preclinical studies in helping guide the drug-selection process.

One other drug that has been discovered also deserves comment: carbovir. This drug is in the very early stages of preclinical evaluation. It is not known whether or when it will reach clinical trial.

Carbocyclic nucleosides have been evaluated as chemotherapeutic agents for the

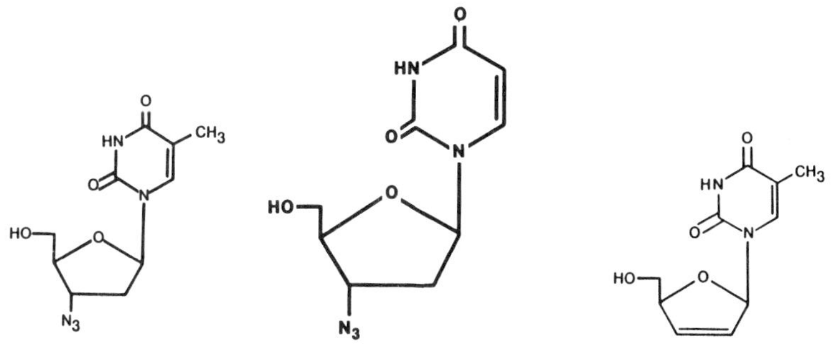

3'-AZIDO-2',3'-DIDEOXYTHYMIDINE
AZT or Retrovir

CS-87; AzddU

2',3'-DIDEOXYDIDEHYDROTHYMIDINE
D4T

FIGURE 4. Structural formulae of 3′-azido-2′,3′-dideoxythymidine (AZT), 3′--azido-2, 3′-dideoxyuridine (AZdU), and 1-(2,3,dideoxy-B-D-glycero-pent-2-enofuranosyl)thymine (d4T).

treatment of viral diseases (herpes) and cancer. The carbocyclic nucleoside is designed to retain the activity associated with a nucleoside and add hydrolytic stability to the molecule. This is one of the first of this class that has been found to be active in cell culture against HIV. Thus, the discovery in the NIH screening program that carbovir is active gives promise that this class of compounds may be useful in the treatment of those infected with HIV. The therapeutic index of carbovir is 2-8-fold lower than that of AZT,[8] depending upon the cell line used. The synthesis of carbovir results in racemic forms of the molecule. Whether one or both forms have antiviral activity has not been reported.

Last, the compound hypericin has been reported to have anti-retroviral activity. Hypericin represents a new class of promising compounds which appear to inhibit animal retroviruses *in vivo* at a step other than DNA chain elongation by the viral reverse transcriptase. Hypericin was first purified from St. John's wort, but can be synthesized chemically.[9,17] In animals, hypericin seems to clearly reduce the amount of detectable retrovirus infection when given once a week. This contrasts dramatically with the schedule used for the administration of nucleoside antiviral agents in animals or man, which typically has been three to four times a day. One cautionary note about hypericin must be stressed. St. John's wort is an ingredient of certain products sold

TABLE 3. Antiretroviral Activity of AZT, AZdU, and d4T in Different Cell Systems[a]

Cell Line/Viral Strain	AZT	AZdU	d4T
PBMC/LAV-1	0.002[b]	0.18	0.009
CEM/LAV-1[c]	0.002	0.013	0.38
Macrophage/HIV-DV	0.0008	0.03	0.16
ATH8/HIV-IIIB	0.32	0.4	—

[a] Results of Schinazi *et al.*[18]

[b] All data expressed as the concentration of nucleoside analogue required to reduce reverse transcriptase activity, p24 antigen expression, number of plaques, or viral cytopathic effect by 50%.

[c] Results of Shannon and Kahlon (Southern Research Institute).[18]

in health food stores. However, the proportion of hypericin present in these products is negligible. Further, severe toxicities might occur from any aberrant use of these health food products.

Like castanospermine, carbovir and hypericin have sparked interest in new classes of compounds that have potential antiviral activity. Whether they or their analogues will undergo full-scale development and eventual clinical trial in HIV-infected persons will be determined within the next year.

CONCLUSION

This brief update has presented information on current research efforts to discover and develop treatments for HIV infections and how to apply the information to a preclinical evaluation of traditional medicines. The information provided represents only a fraction of the active research directed toward the discovery of new drugs targeted to block each step of HIV replication. The continual discovery of new agents to treat HIV infections allows us to offer hope to clinicians that they will have other effective means of therapy for those infected with HIV and those with associated opportunistic infections.

REFERENCES

1. SMITH, D. H., R. A. BYRN, S. A. MASTERS, T. GREGORY, J. E. GROOPMAN & D. J. CAPON. 1987. Science **238:** 1704.
2. TILL, M. A., V. GHETIE, T. GREGORY, E. J. PATZER, J. P. PORTER, J. W. UHR, D. J. CAPON & E. S. VITETTA. 1989. Science **242:** 1166.
3. LIU, P. 1988. Analogues of Castansopermine with Anti-HIV Activity. National Cooperative Drug Discovery Group Meeting for AIDS. Oakland, CA.
4. LIN, T.-S., M. S. CHEN, C. MCLAREN, Y.-S. GAO, I. GHAZOULI & W. H. PRUSOFF. 1987. J. Med. Chem. **30:** 440.
5. MANSURI, M. M., J. E. STARRETT, I. GHASSOULI, M. J. M. HITCHCOCK, R. Z. STERZYCKI, V. BRANKOVAN, T. S. LIN, E. M. AUGUST, W. H. PRUSOFF, J. P. SOMMADOSSI & J. M. MARTIN. 1989. J. Med. Chem. **32:** In press.
6. BABA, M., R. PAUWELS, P. HERDEWIJN, E. DECLERCQ, J. DESMYTER & M. VANDEPUTTE. 1987. Biochem. Biophys. Res. Commun. **142:** 128.
7. SOMMADOSSI, J. P. & R. CARLISLE. 1987. Antimicrob. Agents Chemother. **31:** 452.
8. VINCE, R., M. HUA, J. BROWNELL, S. DALUGE, F. LEE, W. M. SHANNON, G. C. LAVELLE, J. QUALLS, O. S. WEISLOW, R. KISER, P. G. CANONICO, R. H. SCHULTZ, V. L. NARAYANAN, J. G. MAYO, R. H. SOEMAKER & M. R. BOYD.1988. Biochem. Biophys. Res. Commun. **156:** 1046.
9. MERUELO, D., G. LAVIE & D. LAVIE. 1988. Proc. Natl. Acad. Sci. USA **85:** 5230.
10. SUNKARA, P. S., T. L. BOWLIN, P. S. LIN & A. SJOERDSMA. 1987. Biochem. Biophys. Res. Commun. **148:** 206.
11. WALKER, B. D., M. KOWALSKI, W. C. GOH, K. KOZARSKY, M. KRIEGER, C. ROSEN, L. ROHRSCHNEIDER, W. A. HASELTINE& J. SODROSKI. 1987. Proc. Natl. Acad. Sci. USA **84:** 8120.
12. RUPRECHT, R. M., S. MELLANEY, J. ANDERSON & M. BROWNSON. J. Acq. Immun. Defic. Synd. In press.
13. MITSUYA, H. & S. BRODER. 1986. Proc. Natl. Acad. Sci. USA **83:** 1911.

14. HERDEWIJN, P., J. BALZARINI, E. DECLERCQ, R. PAUWELS, M. BABA, S. BRODER & H. VANDERHAEGHE. 1987. J. Med. Chem. **30:** 1270.
15. MITSUYA, H., K. J. WEINHOLD, P. A. FURMAN, M. H. ST. CLAIR, S. NUSINOFF LEHRMAN, R. C. GALLO, D. BOLOGNESI, D. W. BARRY & S. BRODER. 1986. Proc. Natl. Acad. Sci. USA **82:** 7096.
16. BILELLO, J. A., C. MACAULEY, M. BELL, R. A. YETTER, S. SHAPIRO & J. L. EISEMAN. 1988. National Cooperative Drug Discovery Groups Meeting. Oakland, CA.
17. BROCKMAN, H., F. KLUGE & H. MUXFELDT. 1957. Chem. Ber. **90:** 2302.
18. SCHINAZI, R. F., C. K. CHU, B. F. H. ERIKSSON, J. P. SOMMADOSSI, F. D. BOUDINOT, J. GALLO & H. MCCLURE. 1988. National Cooperative Drug Discovery Group Meeting for AIDS. Oakland, CA.
19. FARNSWORTH, N. R., O. AKERELE, A. S. BINGEL, D. D. SOEJARTO & Z. GUO. 1985. Udate le point. Bull. WHO **63:** 965.

The Influence of Different Sexual-Contact Patterns between Age Classes on the Predicted Demographic Impact of AIDS in Developing Countries

R. M. ANDERSON, T. W. NG, M. C. BOILY,
AND R. M. MAY

Parasite Epidemiology Research Group
Imperial College
London University
London SW7 2BB, England

INTRODUCTION

When and where the human immunodeficiency virus (HIV) first began to spread extensively in human communities cannot be determined on the basis of current serologic data. However, it appears probable that rapid spread began in the 1970s. Since that time period, the presence of the virus (HIV-1) has been reported by a majority of countries and the infection plus the disease it induces (AIDS) is now pandemic throughout the world. Since infection with HIV precedes the development of the disease AIDS by many years (current estimates suggest a mean incubation period of around 8-9 years; see Anderson and Medley,[1] and Bacchetti and Moss,[2]) current reports of AIDS cases are but a small fraction of those that will occur over the coming decades.

The World Health Organization (WHO) has identified three distinct patterns of infection and disease on the basis of the predominant risk behaviors for HIV, present in a defined community or country.[3] Pattern I is typified by the majority of cases occurring among homosexual or bisexual men and intravenous drug users. It occurs typically in industrialized countries in North America, Western Europe, Australia, New Zealand, and parts of Latin America. Pattern II is characterized by the majority of cases occurring among heterosexuals and is to be found in areas of Central, Eastern and Southern Africa, and in some areas of Latin America, especially the Caribbean. Pattern III is the disease that occurs in regions in which HIV has only recently been introduced and where the majority of cases of AIDS occur as a result of infected imported blood products and via sexual contact with individuals from pattern I or

[a] This work was aided by financial support from the Overseas Development Agency, U.K., and PANOS.

pattern II areas. Pattern III is observed in parts of Eastern Europe, North Africa, the Middle East, Asia and the Pacific (excluding Australia and New Zealand).

On a global scale the majority of AIDS cases have been reported from pattern I regions (particularly from the United States of America), but serologic surveys suggest that the virus is most widespread in the general population in certain countries that fall within the description of pattern II. Some regions in sub-Saharan Africa are particularly badly affected. The predominant route of transmission of HIV in these areas is via heterosexual contact, prompting governments and international agencies to urgently consider the degree to which the pandemic of AIDS will influence the demography and socioeconomic development of large areas of the world in the coming decades.[3]

As described in a recent publication,[4] precise scientific assessment of this problem is difficult at present because of our limited understanding of the epidemiology of the infection (HIV) and the disease (AIDS), particularly in populations in developing countries. Simple mathematical models that incorporate demographic and epidemiological processes of the transmission dynamics of HIV in heterosexual communities have been developed to aid in the assessment of the potential impact of AIDS.[4-6] These models suggest that the disease is capable of changing population growth rates from positive to negative values over time scales of a few decades. They also predicted that AIDS will have little impact on the dependency ratio of a population, defined as the number of children below age 15 and elderly people over 64 years, divided by the number of adults between 15 to 64 years. Such conclusions, however, are tentative at present because of the many uncertainties that surround parameter assignments and key assumptions concerning transmission.

In this paper we build on earlier work on the construction of demographic and epidemiologic models, to consider various refinements to model structure and parameter definitions. Specifically, we examine three areas: (1) the predicted influence of the infection and the disease on the age structure of populations in pattern II areas of the world, paying particular attention to the dependency ratio and various definitions of this ratio; (2) the significance of different patterns of sexual contact between the age classes of the two sexes; and (3) the impact of control measures, based on education and the use of condoms, on the predicted pattern of the epidemic over the coming decades.

The paper is therefore divided into three major sections which examine the areas identified above. The paper begins with two introductory sections, the first describing model structure and methods of numerical computation, and the second detailing parameter assignments. The paper ends with a brief discussion of the major conclusions derived from model analysis and areas for future research.

MODEL STRUCTURE, ANALYSIS, AND ASSUMPTIONS

Structure

The structure of the model employed in our analysis is similar to that described by May and Anderson[5,6] and Anderson *et al.*[4] It combines descriptions of the basic epidemiologic processes involved in the transmission of HIV with the definition of the demographic processes that determine the pattern of human population growth and age structure.

We consider a closed heterosexual population (no immigration or emigration) where $N_k(a,t)$ denotes the number (or density) of people of sex k($k = 1$ denotes females and $k = 2$ denotes males) of age a at time t. Aside from the stratification by age (a) and sex (k), the population is divided into six subpopulations denoting those susceptible to infection (i.e., uninfected), $X_k(a,t)$; those infected, $Y_{i,k}(a,t)$; those infected who recover and do not develop AIDS (assumed to be noninfectious), $Z_k(a,t)$; and those infected who develop AIDS, $A_k(a,t)$. The infected class, $Y_k(a,t)$ is divided into three subgroups containing individuals of varying degrees of infectiousness[6,7]: $Y_{1,k}(a,t)$, $Y_{2,k}(a,t)$, and $Y_{3,k}(a,t)$.

Sexually mature susceptible persons ("susceptibles") are assumed to acquire infection via sexual contact with an infected partner at a rate $\lambda_k(a,t)$. Newly born infants are assumed to acquire infection vertically from infected mothers. A fraction $(1 - \epsilon)$ of babies born to infected mothers is assumed to acquire the HIV infection. The model does not incorporate transmission via blood transfusions or via contaminated injecting equipment.

The model is compartmental in structure, where susceptibles, on acquiring infection, pass to the first infection class $Y_{1,k}(a,t)$ at a per capita rate $\lambda_k(a,t)$ and leave at a rate $\gamma_{1,k}(a,t)$ to join the second infectious class $Y_{2,k}(a,t)$. They leave this class at a per capita rate $\gamma_{2,k}(a,t)$. In the third class a fraction $\rho_k(a,t)$ "recovers" to join a noninfectious class $Z_k(a,t)$, while the remaining fraction $(1 - \rho_k(a,t))$ develops AIDS and joins the class $A_k(a,t)$. In both cases the per capita rate of leaving $Y_{3,k}(a,t)$ is $\gamma_{3,k}(a,t)$. In the AIDS class individuals die at a rate $\alpha_k(a,t)$. In the present study we assume that $\rho_k(a,t) = 0$ for all values of a,t and k. The average incubation period of the disease AIDS, $T_k(a)$, is defined by the sum of the average durations of stay in the three infected classes $Y_{i,k}(a,t)$, where

$$T_k(a) = \sum_{i=1}^{3} 1/\gamma_{i,k}(a)$$

We assume that the incubation period in those who acquire infection via sexual contact is constant and independent of age and sex. In the case of infants infected via vertical transmission, we assume, on the basis of current evidence,[1,9] that infected individuals ("infecteds") develop AIDS rapidly and are therefore effectively removed from the population soon after birth. The term $\mu_k(a,t)$ defines the background per capita death rate of individuals of sex k, age a, at time t.

The system of equations describing changes in the numbers of individuals, of age a at time t, in each of the five classes is defined as follows:

$$\partial X_k(a,t)/\partial t + \partial X_k(a,t)/\partial a = -(\lambda_k(a,t) + \mu_k(a,t))X_k(a,t)$$

$$\partial Y_{1,k}(a,t)/\partial t + \partial Y_{1,k}(a,t)/\partial a = \lambda_k(a,t)X_k(a,t) - [\gamma_{1,k}(a,t) + \mu_k(a,t)]Y_{1,k}(a,t)$$

$$\partial Y_{2,k}(a,t)/\partial t + \partial Y_{2,k}(a,t)/\partial a = \gamma_{1,k}(a,t)Y_{1,k}(a,t) - [\gamma_{2,k}(a,t) + \mu_k(a,t)]Y_{2,k}(a,t)$$

$$\partial Y_{3,k}(a,t)/\partial t + \partial Y_{3,k}(a,t)/\partial a = \gamma_{2,k}(a,t)Y_{2,k}(a,t) - [\gamma_{3,k}(a,t) + \mu_k(a,t)]Y_{3,k}(a,t)$$

$$\partial Z_k(a,t)/\partial t + \partial Z_k(a,t)/\partial a = \rho_k(a,t)\gamma_{3,k}(a,t)Y_{3,k}(a,t) - \mu_k(a,t)Z_k(a,t)$$

$$\partial A_k(a,t)/\partial t + \partial A_k(a,t)/\partial a = (1 - \rho_k(a,t))\gamma_{3,k}(a,t)Y_{3,k}(a,t) - [\mu_k(a,t) + \alpha_k(a,t)]A_k(a,t)$$

The force, or per capita rate, of infection (via horizontal (= sexual) transmission) $\lambda_k(a,t)$ is defined as

$$\lambda_k(a,t) = \left\{\int_{a_1}^{a_2} c_k(a,a',t)j_k(a,a',t)[\beta_{1,k}Y_{1,k'}(a',t) + \beta_{2,k}(t)Y_{2,k'}(a',t) + \beta_{3,k}Y_{3,k'}(a',t) + q_kA_{k'}(a,'t)]\,da'\right\} \Big/ \left\{\int_{a_1}^{a_2} j(a,a',t)N_{k'}(a',t)\,da'\right\} \tag{1}$$

Here k denotes one sex and k' the opposite sex. In Equation **1**, $N_k(a,t)$ defines the total number of males ($k = 1$) or females ($k = 2$) of age a at time t. It is assumed in this formulation that all infecteds pass into the AIDS class (i.e., $Z_k(a,t) = 0$). The term $\beta_{i,k}(t)$ defines the probability of transmission for sex k (per partnership contact) arising from contacts between susceptibles and infecteds in infectious class $i(i = 1, 2, 3)$. The parameter q_k denotes the proportion of the AIDS class ($k = 1$ for females and $k = 2$ for males) who are sexually active and therefore capable of transmitting the virus. The function $j_k(a,a',t)$ defines the probability that a susceptible of sex k and age a will choose a partner of age a' of the opposite sex at time t. The limits a_1 and a_2 define, respectively, the lower and upper age bounds of sexual activity. The term $c_k(a,a',t)$ denotes the effective mean rate of sexual partner change of age a sex k with individuals of opposite sex in age class a' at time t. As described by May and Anderson[10] and Anderson *et al.*[11] the overall effective rate c (over all age classes) is not simply the mean m_k, but is more accurately described by the equation

$$c_k(t) = m_k(t) + \sigma_k^2(t)/m_k(t) \tag{2}$$

where σ_k^2 is the variance of the rate of sexual-partner change of sex k.

The case or basic reproductive rate of infection (the average number of secondary cases generated by one primary case in a susceptible population[11]), R_0, is approximately given by

$$R_o = (\beta_1 c_1 \beta_2 c_2)^{1/2} T \tag{3}$$

where β_k denotes the average probability of infection arising from contact with the opposite sex over the average incubation period T for sex k. Similarly c_k denotes the effective mean rate of sexual partner change for sex k (it is assumed that the magnitude of T is independent of sex).

For clarity of exposition we denote X_k, Y_{ik}, Z_k, and A_k as the components of a vector $U_k(a,t)$ for a given sex k. The model can now be expressed in a more concise form where

$$\frac{\partial}{\partial t} U_k(a,t) + \frac{\partial}{\partial a} U_k(a,t) = F_k[\lambda_k(a,t),\ \mu(a,t),\ \gamma_{i,k}(a,t),\ \rho_k(a,t),\ U_k(a,t)]U_k(a,t) \tag{4}$$

For the hyperbolic system of Equation **4** to be well posed, we require an initial conditon of the form

$$U_k(a,0) = U_{o,k}(a) \tag{5}$$

where $U_{o,k}(a)$ defines the age distribution in each of the poulation compartments of the vector at time $t = 0$. In a developing country, the introduction of the infection (at time $t = 0$) will result from the arrival of a few infecteds, say in class $Y_{1,k}(a,0)$. We assume that the age distribution in the susceptible population is approximately exponential in form (i.e., $\mu(a,t) =$ constant for all values of a) with $(1 - \epsilon)$ being the proportion of children born that are infected.

The boundary condition, or renewal equation, is given by

$$U_k(o,t) = [X_k(o,t),\ Y_{1k}(o,t),\ o,o,o,o]$$

where

$$X_k(o,t) = 1/2 \int_{b_1}^{b_2} m_1(a,t)X_1(a,t)\,da + 1/2 \int_{b_1}^{b_2} (\epsilon)[m_2(a,t)Y_{11}(a,t) + m_3(a,t)Y_{21}(a,t) + m_4(a,t)Y_{31}(a,t) + m_5(a,t)Z_1(a,t) + m_6(a,t)A_1(a,t)]\,da, \quad \text{and}$$

$$Y_{1,k}(o,t) = 1/2 \int_{b_1}^{b_2} (1 - \epsilon)[m_2(a,t)Y_{11}(a,t) + m_3(a,t)Y_{21}(a,t) + m_4(a,t)Y_{31}(a,t) + m_5(a,t)Z_1(a,t) + m_6(a,t)A_1(a,t)]\,da.$$

The factor 1/2 denotes the assumption of a 1:1 sex ratio of males to females at birth and m_i, $i = 1, 2, 3, 4, 5, 6$ represents fertility rates for each infection compartment. With the assumption that all infecteds progress to AIDS such that $Z_k(a,t) = 0$ for all a and t, then $m_5 = 0$. We also assume that AIDS patients are unable to produce viable offspring such that $m_6 = 0$. For the remaining classes we assume that $m_i(a,t) = m(a)$ for all values of i and t.

Numerical Methods

The first-order hyperbolic system can be solved numerically using an explicit finite difference method, with a backward difference in age and a forward difference in time, by the approximation;

$$\frac{\partial}{\partial t} V \approx (V_{j,n+1} - V_{j,n})/\delta t$$

and

$$\frac{\partial V}{\partial a} \approx (V_{j,n} - V_{j-1,n})/\delta a$$

The resulting finite different scheme can be written as

$$V_{j,n+1} = V_{j-1,n} + (1 - \rho)V_{j,n} + \delta t. f_{j,n}(\lambda_{j,n}, V_{j,n})V_{j,n} \tag{7}$$

where $V_{j,n}$ are compartments of $U_{j,n}$ at $a = j\delta a$, $j = 1, 2, 3 \ldots$, $t = n\delta t$, $n = 1, 2, 3 \ldots$ and $\rho = \delta t/\delta a$ such that $0<\rho<1$. $V_{o,n}$ for $n = 1, 2, \ldots$ is computed from the boundary condition using a guadrature scheme. The system can be integrated along the characteristic direction by using the transformation, t − a = w, $t = s$, such that Equation **4** becomes

$$\frac{\partial}{\partial s} U_k(w,s) = F_k[U_k(s - w,s)]U_k(w,s) \tag{8}$$

Finite differing scheme for Equation **8** can then be written as

$$V_{j,n} = V_{j-1,n} + \delta t[f_{j-1,n}(V_{j-1,n})]V_{j-1,n} \tag{9}$$

The above scheme is easy to implement, explicitly stable, and of order-one accuracy.

Dependency Ratio

The dependency ratio $d(t)$ of a population at time t is typically defined as the size of the population of infants and children ($< b_1$ years of age) plus elderly people ($> b_2$ years of age) divided by the population of productive teenagers and adults (aged b_1 to b_2 years of age).[4]

$$d(t) = \left\{\sum_{k=1}^{2}\left[\left[\int_0^{b_1} N_k(a,t)\,da + \int_{b_2}^{\infty} N_k(a,t)\,da\right]\right]\right\} \Big/ \left\{\sum_{k=1}^{2}\int_{b_1}^{b_2} N_k(a,t)\,da\right\} \tag{10}$$

Typical values for b_1 and b_2 are 15 and 64 years of age, respectively. This definition ignores the extra burden imposed on the working population by AIDS. In reality the core of AIDS patients will itself impose an extra burden on those non-AIDS individuals in the working and productive age groups (ages b_1 to b_2).

To take account of this problem in the context of the AIDS epidemic in a defined country we define a new disease-related dependency ratio D as

$$D(t) = \left\{\sum_{k=1}^{2}\left[\left[\int_0^{b_1} N_k(a,t)\,da + \int_{b_2}^{\infty} N_k(a,t)\,da + W\int_{b_1}^{b_2} A_k(a,t)\,da\right]\right]\right\} \Big/ \left\{\sum_{k=1}^{2}\int_{b_1}^{b_2}[N_k(a,t) - A_k(a,t)]da\right\} \tag{11}$$

Here W denotes a weighting factor ($W > 0$) representing the extra burden imposed by the care of adult AIDS patients. Note that the number of adult AIDS patients is subtracted from the denominator and added in a weighted manner (W) to the numerator. More generally, we could modify the disease-related dependency ratio to take account of any extra burden (over that present in an uninfected population) imposed by AIDS patients among the child-age classes, or infected but non-AIDS patients in the $Y_i(a,t)$ classes ($i = 1, 2, 3$).

The Force or Rate of Infection

The most important assumptions, with respect to determining the pattern of spread of infection within the population, are embodied in the term represented in Equation 1, which defines the per capita rate at which a susceptible individual of sex k and age a acquires infection at time t via sexual contact with an infected person of the opposite sex. If we ignore the age and sex structure of the population and assume that the probability of transmission, β, is constant over the three infected classes and that AIDS patients are not sexually active, then Equation 1 simplifies to

$$\lambda(t) = \beta c\left(\sum_{i=1}^{3} Y_i(t)\right)/N(t) \tag{12}$$

In other words, we have assumed that the per capita rate is proportional to the probability of transmission, β, times the effective average rate of sexual-partner change, c, times the proportion of sexual contacts that are with infected persons, $\sum_{i=1}^{3} Y_i(t)/N(t)$. This form of λ is based on the assumption of homogeneous mixing within the sexually active population. However, a crude allowance is made for heterogeneity in sexual activity within the population by the definition of the effective rate of sexual-partner change, c (see Equation **2**).[10,11] For heterosexual transmission, the complication of unequal transmission probabilities between the sexes and differences in effective average rates of sexual-partner change can be included by the insertion of a subscript k to denote sex (i.e., $k = 1$ is female, $k = 2$ is male) such that

$$\lambda_1(t) = \beta_1 c_1(t)\left(\sum_{i=1}^{3} Y_{i,2}(t)/N_2(t)\right) \quad \textbf{(13)}$$

More generally, as depicted in Equation **1**, we can introduce the added complication of heterogeneity in sexual contacts between the different age classes of the two sexes by the introduction of the function $j_k(a,a't)$, which defines the probability that a susceptible of sex k and age a will choose a partner of age a' of the opposite sex at time t. This formulation allows us to take account of differences by age in the way males and females choose sexual partners. In many developing and developed countries there is a tendency for men to choose female sexual partners of a younger age than themselves. Age- and sex-stratified data on the incidence of HIV infection (proportions seropositive by age and sex) and the incidence of AIDS provide a clear indication of this trend. For example, in Figure 1, which reecords the reported incidence of AIDS by age and sex in Uganda up to July 31, 1988, the age distribution of cases among females is more skewed to the younger age classes than is the equivalent distribution among males.

The assumptions embodied in Equation **1**, however, give rise to a major complication if the transmission probabilities between females to males, and males to females,

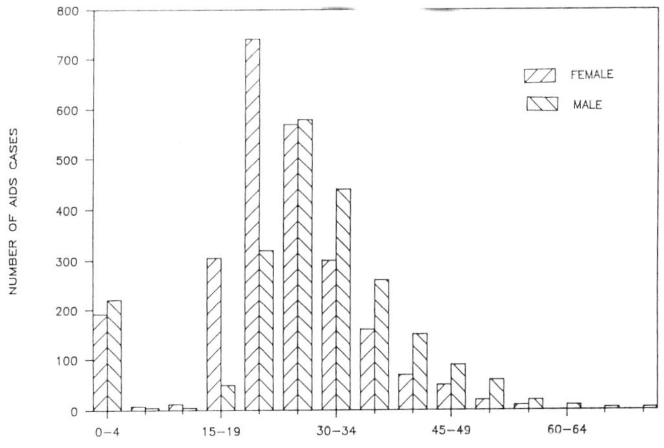

FIGURE 1. Age and sex distribution of reported cases of AIDS in Uganda up to the end of July 1988. (SOURCE: Berkley, Okware, and Naamura.[21]) *Vertical axis:* number of AIDS cases; *horizontal axis:* age group of patients (years).

are not equal (i.e., $\beta_1 \neq \beta_2$). If the transmission probability from males to females (β_1) is greater in magnitude than that for females to males ($\beta_1 > \beta_2$), then more women than men will become infected and die from AIDS. As the epidemic progresses, the sex ratio in the population will therefore shift in favor of males. A problem then arises in the interpretation and definition of the effective rates of sexual-partner change among females ($c_1(a,a',t)$) and males ($c_2(a',a,t)$) as the sex ratio changes. If we assume that the effective rate of sexual-partner change of the men ($c_2(a',a,t)$) remains unchanged, this would imply that the effective rate of partner change among females rises to take account of the increasing bias in the sex ratio towards men as the epidemic unfolds. In other words, a decreasing proportion of women would have to accommodate an unchanged pattern of sexual activity among a growing proportion of men.

At present it is not possible to judge what will happen under such circumstances. However, what is clear when $\beta_1 = \beta_2$ is that the mean rates of sexual-partner change for the two sexes must be formulated as functions of age and time to accommodate changes in the sex ratio of the population (i.e., $c_1(a,a',t)$ and $c_2(a',a,t)$, since the epidemic imposes unequal mortality rates on males and females. This is necessary to ensure that the total number of partnerships made by women in age class a with men in age class a' is equal to the total number of partnerships made by men in age class a' with women in age class a.

With respect to the partner-choice function, $j_k(a,a',t)$, there are three constraints that must be satisfied. These can be expressed as follows:

$$N_1(a,t)c_1(a,a',t)j_1(a,a',t) = N_2(a',t)c_2(a',a,t)j_2(a',a,t) \quad \textbf{(14)}$$

$$\int_0^\infty j_k(a,a',t)\, da' = 1 \quad \text{for all} \quad t > 0 \quad \textbf{(15)}$$

and

$$1 \leq j_k(a,a',t) \geq 0 \quad \textbf{(16)}$$

To satisfy constraint **(14)**, as the age and sex distribution of the population changes during the course of the AIDS epidemic, we can alter either the elements of the partner-choice functions, or change the age-dependent mean rates of sexual-partner change, or alter both. The simplest option is to assume that the partner-choice functions of both sexes ($j_k(a,a',t)$) remain constant through time, to represent an "ideal" pattern of sexual-partner choice in the absence of availability constraints, and that the mean rates of sexual-partner change of a given sex and age class change through time in accord with the availability of partners of the opposite sex in the preferred age classes.

A simple way of achieving this aim[12] is as follows: We assume that the effective mean rate of sexual-partner change of one sex depends on the number of persons of the opposite sex, and that their choice with respect to age depends on the age distribution of the opposite sex. We define

$$c_k(a,a',t) = \bar{c}_k(a,a')\, N_k(a',t)/[N_1(t) + N_2(t)] \quad \textbf{(17)}$$

where the term $\bar{c}_k(a,a')$ is set as an initial condition of sexual activity at the start of the epidemic such that

$$\bar{c}_1(a,a') = c_1(a,a',o)[N_1(o) + N_2(o)]/N_2(a,o)$$

or

$$\bar{c}_2(a',a) = c_2(a',a,o)[N_1(o) + N_2(o)]/N_1(a,o). \quad \textbf{(18)}$$

Having fixed $c_k(a',a,o)$ and $j_k(a,a',o)$ at the start of the epidemic, such that Equations **14**, **15**, and **16** are satisfied, it can be shown that the same equations are satisfied for all values of t, provided that $c_k(a,a',t)$ is as defined in Equation **17** and **18**. The simple idea embodied in these equations is that the ideal partner-choice pattern ($j_k(a,a',t)$) remains unaltered as age and sex distribution change, but that the effective mean rates of partner change of either sex alter as the epidemic changes the age and sex distribution of the population.

PARAMETER ASSIGNMENTS

Demography

At the start of the epidemic ($t = 0$) the total population size is set at 16.6 million people with equal numbers of males and females. The age-specific fertility and mortality rates were set as defined in TABLE 1 to mimic the patterns recorded in a typical sub-

TABLE 1. Age-Specific Fertility and Mortality Rates[a]

Age Class (yr)	Mortality Rate $\mu(a)$ (yr^{-1})	Fertility Rate $n(a)$ (per female/yr)
0-1	0.110	0.0
1-5	0.014	0.0
5-10	0.003	0.0
10-15	0.002	0.0
15-20	0.005	0.079
20-25	0.005	0.368
25-30	0.005	0.392
30-35	0.005	0.311
35-40	0.006	0.226
40-45	0.008	0.105
45-50	0.011	0.014
50-55	0.015	0.0
55-60	0.024	0.0
60+	0.039	0.0

[a] Instantaneous rates are defined as yr.$^{-1}$

Saharan African country with a net population growth rate between 3-4% per annum (set at 3.8% per annum). For ease of representation and numerical solution, the age distribution of the population was divided into a series of classes denoting those less than 1 year of age, those between 1 and 4 years of age, and, thereafter, those aged progressively in 5-year age increments.

The sexually active age classes were assumed to be between 15 years of age to 50 years of age. For the purpose of calculating dependency ratios (see Equations **10** and **11**), the parameters b_1 and b_2 were set at 15 years and 64 years, respectively. At time $t = 0$, the dependency ratio was approximately 1.12, and various values of the weighting factor, W, were applied in different simulations (i.e., $W = 0$, 1, 2 and 3). The value of 1.12 in the uninfected population, as determined by the age-specific mortality rates, is similar to that observed in countries such as Kenya and Uganda (see Table 1 in Anderson *et al.*[4]).

Epidemiology

The assignment of values to the numerous epidemiologic parameters defined in the model is difficult at present because of the many uncertainties that sourround both the key transmission processes and the typical course of infection in individual patients.[1,4,10] Past work on mathematical models of the transmission dynamics and demographic impact of HIV and AIDS has indicated that predicted patterns of population change through time are very sensitive to the magnitudes of certain key parameters.[4] Knowledge about HIV and AIDS in developing countries is very limited at present, hence certain of our parameter assignments are based on published studies of the epidemiology of infection and disease in North America and Europe.

Current estimates of the incubation period of the disease in adults, based on studies of male homosexual and transfusion recipients in developed countries, suggest a mean period of approximately 8–9 years from the point of infection.[2,13] Other studies tentatively suggest that there may be two periods of peak infectiousness, one shortly after infection, and perhaps lasting for 6 months, and the other as patients progress to ARC and AIDS, perhaps lasting for 2 years. In between these two periods, it appears as though many patients are of low or negligible infectiousness. On the basis of this information (admittedly tentative at present and not necessarily representative of infection in African patients), we assume that the rates of progression through the three infectious classes, $Y_i(a,t)$, are 2.0 yr^{-1}, 0.182 yr^{-1}, and 0.5 yr^{-1} (the magnitudes of the γ_{ki} values) for both sexes, giving average duration of stay in each of the three classes ($i = 1, 2, 3$) of 0.5 yr, 5.5 yr, and 2 yr, respectively. The sum of these periods gives an average incubation period of 8 yr. Disease progression in infected infants is known to be more rapid than that in adults and we choose an average incubation period of 2 yr with equal rates of progression via each of the three infected classes. Infected infants are assumed not to contribute to transmission within the general population. Limited studies of the efficiency of vertical transmission in Europe and North America suggest values in the range of 0%–65%, with a mean value around 40%–50%, depending on when the birth occurs during the long and variable incubation period of the disease in the mother. Two recent studies in Africa suggest figures of 50%–60% (see Table 2 in Anderson and Medley.[1]) We choose an ϵ value of 0.5 to represent a 50% efficiency of transmission to babies born to mothers in any of the infected classes (i.e., the $Y_{1,i}(a,t)$ class and the $A_1(a,t)$ class.)

TABLE 2. Probabilities $j_k(a,a')$ for a Person of Age a to Chose a Sexual Partner of the Opposite Sex of Age a'.

Age Group (yr)	a' 15-20	20-25	25-30	30-35	35-40	40-45	45-50
a			k = 1, female choice of males				
15-20	0.2548	0.3345	0.1363	0.1033	0.0769	0.0558	0.0385
20-25	0.2548	0.1713	0.3255	0.0968	0.0704	0.0493	0.0319
25-30	0.2548	0.1630	0.1215	0.3341	0.0621	0.0409	0.0236
30-35	0.2548	0.1528	0.1110	0.0780	0.3601	0.0305	0.0132
35-40	0.2548	0.1394	0.0979	0.0648	0.0385	0.4046	0.0000
40-45	0.2548	0.1227	0.0812	0.0481	0.0218	0.0006	0.4708
45-50	0.2548	0.2039	0.1624	0.1294	0.1031	0.0819	0.0646
			k = 2, male choice of females				
15-20	0.2548	0.2039	0.1624	0.1294	0.1031	0.0819	0.0646
20-25	0.4178	0.1713	0.1298	0.0968	0.0704	0.0493	0.0646
25-30	0.2138	0.4087	0.1215	0.0884	0.0621	0.0409	0.0646
30-35	0.2034	0.1525	0.4195	0.0780	0.0516	0.0305	0.0646
35-40	0.1902	0.1394	0.0979	0.4521	0.0385	0.0173	0.0646
40-45	0.1735	0.1227	0.0812	0.0481	0.5092	0.0006	0.0646
45-50	0.1517	0.1009	0.0594	0.0264	0.0000	0.5970	0.0646

We assume that the life expectancy of an AIDS patient is approximately 1 year ($\alpha = 1$ yr^{-1}) and that all infected persons progress to AIDS (with a mean incubation period $T = 8$ yr). The fraction who will progress is uncertain at present, but a growing body of evidence suggests that it will be a very high proportion (if not unity) of those infected.[2]

Estimates of the magnitude of the transmission probability (defined per partnership) vary widely among different studies (see Table 2 in May and Anderson[14] and Tables 1 and 2 in Johnson and Laga.[15]) In one of the most detailed studies, Peterman *et al.*[14] arrive at the rough estimates of $\beta_1 \approx 0.2$ (male to female) and $\beta_1 \approx 0.1$ (female to male). In numerical simulations in which we set $\beta_1 = \beta_2$, we use a value of 0.1 per partnership and assume that this is related to periods of infectiousness during the average incubation period of 8 years. Indirectly, rough estimates of the parameter combination βc can be obtained from a knowledge of the doubling time of the epidemic (longitudinal data on the incidence of either HIV infection or AIDS) in its early stages (assuming that $\beta_1 c_1 = \beta_2 c$).[4,10] As described by May and Anderson,[14] the relationship between βc and the doubling time, t_d, is given approximately by

$$\beta c \approx [\ln(2)/t_d] + 1/D \tag{19}$$

where D is the average period over which individuals may be capable of transmitting the infection (i.e., $D \approx 8$ yr). Published data on doubling times of the epidemic in sub-Saharan African countries suggest values in the range of 1 to 3.5 years during the early stages of the epidemic (see Table 2 in Anderson *et al.*[4]). A value of $t_d = 1$ yr, with D set at 8 yr, yields an estimate of βc of approximately 0.82 yr^{-1}. At t_d value of 3.5 yr yields an estimate of βc of approximately 0.32 yr^{-1}. With a β value of 0.1, these figures produce estimates of c, the effective average rate of sexual-partner change, of 8.2 and 3.2, respectively. A recent review of rates of sexual-partner change in developed and developing countries revealed an interesting relationship between the mean and variance of the distributions of such rates in a variety of communities.[6] A body of empirical data suggests that the mean, m, is related to the variance, σ^2, by a simple power law of the form

$$\sigma^2 = am^b \tag{20}$$

where a and b are coefficients ($a = 0.555$ and $b = 3.231$ in the review of Anderson and May[6]). The estimates of c derived above (i.e., values of 8 for a doubling time of 1 yr, and 3 for a doubling time of 3.5 yr), in conjunction with Equations **20** and **2** (which defines the relationship between c, m and σ^2), give the approximate results that doubling times of the order of 1 to 3.5 yr suggest mean rates of sexual-partner change of between 1.3 to 2.2 new partners per year. It must be stressed that these estimates are extremely crude and that their derivation is only made in the absence of good quantitative data on sexual habits in African countries. A few preliminary studies do suggest higher rates of sexual-partner change among heterosexuals in certain African communities than those reported in studies carried out in Europe and North America (see Konings *et al.*[17] and Table 4 in Anderson *et al.*[18]). In our numerical studies we examine population trends with values of βc in the range of 0.4 to 1.0 in different simulations.

The Choice of Sexual Partners

As indicated in the previous section, current knowledge of the distribution of rates of sexual-partner change in developed countries is extremely limited at present. The data that are available simply record summary statistics of the distribution, such as the mean and the variance per unit of time.[17] We are not aware of any data that allow us to estimate the form of the "partner choice by age" function $j_k(a,a',t)$ [note that we set $j_k(a,a',t) = j_k(a,a',o) = j_k(a,a')$]. To simplify matters, we choose values for a discrete approximation of the function based upon the division of the age variable into discrete age classes denoting 5-year age spans (see TABLE 1 for the precise divisions in the age range from 15 to 50 years). Our aim is to crudely mirror the trend recorded in FIGURE 1 (AIDS cases in Uganda stratified by age and sex), in which males appear, on average, to choose female sexual partners of a younger age than themselves. We examine two cases. The first is termed *restricted* mixing, and represents a pattern in which individuals only choose sexual partners from their own age class (the diagonal elements of the partner-choice matrix set at unity in value, all other elements set to zero). The second is termed *preferred* mixing and represents a pattern in which males, on average, choose female partners younger than themselves. For the purpose of illustration TABLE 2 records the elements of the partner choice matrices employed in simulations of the second pattern of behavior. The matrices satisfy the constraints in Equations **14**, **15**, and **16**. They are but a crude mirror of the pattern in which males choose sexual partners of a younger age. In calculating the elements of the two matrices, the terms in the male-choice-of-females matrix were set first and then the elements of the female-choice-of-males matrix were derived after fixing the values in the first column of the matrix. The remaining elements were calculated on the basis of the contraints defined in Equations **14**, **15**, and **16**.

TEMPORAL CHANGES IN POPULATION SIZE AND STRUCTURE

General Trends

This section examines the predicted impact of the HIV epidemic, as it progresses through time from the point of introduction, on the dependency ratio of the population. As discussed in the section on model structure, we consider changes in the ratio D (Eq. **11**), making different assumptions about the magnitude of the weighting factor W, which denotes the extra burden imposed by the care of AIDS patients in the adult age classes. However, before proceeding to consider this problem we first detail some general results concerning model predictions of the impact of AIDS on population size and the distribution of infection in the different age classes of the population. We also examine the impact of unequal transmission probabilities for HIV from male to female and vice versa ($\beta_1 \neq \beta_2$). In certain of the numerical simulations presented in this section, the doubling time of the epidemic in its early stages was set at t_d = 2.5 yr and the age-dependent partner-choice matrix was as defined in TABLE 2. For the cases $\beta_1 = \beta_2$ and $\beta_1 \neq \beta_2$, a doubling time of 2.5 yr and an average period over which individuals may be infectious of 8 yr results in an R_0 value of approximately 3.2 (i.e., in the early stages of the epidemic it is assumed that for transmission by sexual contact each primary case of infection gives rise to 3.2 secondary cases). In these circumstances, when $\beta_1 - \beta_2$ the value of βc is set at 0.402. We also examine the case in which the transmission probability from infected males to susceptible females is three times that from infected females to susceptible males such that $\beta_1 c_1 = 3\beta_2 c_2$. In this case, to give a doubling time of 2.5 yr, and an R_0 value of 3.2, $\beta_2 c_2$ is set at 0.23 yr^{-1}.[14] In other simulations, we set the doubling time of the epidemic (in its early stages) at 1.5 yr to give an R_0 value of 4.7. With $\beta_1 c_1 = \beta_2 c_2$ this gives a βc value of 0.587 yr^{-1}. When $\beta_1 c_1 = 3\beta_2 c_2$, a $\beta_2 c_2$ value of 0.339yr^{-1} is obtained. In all simulations, we ignore the complications introduced by two peaks of infectious ness during the incubation period. We consider an average value of β_k over the average incubation period, and focus on the effects of differences in the magnitude of β_k between the two sexes.

Each numerical simulation was run over a time period of 100 years after the introduction of the infection. The complexity of the model's structure generates a large quantity of numerical information over the long simulation time period, representing changes by age and sex of the numbers of susceptibles, infecteds, and persons with AIDS as the epidemic develops. We summarize this information in graphic form by considering (1) changes through time in the total population size, the total number of cases of AIDS and the proportion of infected persons; (2) age- and sex-stratified changes in population size, AIDS cases, and HIV-infected persons; and (3) changes through time in the dependency ratio, D, of the population.

With the parameter assignments detailed in the preceding section and in the paragraphs above, the epidemic is able to change a positive net population growth rate of 3.8% per annum prior to the introduction of the virus to a negative rate over a time scale of approximately 50 to 60 years. An illustration of this point is presented in FIGURE 2a, where temporal changes in total population size are recorded for an R_0 value of 3.2 in simulations in which $\beta_1 c_1 = \beta_2 c_2$ and $\beta_1 c_1 = 3\beta_1 c_2$. Note than when the probability of transmission is higher from infected male to susceptible female than vice versa, the disease has a greater impact on population growth and decline. This is because of the impact of high infection among females on the reproductive

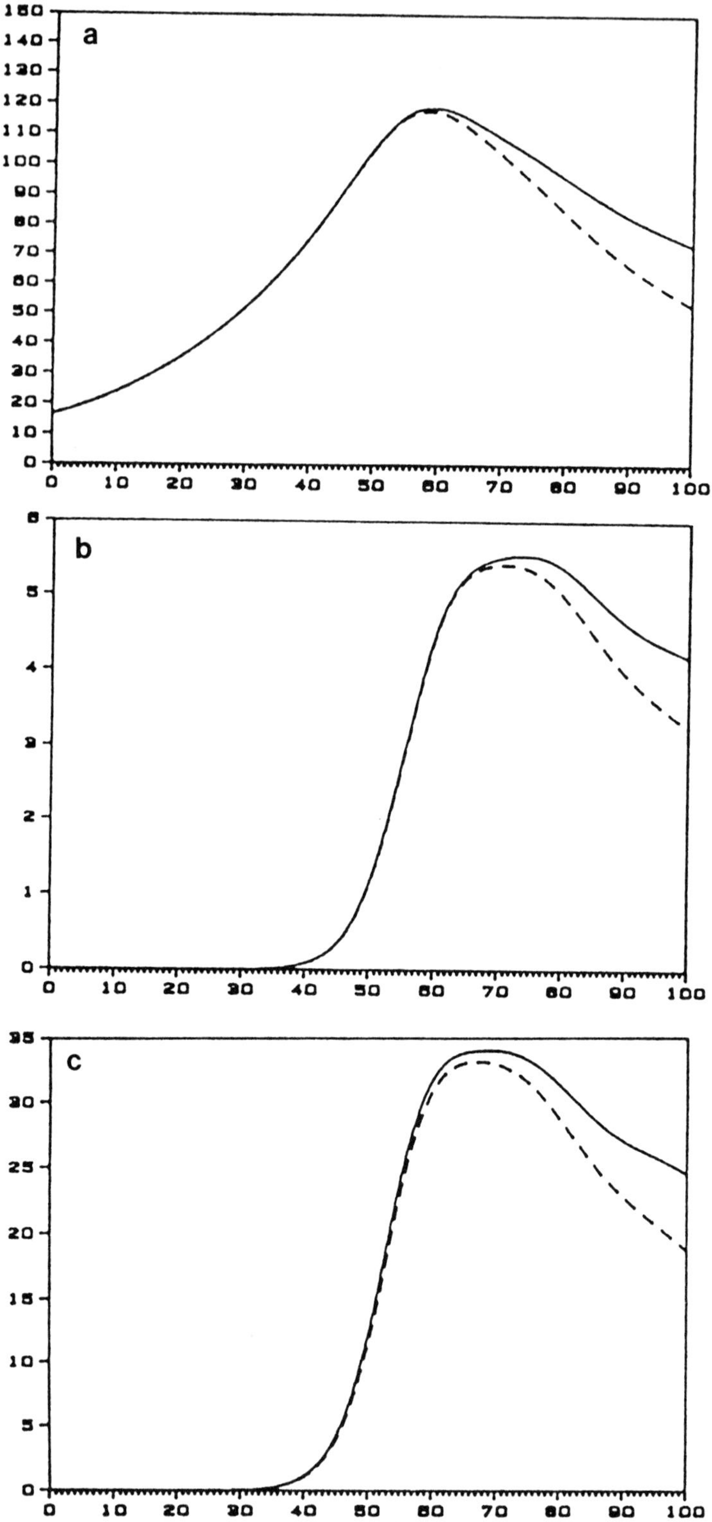
a
0 10 20 30 40 50 60 70 80 90 100 110 120 130 140 150
0 10 20 30 40 50 60 70 80 90 100
b
0 1 2 3 4 5 6
0 10 20 30 40 50 60 70 80 90 100
c
0 5 10 15 20 25 30 35
0 10 20 30 40 50 60 70 80 90 100

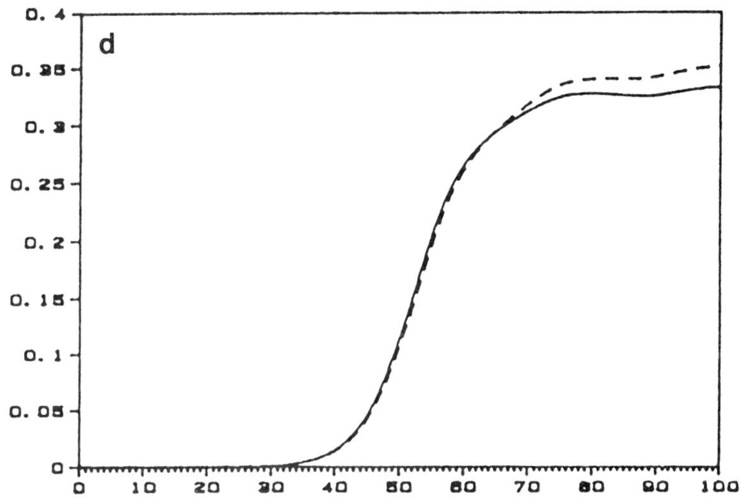

▲
◀ **FIGURE 2.** The influence of unequal transmission probabilities from male to female and female to male. The results from two simulations are recorded in four graphs with $\beta_1 c_1 = \beta_2 c_2$ (*solid line*) and $\beta_1 c_1 = 3\beta_2 c_2$ (*broken line*). Parameter values were set as described in the text with $R_0 = 3.2$ and $t_d = 2.5$ yr. *Vertical axes:* (**a**) Changes in total population size (millions); (**b**) changes in the number of persons with AIDS (millions); (**c**) changes in the total number infected (millions); and (**d**) changes in the proportion infected. *Horizontal axes:* time in years.

potential of the population. FIGURES 2b, c, and d record temporal trends in the number of AIDS cases, the number of infected persons, and the proportion infected, respectively, for both sets of values. Note how slowly the epidemic progresses over the first 20 to 40 years, followed by a rapid "explosion" over the subsequent 10 years. In the case where $\beta_1 c_1 = 3\beta_2 c_2$, the proportion of females infected is higher, but not by a factor of 3 (FIG. 3). This is because of the assumptions made in the transmission term that decrease the effective rate of sexual-partner change among males as the sex ratio changes in the population by virtue of a larger number of female deaths as a result of AIDS (due to the mixing by sex and age function).

If the case reproductive rate of infection, R_0, is increased to a value of 4.7 (a doubling time of 1.5 yr), the epidemic develops more rapidly and the net population growth rate changes from positive to negative after about 25 years after the introduction of the infection (FIG. 4, where $\beta_1 c_1 = \beta_2 c_2$). In all cases, note that the peak in the number infected with HIV precedes the peak in the number of persons with AIDS by many years because of the long incubation period of the disease.

A more detailed picture of the pattern of the epidemic is obtained by plotting changes in the age distribution of the population through time. We examine the parameter set that induces the most severe change in population size and age structure, where the doubling time is set at 1.5 yr ($R_0 = 4.7$) and $\beta_1 c_1 = 3\beta_2 c_2$. Temporal changes in the age distributions of the total population, females and males, are recorded in FIGURES 5 and 6a and b, respectively. Note that the rather jagged pattern in the age distribution as the epidemic develops is induced by the nonlinearities inherent in the choice of sexual partners by age function, $j_k(a,a't)$. The most important points illustrated by these figures are (1) the differential impact on males and females induced by the unequal transmission probabilities and (2) the dramatic predicted impact of

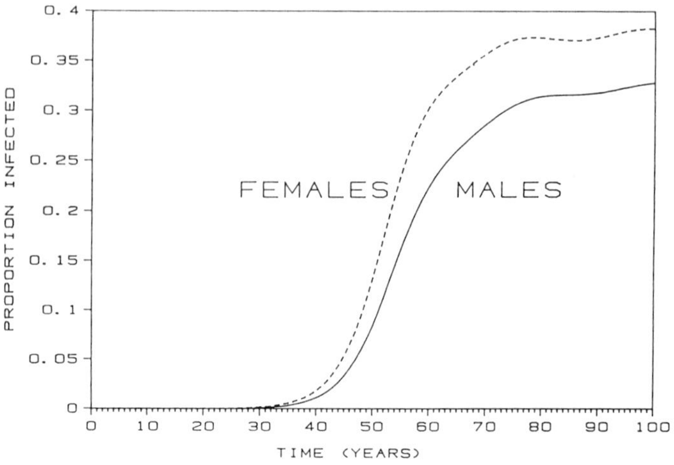

FIGURE 3. Changes in the proportion of females (*broken line*) and males (*solid line*) infected through time. Parameter values: $\beta_1 c_1 = 3\beta_2 c_2$, $R_0 = 3.2$, $t_d = 2.5$ yr.

the disease on both population size and age distribution. Further detail is provided in FIGURES 7 and 8, in which temporal changes in the age distribution of persons with AIDS and HIV-infected individuals are recorded, respectively. The U-shaped patterns of these distributions are created by the combination of vertical (mother to unborn infant) and horizontal (by sexual contact) transmission processes that determine the spread of HIV infection. A clearer picture of the age distributions of females and males with AIDS is presented in FIGURE 9, where the age distributions by sex are compared at three points in time (t = 20, 50, and 90 yr).

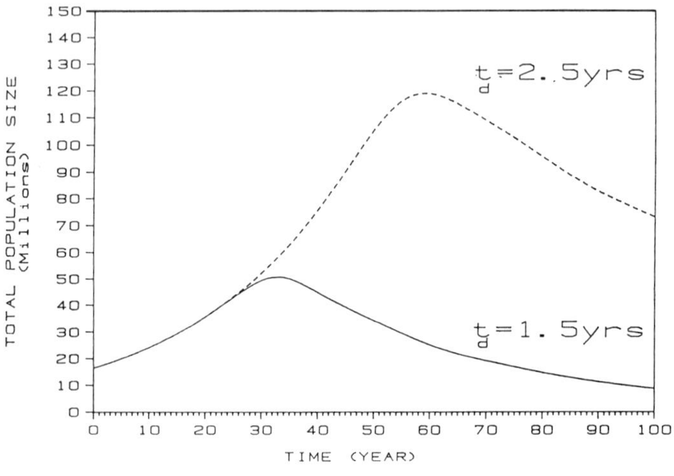

FIGURE 4. Changes in total population size through time for simulations with $\beta_1 c_1 = \beta_2 c_2$ and doubling times (t_d) of 2.5 years (top line in the early stages) and 1.5 years.

Dependency Ratio

We again consider the case where doubling time is set at 1.5 yr in the early stages of the epidemic such that $R_0 = 4.7$. FIGURE 10 compares the two definitions of the ratio—the dependency ratio $d(t)$ (Eq. **10**) and the disease-related dependency ratio $D(t)$) (Eq. 11). Here temporal changes in $d(t)$ and $D(t)$ are recorded for the case where $\beta_1 c_1 = \beta_2 c_2$, and for different values of the weighting factor W [in the case of $D(t)$]. Note that $d(t)$ changes little through time[4] because of the counterbalancing effects of AIDS-related deaths in young infants as a result of vertical transmission, and AIDS-related deaths among adults due to horizontal (= sexual) transmission.

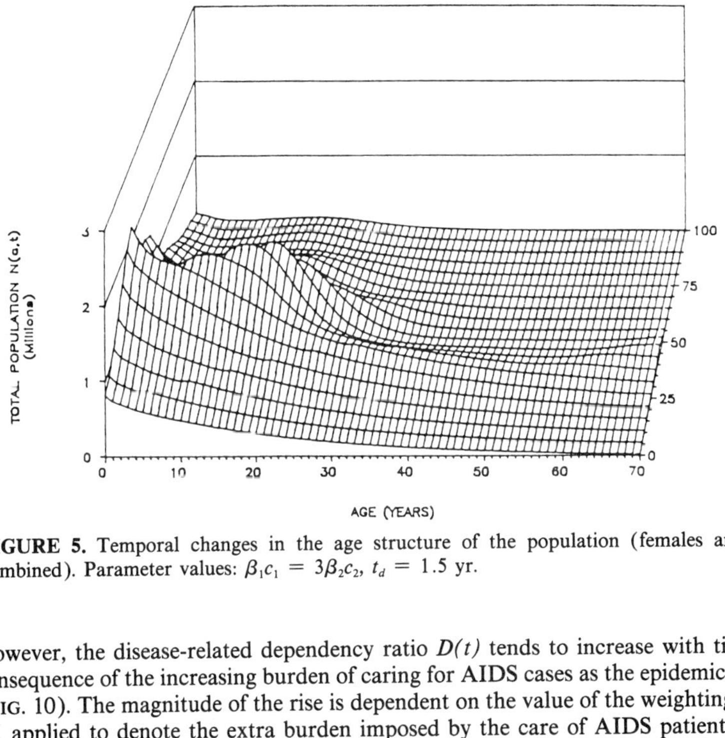

FIGURE 5. Temporal changes in the age structure of the population (females and males combined). Parameter values: $\beta_1 c_1 = 3\beta_2 c_2$, $t_d = 1.5$ yr.

However, the disease-related dependency ratio $D(t)$ tends to increase with time as a consequence of the increasing burden of caring for AIDS cases as the epidemic unfolds (FIG. 10). The magnitude of the rise is dependent on the value of the weighting factor, W, applied to denote the extra burden imposed by the care of AIDS patients.

A slightly different picture emerges when we consider temporal changes in the disease-related dependency ratio, $D(t)$, with unequal transmission probabilities ($\beta_1 c_1 = 3\beta_2 c_2$, $R_0 = 4.7$, and $t_d = 1.5$ yr) (FIG. 11). For a zero weighting factor ($W = 0$), the value of $D(t)$ decreases as the epidemic progresses because of the greater impact of the infection on the female segment of the population (transmission greater from males to females than vice versa) and its subsequent effects on the rate of production of infants. In general, for both cases and for the various definitions of the ratio, the simulation suggests only minor changes through time. Note, however, that minor changes in the ratio can imply major changes in the number of dependents.

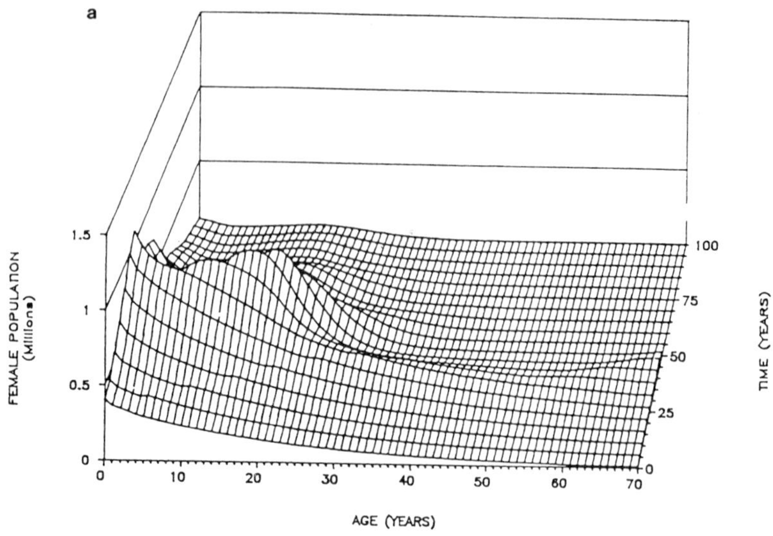

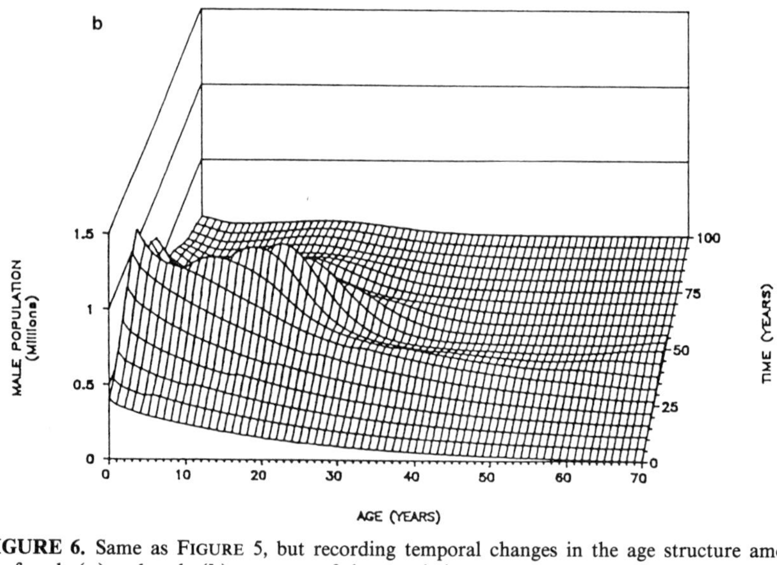

FIGURE 6. Same as FIGURE 5, but recording temporal changes in the age structure among the female (**a**) and male (**b**) segments of the population.

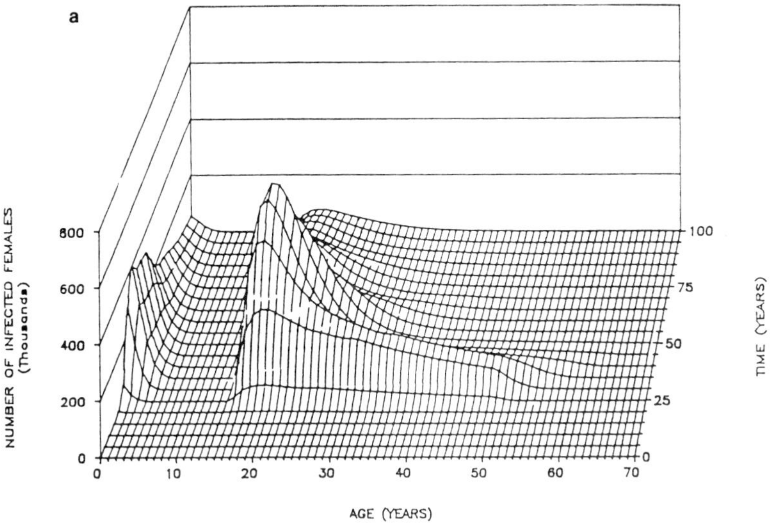

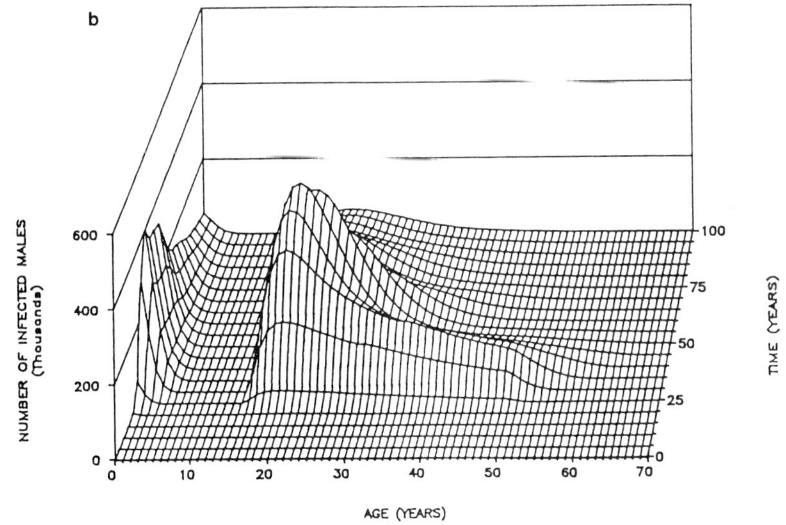

FIGURE 7. Same as the simulations recorded in FIGURE 5, but recording changes in the number of persons infected with HIV in the female (**a**) and male (**b**) segments of the population.

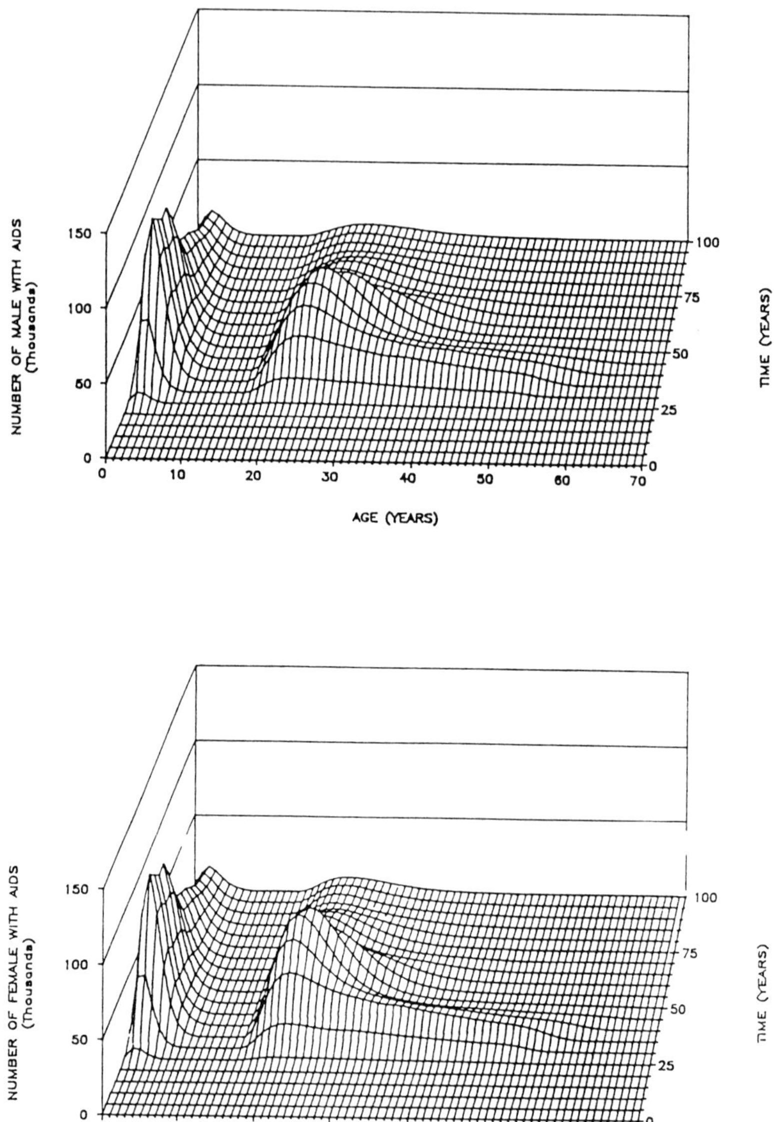

FIGURE 8. Same as the simulations recorded in FIGURE 5, but recording changes in the number of persons with AIDS in the female (**a**) and male (**b**) segments of the population.

PATTERNS OF SEXUAL CONTACT BETWEEN AGE CLASSES

In the preceding section we consider the predicted demographic impact of AIDS employing an age-structured sexual-partner choice matrix $j_k(a,a',t)$ to denote the probability that a person of age a chooses a sexual partner of the opposite sex of age a' at time t. An arbitrary matrix was chosen (TABLE 2) to reflect the tendency of males in many African societies to chose female sexual partners younger than themselves. Time-dependency was added to take account of the changing age and sex structure of the population as the epidemic develops. The age and sex structure are influenced by the form of the function $j_k(a,a',0)$ and by the magnitudes of the transmission probabilities for sexual contact between infected males and susceptible females and vice versa (the β_k values). In this section we compare the predictions presented in the previous section with a new set generated by the model under the assumption that individuals in each age class only choose sexual partners of the opposite sex in the same age class as themselves. This is performed to highlight the significance of the age and sex partner-choice function to the predicted pattern and impact of the epidemic. In the "discretized" version of the function $j_k(a,a',0)$, the diagonal elements of the separate matrices for males and females are unity in value, while all other elements have a value of zero.

A comparison between two types of partner-choice matrices (termed "preferential" and "restricted") is made in FIGURE 12, where the predicted temporal changes in total population size are recorded (for $\beta_1 c_1 = \beta_2 c_2$; $R_0 = 4.7$ and $t_d = 1.5$yr). Note the very substantial differences in the predicted impacts where mixing preferential by age between the sexes generates a much more severe effect on population growth. This arises via the choice-of-mixing matrix, in which men chose female partners younger than themselves. This gives rise to an age distribution of infection and disease skewed to younger age classes of women when compared with the same distribution among males. A female distribution skewed to young age classes has a much greater impact on net fertility than an equivalent distribution among females shifted more to older age classes. Note that if we constructed the matrix $j\ (a,a',0)$ to mirror male choice of females older than themselves, the "preferential"-choice matrix assumption would result in less demographic impact than the "restricted"-mixing assumption.

The second point to note is that partner choice restricted within age cohorts generates a much "smoother" epidemic than that generated by the "preferential" matrix. This is illustrated in FIGURE 13, where temporal changes in the age distribution of persons with AIDS and the total population size are recorded for the within-age-group-mixing assumption (this figure is to be compared with FIGURES 3 and 6).

A further point of interest concerns the comparative influences of preferential choice of sexual partners by age, and unequal transmission probabilities of infection between male and females, and females and males, on the predicted demographic impact of the disease AIDS. In FIGURE 14 we record temporal changes in total population size (for within-age-group mixing) for four different sets of female-to-male and male-to-female transmission probabilities. In each, $R_0 = 4.7$, $t_d = 1.5$ yr, but we alter the ratio $\beta_1 c_1 / \beta_2 c_2$ from 1, to 3, to 6 and to 9. We therefore reflect increasing bias towards more efficient transmission of infection from infected male to susceptible female, when compared with that from infected female to susceptible male. Note that a rising bias, although increasing the demographic impact somewhat due to the influence on net fertility of higher levels of infection among females than males, has much less effect than that recorded by changing the mixing matrix from within-age-group to preferential choice.

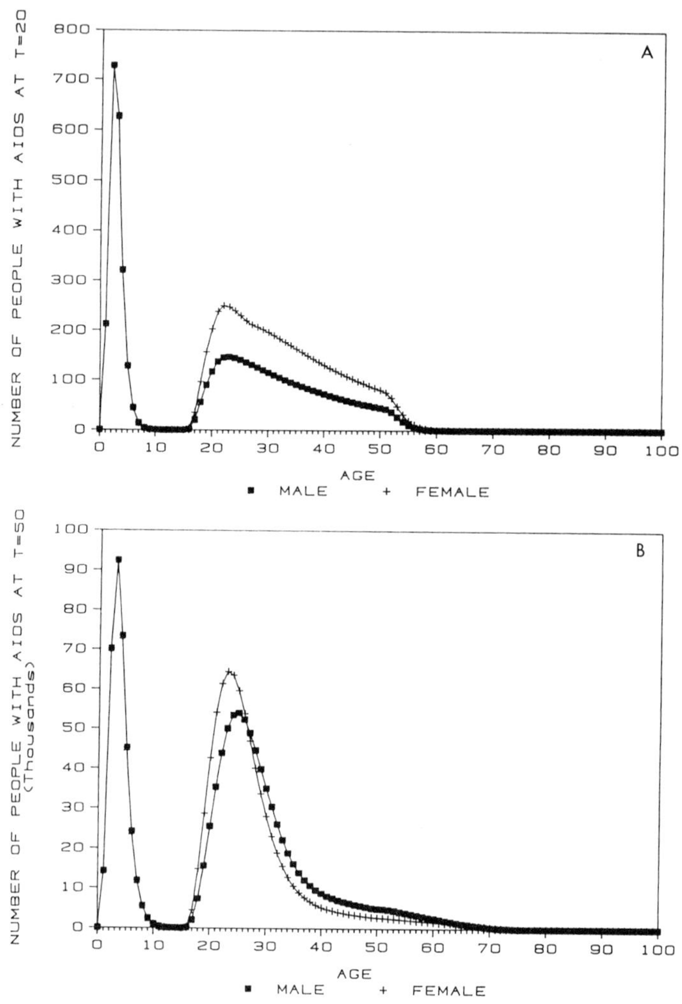

Finally in this section we refer to temporal changes in the disease-related dependency ratio, $D(t)$. As recorded in FIGURE 15, the ratio changes little as the epidemic progresses unless we apply a heavy weighting ($W = 3$) to the cases of AIDS among adult patients.

THE IMPACT OF CONTROL MEASURES INTRODUCED AT DIFFERENT TIMES AFTER THE START OF THE EPIDEMIC

Options for the control of HIV and AIDS are limited at present. Aside from the treatment of AIDS patients with zidovudine (which appears to increase life expectancy

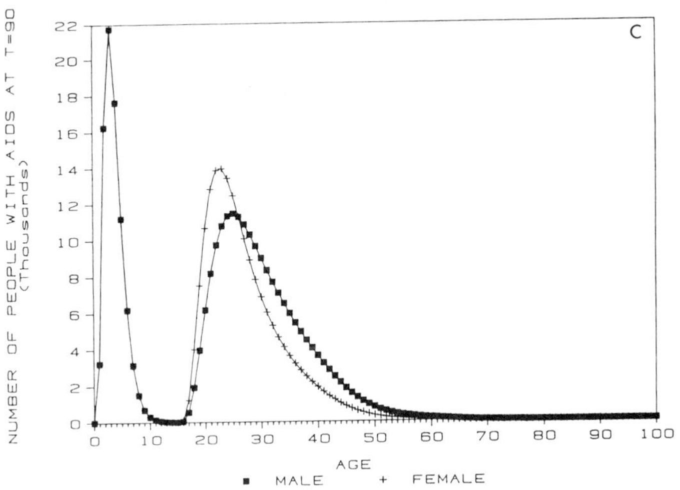

▲ FIGURE 9. A comparison of the age distribution of AIDS cases in males and females at three different time points in the course of the epidemic: (**A**) $t = 20$ yr; (**B**) $t = 50$ yr; and (**C**) $t = 90$ yr. Parameter values: $\beta_1 c_1 = 3\beta_2 c_2$, $t_d = 1.5$ yr.

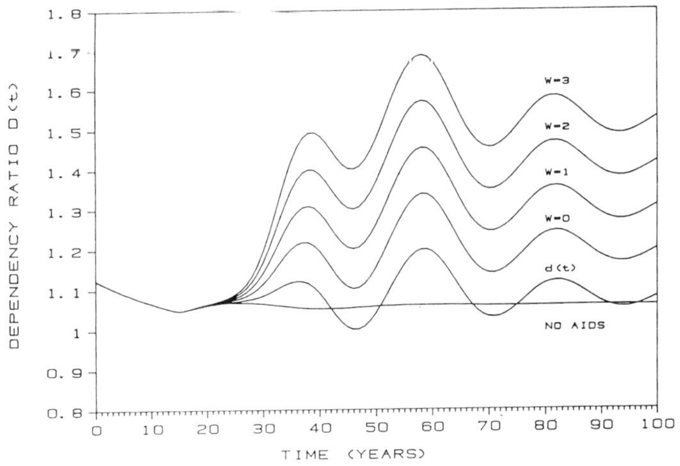

FIGURE 10. Temporal changes in the disease-related dependency ratio, $D(t)$ (see Equations **10** and **11** in the text) for $\beta_1 c_1 = \beta_2 c_2$ and $t_d = 1.5$ yr. The graph shows five different simulations with the old definition of the dependency ratio [Eq. **10**, $d(t)$] and the new definition with the weighting factor, W, set at 0, 1, 2 and 3.

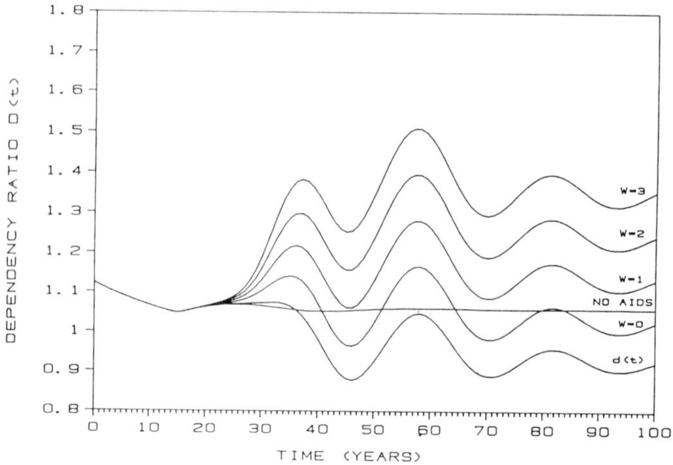

FIGURE 11. Similar to FIGURE 10 but with parameter values, $\beta_1 c_1 = 3\beta_2 c_2$, $t_d = 1.5$ yr and recording changes in $D(t)$ for $W = 0$, 1, 2, and 3.

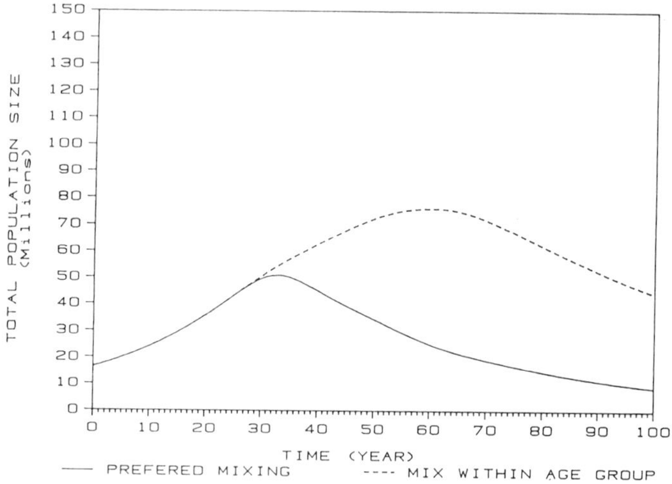

FIGURE 12. Temporal changes in total population size under the preferential mixing function assumption (*bottom line*) and the mixing-within-age class function (*top line*). Parameter values: $\beta_1 c_1 = \beta_2 c_2$, $t_d = 1.5$ yr.

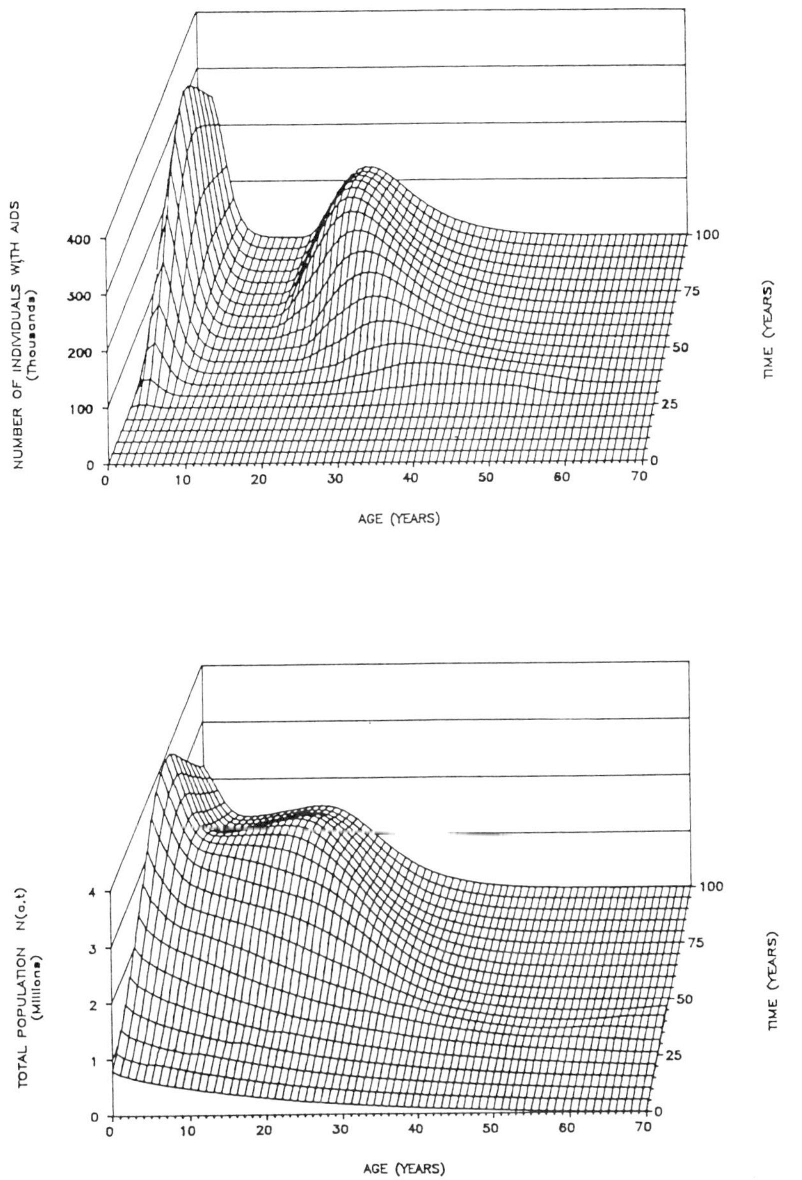

FIGURE 13. Temporal changes in the age distribution of persons with AIDS (*top*) and total population (*bottom*) for an age and sex choice function in which people only choose sexual partners from their own age class. Parameter values: $\beta_1 c_1 = \beta_2 c_2$, $t_d = 1.5$ yr.

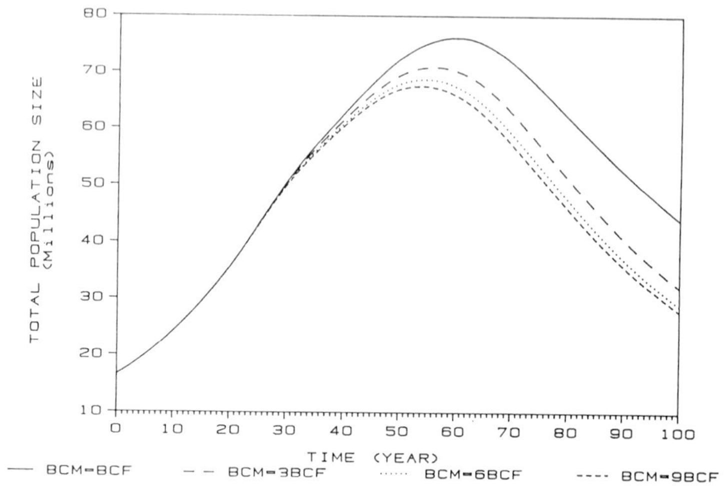

FIGURE 14. The influence of unequal transmission probabilities (β_k values) between males and females on temporal changes in total population size. Parameter values: t_d = 1.5 yr. From the top line to the bottom line, respectively, the ratio $\beta_1 c_1 / \beta_2 c_2$ is 1,3,6, and 9.

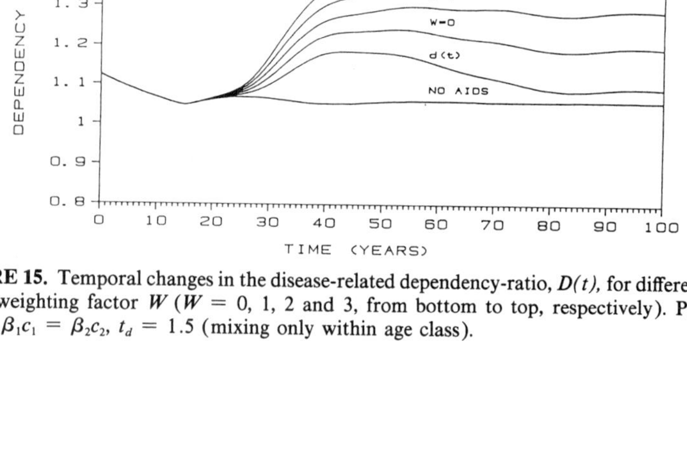

FIGURE 15. Temporal changes in the disease-related dependency-ratio, *D(t)*, for different values of the weighting factor *W* (*W* = 0, 1, 2 and 3, from bottom to top, respectively). Parameter values: $\beta_1 c_1 = \beta_2 c_2$, t_d = 1.5 (mixing only within age class).

to a limited degree[19]), the absence of an effective vaccine to prevent infection by HIV means that control efforts must center on education, a reduction in high-risk behaviors, the use of condoms, and the screening of blood and blood products. By means of numerical studies of model behavior, we consider one aspect of control, namely, the influence of the timing of control measures (after the start of the epidemic) that reduce the net rate of transmission through sexual contact. This is achieved in the numerical simulation by a sustained reduction in the quantities $\beta_1 c_1$ and $\beta_2 c_2$ at a particular time point after the start of the epidemic. Specifically, we consider the case where both $\beta_1 c_1$ and $\beta_2 c_2$ are halved in magnitude at time points 10, 20, and 30 years after the introduction of the virus. Prior to control, the doubling time is set at 1.5 years ($R_0 = 4.7$) and $\beta c_1 = 3\beta_2 c_2$. It is assumed that the reduction in the quantities $\beta_k c_k$ is achieved by an increased use of condoms (influencing β_k) and/or by a reduction in the effective average rate of sexual-partner change (c_k).

As illustrated in FIGURE 16 the numerical studies reveal that the timing of the introduction of control has a very substantial impact on the course of the epidemic. FIGURE 16 records temporal trends in the age distributions of persons with AIDS for three separate simulations in which a 50% reduction in $\beta_1 c_1$ and $\beta_2 c_2$ occurred at 10 yr, 20 yr, and 30 yr after the introduction of HIV into the population. A number of points are of interest in this figure: First, when control is introduced after 10 years, the epidemic takes off extremely slowly and is unable to change the population growth rate from positive to negative (over a 100-year time span) (compare this figure with FIGURE 14). The disease can reverse the sign of the population growth rate when control is not introduced and when it is introduced at 20 or 30 years after the start (over the 100-year time span). A clearer picture of this is provided in FIGURE 17, where temporal trends in total population size are recorded for each simulation. The second major point, which is linked to the first, concerns the timing of control on the total number of persons with AIDS in the population. When control is introduced early on (10 years after the introduction of HIV), the disease fails to regulate human population growth and, although the proportion of persons with AIDS is smaller than it is when control is not introduced, the total number of people with AIDS is in fact larger (due to increased total population size). This trend is illustrated in FIGURE 18, which records temporal trends in the number of persons with AIDS for the different simulations.

The third and final point concerns the impact of changes in behavior on the disease-related dependency ratio, $D(t)$. As illustrated in FIGURE 19, changes in behavior at each time point (10 yr, 20 yr, and 30 yr) tend to decrease the ratio when the weighting factor applied to represent the care of adult AIDS cases (W) is low, but increase the ratio when the weighting is high.

DISCUSSION

The model described in the opening section of this paper is a very simple caricature of the many demographic, epidemiologic, and behavioral processes that determine the spread of HIV in a given country. In its formulation, and the investigation of its properties, it is not our intent to make firm predictions about future trends. At present, the paucity of information on key epidemiologic variables blocks this objective. Our aim is somewhat different, namely, to further understanding of how different processes influence the potential demographic impact of AIDS and its pattern of spread within

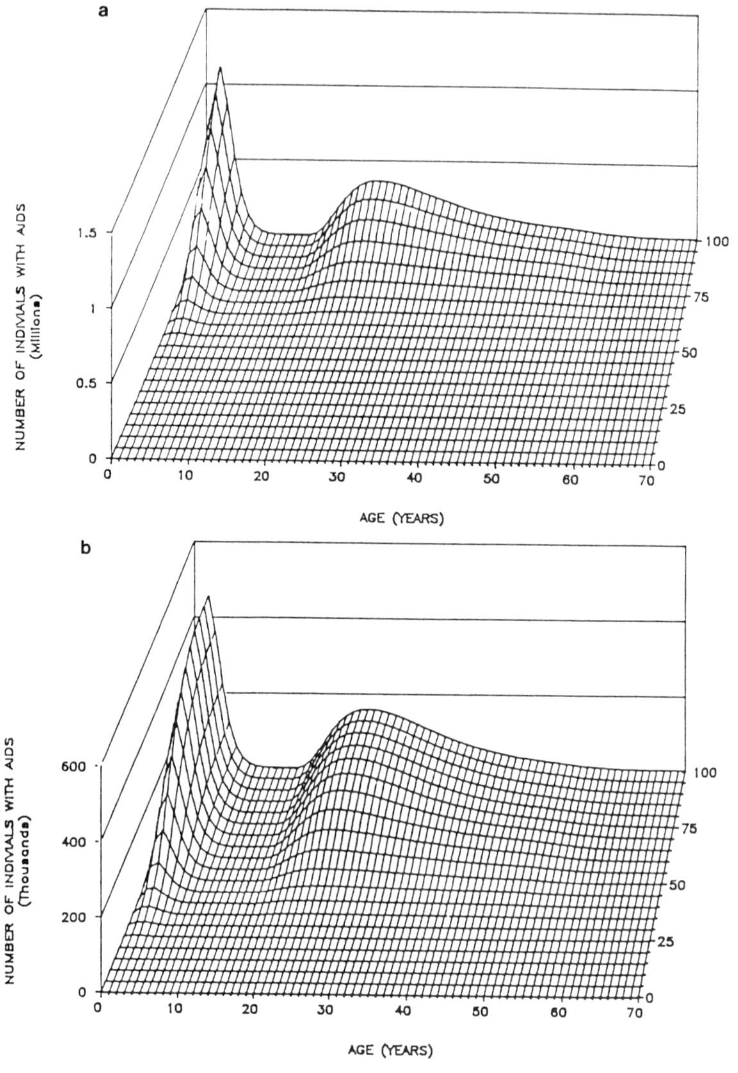

a population. To this end, we described the investigation of three different aspects of the interaction between demographic and epidemiologic processes. The major conclusions that emerged from these numerical studies may be summarized as follows. First, the manner in which we define a dependency ratio, to reflect the impact of AIDS on the fraction of dependents to working adults in a population, influences temporal projection. If the definition takes account of the extra burden imposed by the care of large numbers of AIDS patients (whether adults or children), the ratio is likely to increase as the epidemic spreads. In line with the conclusions of an earlier study[4] the degree to which the ratio is likely to increase is relatively small. However, a small increase can imply a significant change with respect to the number of dependents that must be supported by the adult working population.

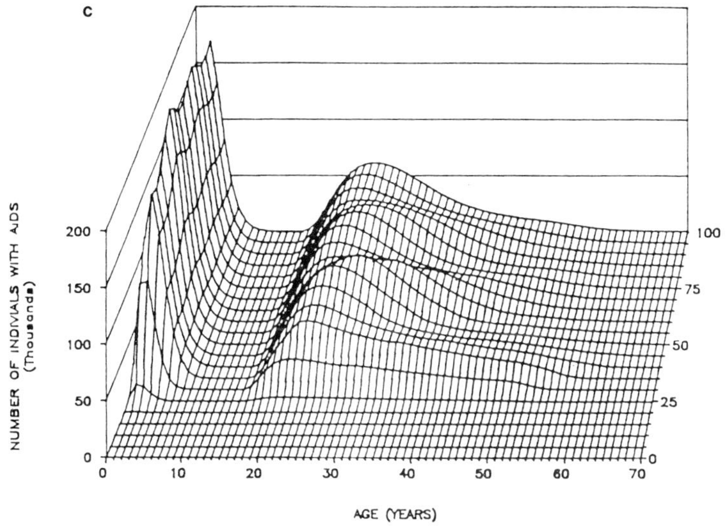

▲

◀ **FIGURE 16.** Temporal changes in the age distribution of persons with AIDS under the assumption that behavioral changes reduced transmission by 50% at time points from the start of the epidemic of 10 years (**a**), 20 years (**b**), and 30 years (**c**). Parameter values: $\beta_1 c_1 = 3\beta_2 c_2$, $t_d = 1.5$ yr (preferential mixing).

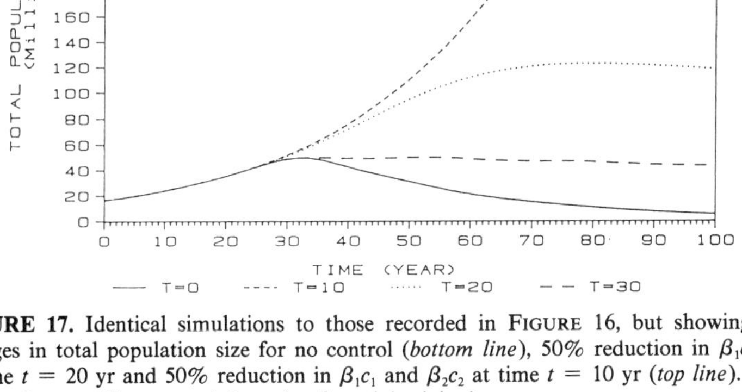

FIGURE 17. Identical simulations to those recorded in FIGURE 16, but showing temporal changes in total population size for no control (*bottom line*), 50% reduction in $\beta_1 c_1$ and $\beta_2 c_2$ at time $t = 20$ yr and 50% reduction in $\beta_1 c_1$ and $\beta_2 c_2$ at time $t = 10$ yr (*top line*). Parameter values: $\beta_1 c_1 = 3\beta_2 c_2$, $t_d = 1.5$ yr. (preferential mixing).

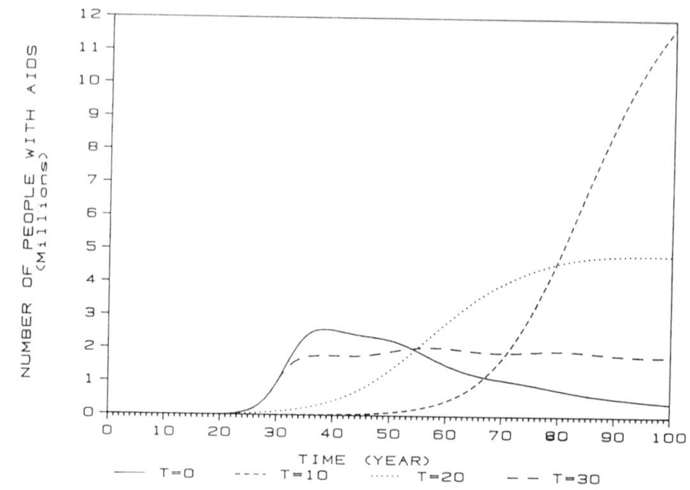

FIGURE 18. Identical to FIGURE 17, but recording changes in the number of persons with AIDS.

A number of variables and processes influence the degree to which an epidemic of AIDS will influence the net growth rate of a human community. Because of the long incubation period of the disease, the epidemic builds in magnitude over many decades. The magnitudes of the population growth rate prior to the introduction of HIV and the basic reproductive rate of infection (R_0) determine whether or not the epidemic will exert a negative change on population growth rates and on what time scale. However, aside from these variables, three other factors will play a very important role, particularly in Africa. They are the degree to which the transmission probability of HIV via sexual contact between infected and susceptible partners differs according to whether the infected individual is male or female, the structure of the sexual-partner choice by age function, and the degree of heterogeneity in sexual activity within the population. If the likelihood of transmission between an infected male and a susceptible female is greater than the reverse direction, as seems to be the case in practice,[15] then for a fixed overall intensity of transmission (a given value of R_0), the demographic impact of the disease will be greater. This is because of the impact of differential mortality among females on the net fertility of the population. Interestingly, a three-fold difference in the magnitude of the transmission probability from male to female and female to male does not result in a three-fold difference in the proportion infected in each sex. This is because the extra mortality induced among females results in a decrease in the female/male sex ratio in the population, and concomitant changes in the effective average rates of sexual-partner change within the different age classes.

The impact of the partner choice by age function is somewhat similar, but our numerical studies suggest that it is of greater importance. If older males tend, on average, to chose female sexual partners of a younger age than themselves, then the impact of AIDS on net fertility is greater than if the reverse were true. In Africa, the data that are available (see FIGURE 1, for example) seem to suggest that men do choose female partners younger than themselves. Our model provides a good mimic of the observed age and sex distribution of cases of AIDS depicted in FIGURE 1 for Uganda (up to July 1988). Interestingly, the influence of differential sexual-partner choice by age appears of greater importance in determining the demographic impact of AIDS than are differences in the transmission probabilities of infection between the sexes.

Heterogeneity in sexual activity within and between age classes was not incorporated in our model. This is an important area for model development in the future. In general, however, we can make the following speculations about its likely impact on the basis of studies of the influence of heterogeneity in sexual activity in models of HIV spread among male homosexual communities.[11,18,20] For a fixed mean rate of sexual-partner change, increasing variability in sexual activity within a population is likely to decrease the demographic impact of AIDS. This tendency will be enhanced as we move from assumptions of proportionate mixing (partners chosen at random by individuals in each activity class) to assumptions where an individual chooses partners more frequently than random from the same sexual-activity class to which he or she belongs (preferred mixing, class based on the rate of sexual-partner change per unit of time).

For any given population we are not able to assess whether the balance between the countervailing forces of age-preferential partner choice, unequal transmission probabilities between the sexes, and heterogeneity in sexual activity is such that AIDS is, or is not, capable of turning positive population growth rates (of 3-4% per annum) negative over time scales of a few decades. In future epidemiologic and anthropological research, quantitative data are urgently required on patterns of sexual behavior.

The final area addressed in our numerical studies concerned the impact of changes in sexual behavior (a reduction in transmission) on epidemiologic and demographic trends. The obvious conclusion to emerge was that the sooner such changes are introduced, the greater the impact on slowing the course of the epidemic and lessening the demographic effects of AIDS. In certain simulations, however, the change in sexual behavior was sufficient to result in continued growth of the human population (over a 100-year time span). The consequence was an overall increase in the total number of persons with AIDS (although a decreased proportion of the population compared with that in the simulation in which no changes of behavior occurred) as a result of population growth and a very slowly developing epidemic. It should be noted, however, that this conclusion is based on the assumption of unchanging fertility patterns (in those not infected with HIV) over a 100-year time span. With a 3-4% annual growth rate, the population would double in size every 20 years. This is unlikely to occur in practice since constraints other than AIDS will restrict population size, such as resource limitation. The central message generated by these numerical studies is the urgency of inducing behavioral changes as soon as possible within the time course of what is likely to be a protracted epidemic.

SUMMARY

A model is developed to describe the spread of HIV within heterosexual communities and the demographic impact of AIDS. The model combines epidemiologic and demographic processes and is designed to mirror the impact of AIDS in sub-Saharan Africa. Refinements on past work in this area include unequal probabilities for transmission from females to males and from males to females, the inclusion of an age- and sex-dependent sexual-partner choice function and distributed incubation

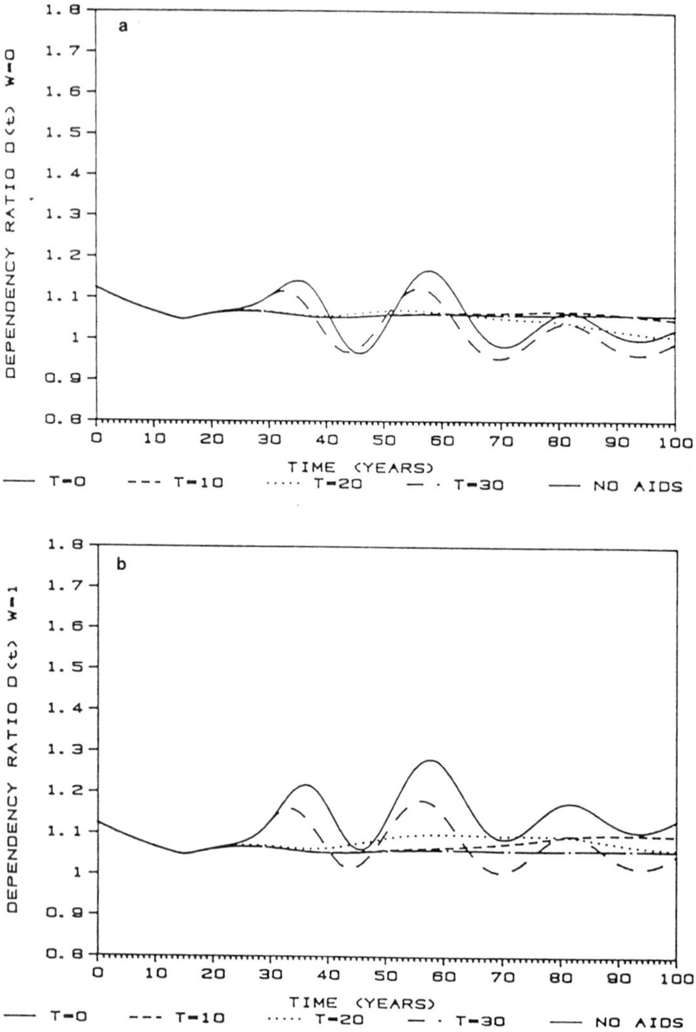

plus infectious periods. Numerical studies suggest that unequal transmission probabilities (weighted to a greater probability from males to females than vice versa), and the tendency of males to choose sexual partners of the opposite sex younger than themselves, both act to increase the demographic impact of AIDS over that predicted with equal transmission between the sexes and partner choice restricted within given age classes. Analyses support the conclusions of past work that the epidemic will only have a small detrimental impact on the dependency ratio of a population (the ratio of dependents to working adults) even when a weighting is added to take account of the extra burden imposed by the care of adult AIDS patients. However, a small increase in the ratio can imply a significant rise in the number of dependents within

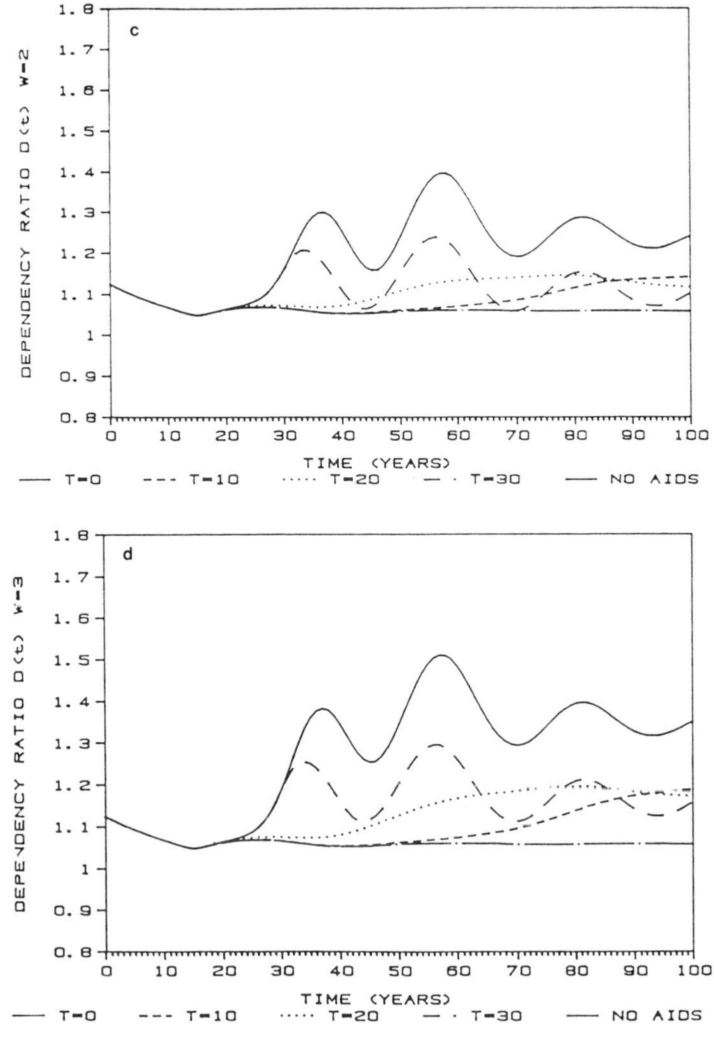

▲
◄ **FIGURE 19.** Temporal changes in the disease-related dependency ratio, $D(t)$, under the impact of changes in behavior induced at 10, 20, and 30 yr after the start of the epidemic, and no changes at all. Parameter values: $\beta_1 c_1 = 3\beta_2 c_2$, $t_d = 1.5$ yr (preferential mixing). Graphs (**a**) to (**d**) record, respectively, different weighting factors, W, applied to take account of the care of AIDS patients with $W = 0$ (**a**), 1 (**b**), 2 (**c**), and 3 (**d**).

the population. Simulation studies of the impact of changes in behavior to reduce transmission highlight to the need to induce such changes as early as possible in the course of the epidemic in order to minimize its impact. Directions for future research are discussed emphasizing the need to acquire quantitative data on sexual habits and to construct models to represent heterogeneity in sexual behavior.

REFERENCES

1. ANDERSON, R. M. & G. F. MEDLEY. 1988. Epidemiology of HIV infection and AIDS: Incubation and infectious periods, survival and vertical transmission. AIDS 2 (Suppl.1): 557-563.
2. BACCHETTI, P. & A. R. MOSS. 1988. Incubation periods of AIDS in San Francisco. Nature **338:** 251-253.
3. CHIN, J. & J. M. MANN. 1988. The global patterns and prevalence of AIDS and HIV infection. AIDS 2 (Suppl.1): S247-S252.
4. ANDERSON, R. M., R. M. MAY & A. R. MCLEAN. 1988. Possible demographic consequences of AIDS in developing countries. Nature **332:** 228-234.
5. MAY, R. M., R. M. ANDERSON & A. R. MCLEAN. 1988. Possible demographic consequences of HIV/AIDS epidemics: I. Assuming HIV infection always leads to AIDS. Math. Biosc. In press.
6. ANDERSON, R. M. & R. M. MAY. 1988. Epidemiological parameters of HIV transmission. Nature **333:** 514-518.
7. ANDERSON, R. M. 1988. The epidemiology of HIV infection: Variable incubation plus infectious periods and heterogeneity in sexual activity. J. Roy. Stat. Soc. A. **151:** 66-93.
8. MAY, R. M., R. M. ANDERSON & A. R. MCLEAN. 1988. Possible demographic consequences of HIV/AIDS epidemics: II. Assuming HIV infection does not necessarily lead to AIDS. Lecture Notes in Biomathematics. **100:** 419-442.
9. ROGERS, M., P. A. THOMAS, E. T. STORCHER & M. C. NOA. 1987. AIDS in children: Report of the CDC national surveillance. Pediatrics **78:** 1008-1014.
10. MAY, R. M. & R. M. ANDERSON. 1987. Transmission dynamics and HIV infection. Nature **326:** 137-142.
11. ANDERSON, R. M., G. F. MEDLEY, R. M. MAY & A. M. JOHNSON. 1986. A preliminary study of the transmission dynamics of the human immunodeficiency virus (HIV), the causative agent of AIDS. IMA J. Math. Appl. Med. Biol. **3:** 229-263.
12. MCLEAN, A. R. & R. M. ANDERSON. 1989. In preparation.
13. MEDLEY, G. F., R. M. ANDERSON, D. R. COX & L. BILLARD. 1987. Incubation period of AIDS in patients infected via blood transfusion. Nature **328:** 719-721.
14. MAY, R. M. & R. M. ANDERSON. 1988. The transmission dynamics of human immunodeficiency virus (HIV) Phil. Trans. Roy. Soc. Lond., B. **321:** 565-607.
15. JOHNSON, A. M. & M. LAGA. 1988. Heterosexual transmission of HIV. AIDS 2(Suppl 1): 549-556.
16. PETERMAN, T. A., R. L. SLONEBURNER, J. R. ALLEN, H. W. JAFFE & J. W. CORRAN. 1988. Risk of human immunodeficiency virus transmission from heterosexual adults with transfusion associated infections. JAMA **259:** 55-58.
17. KONINGS, E., R. M. ANDERSON, D. MORLEY, T. O'RIORDAN & M. MEEGAN. 1988. Rates of sexual partner change among two pastoralist southern nilotic groups in East Africa. AIDS **3:** 245-247.
18. ANDERSON, R. M., S. P. BLYTHE, S. GUPTA & E. KONINGS. 1989. The transmission dynamics of human immunodeficiency virus type I in the male homosexual community in the United Kingdom: The incidence of changes in sexual behavior. Phil. Trans. Roy. Soc. B. **325:** in press.
19. DOURNON, E., S. MALHERON, W. ROZENBAUM *et al.* 1988. Effects of zidovudine in 365 consecutive patients with AIDS or AIDS-related complex. Lancet **ii:** 1927-1302.
20. BLYTHE, S. P. & R. M. ANDERSON. 1988. Heterogeneous sexual activity models of HIV transmission in male homosexual populations. IMA J. Math. Appl. Med. Biol. **5:** 237-260.
21. BERKLEY, S., S. OKWARE & W. NAAMARA. 1989. Surveillance for AIDS in Uganda. AIDS **3:** 79-85.

Social Science and the Improvement of Tropical Disease Control Programs

BURTON SINGER

Department of Epidemiology and Public Health
School of Medicine
Yale University
New Haven, Connecticut 06510

INTRODUCTION

There is a growing consensus that a pervasive and mutually beneficial integration between social science research and tropical disease control is long overdue. Technological innovations—whether they be sophisticated forms of chemotherapy, such as ivermectin for onchocerciasis or Melfloquine for malaria, or simply drainage and redirection of water sources—have provided at most necessary, but certainly not sufficient components of successful intervention campaigns. Social, economic, and political issues have been of equal if not greater importance than technological innovation in the implementation of effective control programs. Thus it is important to understand the essential ingredients of successful programs in the past and to use them as a guide to research needs and intervention objectives in the future.

Successful tropical disease control programs in the past have virtually all had horizontal (decentralized) organizational structures with local personnel engaged in community-wide cooperative ventures.[1–5] *Sustained* local self-reliance, guided by understanding of biology, ecology, and socioepidemiology of the disease(s) in question, has been the central feature of successful programs. The principal challenges for the future are:

(i) The conversion or modification of many existing programs from a vertical to a more horizontal organizational structure and the gradual facilitation of self-reliant locally operated control strategies;

(ii) The design and implementation of control strategies targeted at highly mobile populations which lack social cohesion and are often engaged in the opening of new "frontier" lands.

Accompanying each of these broad challenges is an extensive array of socioeconomic problems, many of which require innovative research prior to, or in combination with, program implementation. Indeed, coordinated research and sustained communication between local educational institutions and control program personnel is an important feature of any potentially successful response to challenges (i) and (ii).

The purpose of this paper is to illustrate some new conceptual and methodologic innovations in the social sciences that can play a role in developing responses to challenges (i) and (ii). Our list is by no means exhaustive; however, it can serve to focus, and in many instances initiate, the much-needed dialogue between public health officials, field personnel, and the social science research community. An almost immediate corollary of the integration we are suggesting would be the creation of new academic specialties in the social, economic, and political aspects of tropical public health.

In the second section of this paper we discuss qualitative anthropological evidence as the basis for understanding patterns of utilization of extant health care systems prior to the introduction of proposed new technology or organizational modifications. Recently developed computerized retrieval systems tailored to the problems of objective analyses of large bodies of spoken text represent an important step in placing qualitative analysis on a more rigorous foundation.

In the third section strategies for performance evaluation of complex programs are considered. Primary health care systems and malaria control programs with multiple forms of intervention are prototypical of this situation.

Colonization and political unrest frequently give rise to mass migrations of socially heterogeneous populations, which, in turn, initiate unanticipated epidemics.[6–8] Rapid response to such epidemics requires identification of subpopulations that are at especially high risk of acquiring infection. Migration surveys on highly mobile populations[9] often contain fine-grained demographic and behavioral data; however, the challenge is to analyze those data in a manner that will succinctly reveal those subpopulations that require special targeting by control program personnel. In the fourth section of the paper we outline statistical analysis strategies applicable to very heterogeneous populations and that facilitate identification of high-risk subpopulations, defined by a multiplicity of behavioral and ecological conditions.

ANTHROPOLOGICAL (MICRO-APPROACH) EVIDENCE

An important step in understanding the baseline environment where any disease control modifications might be contemplated is the conduct of demographic surveys, the recording of detailed impressions of a community by participant observers, and the conduct of only partially *a priori*-structured in-depth interviews with village residents and extant control program personnel. The importance of the sociocultural setting—ascertained by in-depth interviews—in planning intervention can be seen by examination of the pattern of utilization of health-care services in a rural Malian village.[10]

FIGURE 1 indicates that villagers classify illnesses into five categories, only one of which leads them to utilize a Western-like (or cosmopolitan) health care system. Illnesses resulting from infected water and microbes, as well as onchocerciasis, were usually treated by the cosmopolitan medicine programs. However, most acute symptoms were identified with illnesses caused by black magic, spirits and witchcraft, and they resulted in treatment by traditional healers. Chronic illnesses were viewed as "given by God," with treatment—if sought at all—coming from Islamic medicine. Clearly, any intervention targeted at control of a disease such as trypanosomiasis, for example, must be introduced as part of an effort to switch from traditional healers (folk medicine) to cosmopolitan medicine.

Associated with health-care utilization patterns are perceptions of causality for commonly occurring diseases. Onchocerciasis, for example, is quite common in Boguineda, Mali; and the diversity of villagers' perceptions about its origin is shown in

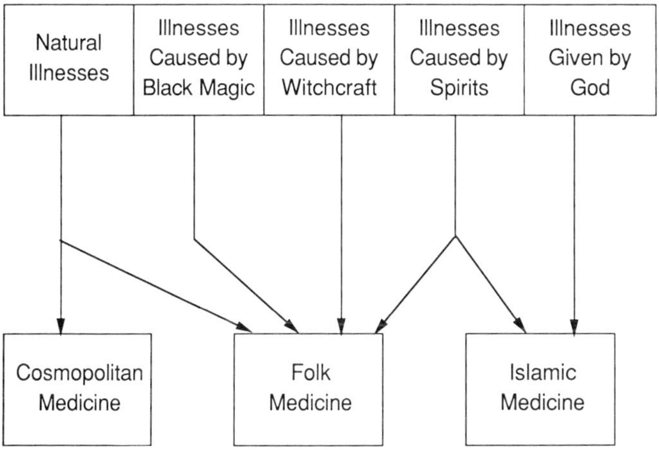

FIGURE 1. Indigenous groups of illnesses and corresponding choice of health care systems in rural Mali. After Hielscher and Sommerfeld.[10]

FIGURE 2, which represents a composite of opinions drawn from laymen and traditional healers. Any control program aimed at either fly control or Ivermectin distribution must confront the diversity of perceived origins of onchocerciasis, if compliance with, and acceptance of, the treatment is to occur.

FIGURES 1 and 2 were derived from informal interviews, partially structured individual interviews, and partially structured group interviews.[10] Evidence of this kind has often been criticized by those engaged in formal survey research and by biologists and epidemiologists as being far too subjective and excessively variable in content to be *widely regarded* as an important evidential base.[11] This negative point of view seems to be a consequence of the difficulty of systematizing the process of extracting regularities from informal spoken and written text. The deeper root of the problem has been a lack of formal algorithms for decomposing substantial bodies of text into more primitive components that could be analyzed in a relatively objective fashion. Recent advances in linguistics[12,13] and in automated text processing[14,15] suggest, however, that substantial progress has been made in providing a more rigorous underpinning to the production of "evidence" from informal interviews.

In order to understand the capabilities and potential of recent advances in more rigorous qualitative analysis methods, we briefly outline the characteristics and structure of GATOR (the Generalized Automatic Text Organization and Retrieval System).[14] The motivation for development of GATOR arose from the fact that *spoken* text rarely evolves in an orderly linear fashion, a presumption of most extant computer-assisted indexing systems. Interviews usually consist of clusters of ideas, each of which an investigator would like to index. Blocks of text containing a given idea often overlap with blocks containing either disjointed or closely related ideas. Thus a system was needed that could isolate blocks of text, index them and order them into groups, and to identify subjects in response to both qualitative (e.g., married or unmarried) or quantitative (e.g., households with two or more children) questions. It would be necessary to locate and display—at a terminal—everything an interviewee said that related to a specific topic and to display or print the corresponding information for all interviewees side-by-side so that any regularities (or patterns) could be readily discerned.

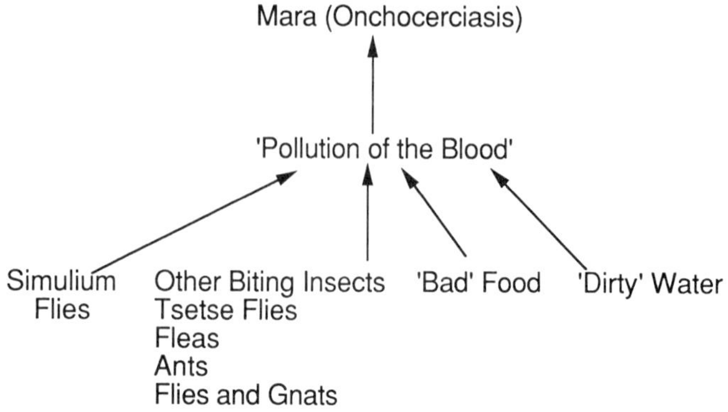

FIGURE 2. Some causational concepts for mara (onchocerciasis) in a rural Malian village. After Hielscher and Sommerfeld.[10]

GATOR requires that an investigator code a text to be analyzed with appropriate key words. It is assumed that extensive recoding and modification of key words to guide the automated retrieval will be a routine interactive part of the analysis of interviews. This intensive interaction between the user and the retrieval system is a simple consequence of the fact that no available software system can reliably *interpret* text. The role of such retrieval systems in understanding the patterns of utilization of health services or perceptions of disease causality is that they permit rapid examination of the full range of material collected from hundreds of hours of tape-recorded interviews. This greatly reduces the probability that a few "choice" interviews might be used in a biased fashion while other less memorable (to the interviewer) materials would tend to be forgotten. By sorting interview text and quantitative data on a diversity of variables and by having immediate access to an array of quotations from each interviewee in a defined subgroup, pattern discovery is facilitated.

Although GATOR and an analogous system, the ETHNOGRAPH,[15] may be regarded as important engineering advances for the systematic exploration of spoken and written text, deeper understanding of the organization of ideas within such text requires a linguistic-theoretic base.[12,13] Nevertheless, analysis of materials routinely collected by anthropologists and sociologists engaged in baseline community studies using the aforementioned automated retrieval systems can be an important step toward providing more rigorously defensible evidence to guide the design of tropical disease control strategies.

PROGRAM EVALUATION

There are four common features of tropical health and disease control programs that make traditional epidemiologic evaluation difficult, if not impossible. These are:

(i) The program contains multiple components, some of which are interventions aimed at source reduction (vector and/or intermediate host control), while the remaining "treatments" are targeted at the human population.

(ii) Voluntary self-selection by humans to utilize a formally defined program is a condition of entry.

(iii) There is considerable heterogeneity in the reasons for individuals' volunteering or declining to take advantage of the program.
(iv) A control group from the target population cannot be assembled.

Point (i) implies that multiple criteria should be introduced to evaluate programs. Point (iv) means that program outcomes must be compared with the *natural* history of transmission in the same or very similar locations assembled at earlier times and in the absence of the program being evaluated. In order to focus the ideas let me initially restrict the discussion to malaria control programs. This is admittedly a much simpler setting than evaluation of comprehensive primary health care systems and/or a *mix* of disease-specific control programs. However, all of the methodologic issues that must be faced with more complex programs already manifest themselves in the narrower domain of malaria control.

Any evaluation of a malaria control program must stipulate specific goals and a finite follow-up period during and after which a performance assessment will be carried out.[16] Since eradication seems to be an increasingly infeasible target, we consider reductions in prevalence that are sustained or improved upon. They can arise from two sources defined by the type of target of the intervention: those kinds of intervention that act on humans and those that act on vectors. Within each of these broad categories we may have the following sets of available interventions:

A. Interventions Acting on Humans

A.1: Distribution of antimalarial drugs
A.2: Distribution of and education about use of bed nets
A.3: Assistance with and education about house screening
A.4: Education about rapid seeking of diagnosis and treatment after initial symptoms

B. Interventions Acting on Vectors

B.1: Water source drainage and maintenance
B.2: Vegetation clearance
B.3: Use of larvicides
B.4: Use of chemical sprays (DDT, Malathion)

It is necessary to evaluate not only the performance of this mix of eight forms of intervention in terms of prevalence reduction in a community, but also the performance of each component. Individual component evaluation provides the basis for sequential surveillance and adaptive modification or improvement of the program over time so that a program can evolve to reach goals that an initial (or pilot stage) program may not be able to attain.

A strategy for evaluation consists of:

(i) Introducing indices of possible problems with (or sources of difficulty for) each component of the program (i.e., A.1-A.4 and B.1-B.4).
(ii) Installing what is deemed at the start to be a potentially effective program;
(iii) Monitoring prevalence over time for a year and evaluating whether there is any improvement (reduction in prevalence relative to the baseline year[s]);
(iv) Improving one or more of the component interventions based on their indices of possible problems for the first year;
(v) Continuing to monitor prevalence for another year under the modified program;
(vi) Repeating this adaptive examination of indices of potential problems, modification (improvement) of component interventions, and monitoring of outcome until major reductions in prevalence have been achieved and original goals are met or closely approximated. This kind of adaptive strategy has

previously been discussed for evaluation of methadone maintenance programs aimed at rehabilitation of chronic heroin addicts.[17,18]

TABLE 1 contains an idealized set of indices of potential problems for a malaria control program with the eight components, A.1-A.4 and B.1-B.4. Values for these indices in a specific program must, of necessity, be very community-specific. Indeed, the frequent impossibility of assembling a matched control group (population) as part of a program evaluation is a consequence of enormous inter-community variability in: (1) vector breeding, biting, and resting behavior; (2) human activity in terms of exposure to *Anopheles* vectors; and (3) cultural norms and their influence on patterns of utilization of available health services.

An interesting and quite early example of an evolution of this kind of adaptive/evaluative malaria control program occurred as part of the Roan Antelope Copper Mine development in Luanshya, Northern Rhodesia, from 1929 through 1934.[5] The Roan control program contained components A.1-A.4 and B.1-B.3; however, primary emphasis was placed on vector control and source reduction (i.e., B.1-B.3). FIGURE 3 shows the prevalence of malaria and total sickness reports over time from the 1929

TABLE 1. Performance-Based Ratings of Malaria Control Programs according to Indices of Potential Problems

Possible Problem with Intervention	Intervention	Rating Index[a] Range for Program Outcome Assessed to Be:			Factors Associated with Poor Performance
		Good	Fair	Poor	
Noncompliance	A.1—Antimalarial drugs	a > 80	20-80	<20	Inadequate community education; inadequately trained medical staff
Noncompliance	A.2—Bed nets	b > 60	30-60	<30	Inadequate community education
Noncompliance	A.3—House screening	b > 85	30-85	<30	Inadequate education and training
Inadequate coverage	A.4—Education	c > 85	50-85	<50	Poor contact strategy
Inadequate coverage	B.1—Drainage	d < 10	10-70	>70	Improper drainage/lack of trained field staff
Inadequate coverage	B.2—Vegetation clearance	d < 10	10-70	>70	Previously unsuspected breeding sites/incomplete cutting
Inadequate coverage	B.3—Larvicides	d < 10	10-70	>70	Low oil supply/insufficient effort by staff
Noncompliance	B.4—Chemical sprays	b > 70	30-70	<30	Inadequate education/poor relationship between program staff and household heads

[a] Rating Index: a = percent of compliance among those self-selecting for treatment; b = percent of households in compliance; c = percent with symptoms volunteering for treatment; $d = \text{maximum over surveillance sites of } \frac{\text{mean mosquito catch in current year}}{\text{mean mosquito catch in baseline year}} \times 100.$

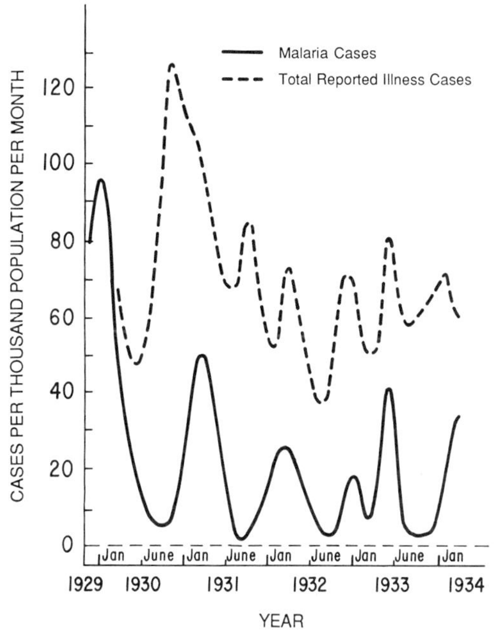

FIGURE 3. Chart showing reduction of malaria and overall illness on Roan Mine site from November 1929 through March 1934. After Watson.[5]

baseline surveys through the introduction of annual adaptive program improvement in the years 1931–1934. Increasing the number of mosquito-catching sites, evaluating mosquito counts and their geographic distribution, systematically controlling and/or draining river and swamp areas, and sustained weekly oiling of damboes were the tactics primarily responsible for the substantial declines in malaria in 1931 and 1932. An evaluation of the reductions in overall sickness at the same site would require consideration of a more comprehensive set of interventions targeted at yellow fever, African trypanosomiasis, and poor nutrition, to name only a few of the challenges confronting health workers in Luanshya.

The comparison of what is subsequently defined as a successful program with earlier versions tried out in the adaptive development process can be viewed as an evaluation with historical controls. The use of performance-based ratings—essentially of the program organization and implementation—together with outcome assessment represents a rather coarse level of detail about the program, but one that should be feasible to carry out on a wide scale. Deeper understanding of program mechanics would entail measuring and modeling the self-selection and compliance associated with components A.1-A.4 and B.4. It should also be pointed out that the Roan Antelope Copper Mine community represents a *relatively* straightforward program evaluation problem due to the fact that the company-sponsored source reduction and health interventions were the only source of malaria control. In addition the local population was not very mobile and its social cohesion facilitated community participation in the control efforts.

A vastly more complex situation is presented by the epidemic malaria resulting from colonization of the Amazon[6] or from the mobile populations in Northern Thailand.[19] In both settings one must assess the contribution of a formally defined program to disease reduction in an environment where substantial uncontrolled drug distribution is occurring simultaneously and where drug-resistant parasites are an increasingly serious problem. Rigorous program evaluation in this context lies in the future and has much in common, conceptually and methodologically, with the evaluation of family planning programs.[20] Finally, we mention two research questions associated with the performance-based rating strategy discussed above that deserve considerable attention. These are:

1. In the development of successful complex programs, can the existing multistage selection methods[21] be adapted and exploited, so that the highest achievable performance levels can be reached as early as possible after the initiation of the development process? This would lead to rapid detection of the conjunction of interventions, and their mode of implementation, that characterizes the conditions of successful operation.

2. Would a hybrid strategy of multistage selection and randomized trials on portions of a program (e.g. randomizing education and interpersonal contact strategies aimed at achieving compliance on use of bed nets and acceptance of chemical sprays) provide a more effective program development and evaluation strategy than the current more informal methods?

COMPLEX CAUSES AND DATA ANALYTIC STRATEGIES FOR CHARACTERIZING HETEROGENEOUS POPULATIONS

Dramatic increases in transmission of malaria in Rondônia, Brazil[6,22,23] and in Chagas' disease[8] in northwestern Argentina during the past few years are two instances of an ever-increasing problem of rapid rise in disease resulting from migration to and settlement of frontier-like lands by nonindigenous populations. In both cases there is a substantial variation in disease incidence and prevalence among the migrants, with the sources of variation distributed among complex *combinations* of conditions. These combinations *appear* thus far to be subtle mixtures of socioeconomic characteristics of migrants and ecology of the settlement areas. The word *appear* is of particular importance here because the existence of very rich-in-detail household surveys (as in the Machadinho project in Brazil[22]) presents a major data analytic challenge for isolating multi-dimensional combinations of conditions that are associated with high *P.falciparum* (in Brazil) prevalence in the migrant population of non-immune persons.

The problem of identifying combinations of conditions associated with high prevalence is important for at least two reasons:

(i) In the initial stages of migration-initiated epidemics, complete coverage of the exposed population by a control program effort is usually impossible. What is required is rapid assessment—by means of surveys of migrants—of a substantial list of potential risk factors and identification of subpopulations at greatest risk for malaria. This immediately suggests more feasible control strategies targeted at the highest-risk subpopulations.

(ii) Migration-initiated epidemics are often unanticipated consequences of economic development programs. Clear documentation of the negative health consequence of such programs can facilitate the increase of health considerations in the planning process by development banks.[24]

Initial analyses[22] of data from the Machadinho project suggest that those most likely to be found positive for *P.falciparum* are characterized by economic circumstances defined in turn by: bundles of commodities owned, nature and location (relative to the forest) of a homesite, nature and location (in the forest or not) of work activity, proximity to the breeding sites of *A. darlingi* (the principal vector of transmission), level of education, background history (defined by such variables as "place of origin prior to migration to Rondônia"), and work characteristics at the place of origin. Sharp delineation of the combinations of conditions—based on these variables—that characterize the highest-risk subpopulations is confounded by the extreme heterogeneity of the migrants. A useful, but as yet underutilized tool for the characterization of special risk groups within heterogeneous populations is the family of Grade-of-Membership (GOM) models. We summarize the essential features of GOM constructions and their interpretations, referring the reader to technical references[25-27] for details about implementation.

Defining subpopulations of a heterogeneous population on the basis of multiple characteristics simultaneously is, on the face of it, a standard problem of cluster analysis. However, when many individuals are identified with multiple risk conditions, no combination of which occurs with high frequency in the full population, then the assignment of individuals to crisply defined categories becomes impossible. A more appropriate strategy is to construct—in a data-intrinsic manner—a small set of "ideal profiles" (or categories), each defined by a multiplicity of conditions, and then to associate with each individual a set of "degree-of-similarity scores" or Grades of Membership (GOM scores) relative to these profiles. The GOM scores are interpreted as degrees of similarity of the set of characteristics of an individual to the set of characteristics that define each profile.

For example, suppose that a population of migrants is to be described by their distribution on the following variables:

1. Economic status (based on commodities owned)........ High__, Low__
2. Primary work activity in forest .... Yes__, No__
3. Engaged in farming .... Yes__, No__
4. Planted coffee trees.................................... Yes__, No__
5. Planted more than 100 coffee trees....................... Yes__, No__
6. Planted cacao trees...................................... Yes__, No__
7. Working for someone .... Yes__, No__
8. Supervising others...................................... Yes__, No__
9. House closed in by 4 walls .... Yes__, No__
10. House with protective screening .... Yes__, No__
11. House within 1 mile of forest............................ Yes__, No__
12. Number of years in Amazon........................... ________
13. Education............................... None__, 0-4 yrs__, >4yrs__

This is only a partial list of variables that can characterize the degree of exposure of a migrant to the Amazon to malaria. It is presented here to illustrate a methodology. For a more comprehensive discussion of variables associated with exposure to malaria in the Amazon, the reader should consult Reference 22.

Now consider a profile defined by:

I. Low economic status *and* working in the forest *and* a house within 1 mile of the forest *and* a house not closed-in by 4 walls *and* less than 4 years of education *and* less than 1 year in the Amazon

and a second profile defined by

II. High economic status *and* not working in the forest *and* supervising others *and* a house closed-in by 4 walls *and* a house with protective screening *and* 3 years in the Amazon *and* more than 4 years of education.

Profile I defines a population within which the prevalence rate for *P. falciparum* malaria is very high, while profile II defines a population at minimal risk. Neither of these profiles characterizes many people. Thus there is a need to associate GOM scores with individuals so that their degree of similarity (based on responses to questions 1-13) to each of the profiles may be represented quantitatively. An individual with GOM scores $(g_I, g_{II}) = (7/8, 1/8)$ has most but not all of the characteristics of profile I (that is, he/she loads 7/8 on profile I and only 1/8 on profile II). An individual with GOM scores (1/2, 1/2) is exactly intermediate between the two profiles. If high prevalence is associated with persons for whom g_I exceeds 3/4, then this defines a high-risk subpopulation to be targeted by a control program.

A Grade-of-Membership representation for our prototype migrant population consists of the logical AND statements defining the profiles (that is, complex combinations of conditions) and a pair of GOM scores for each individual. We hasten to add that, depending upon the community, three or four "ideal profiles" might be relevant with each individual having, respectively, 3 or 4 GOM scores indicating his/her degrees of similarity to the profiles. What makes crisp classification impossible is that in highly heterogeneous populations (in our example suppose that 35% of the population have $1/4 < g_I < 3/4$; hence, $3/4 > g_{II} > 1/4$) many people cannot be neatly placed into the categories, I and II, that are best supported by the data.

Grade-of-Membership representations are quite suitable for the rapid ascertainment of high-risk subpopulations that a control program would target in attempting intervention in the presence of high mobility and lack of social cohesion. However, it is important to understand that this kind of representation is much coarser (but nevertheless well suited to rapid assessment) than a more physically detailed transmission model. Indeed, if interest focuses on a deeper scientific understanding of malaria transmission in an environment of unstable population movements, such as occurred in the colonization of Rondônia, then a dynamic system corresponding to the schematic diagram in FIGURE 4 represents the minimal level of complexity that must be introduced.

Within this admittedly simplified caricature of transmission dynamics we consider a village wherein residents are exposed to a vector population within a 1.5-2-mile radius of breeding sites of the "village vector." Some fraction of the village residents

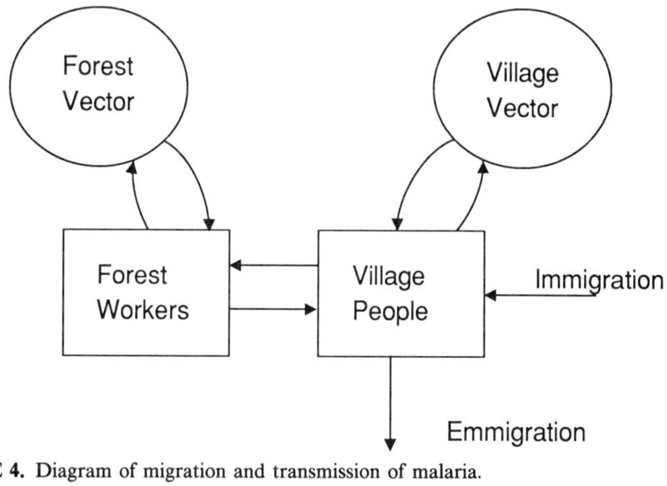

FIGURE 4. Diagram of migration and transmission of malaria.

work in the forest and are exposed to a different insect population whose biting rate in man is much higher than that of the village vector. Thus the forest workers, by virtue of their movement back and forth from the village, provide an increased reservoir of parasites to be transmitted to nonforest workers by the village vector. Immigration to the village area by nonimmune persons represents a dangerous potential for new transmission. Emigration by those who may become disenchanted—as in Rondônia[6,23]—with a previously unanticipated malarious environment actually serves to establish fresh foci of transmission at new settlement sites. A rigorous analysis of this kind of system focusing on the potential consequences of different control strategies is highly important and should be carried out. Among many questions deserving attention is whether or not rigorous distribution to and utilization of antimalarial drugs by the forest workers alone would be a manageable control target (rather than attempting comprehensive coverage of all persons in the area) that could lead to substantially reduced prevalence in an environment of ongoing in- *and* out-migration. Incorporating a more refined set of risk variables into this kind of transmission model would, ultimately, lead to a unified socioepidemiologic characterization of malaria transmission in a very complex setting. This, however, is the prototypical situation for understanding migration-initiated epidemics of Chagas' disease and the very much more complex (relative to malaria) African trypanosomiasis epidemics.[28,29]

DISCUSSION

We have focused on three methodologic strategies that can facilitate an integration of socioepidemiologic research and the design of more effective strategies for tropical disease control. This admittedly selective discussion has, however, confined attention to methods for improving and evaluating the *effectiveness* of control programs. The equally important complement of program development and implementation is cost. A full discussion of cost assessment, even for malaria control programs alone (to say nothing of overall primary health care systems) is a major topic for future research and one that clearly warrants substantial attention. Although quite detailed cost assessments for the Roan Antelope Copper Mine and other early malaria control programs[5] are available, a fine-grained and systematic method for such cost assessments[30,31] is of much more recent vintage. Extension and adaptation of the ideas in this literature to cost assessment of other tropical disease control programs lies in the future.

A second topic not treated in the present paper, but very important for disease control, is the organizational structure and modes of interaction between program personnel and a community at large which facilitate sustained local self-reliance in maintaining community health. The malaria control programs in Pondicherry, India[3] represent an excellent example of such a situation. However, a deeper understanding of the social network structures that facilitate effective horizontal programs will require community studies and analytic strategies analogous to those used, for example, in network studies of urban communes.[32] Understanding the organizational and behavioral principles that underlie the success of a community like Pondicherry is a major challenge for social research and one in which the impact of results could be immediate and profound. The growing literature on evolution of cooperation[33,34] may also be adapted and refined to establish a much needed theoretical underpinning to guide the implementation of locally maintained and cooperative programs.

A final topic omitted from the present paper, but one that warrants much attention in the future, is the coordination of health interventions with economic development programs. The proper coordination of disease control, primary health care and, for example, improvement of agricultural capabilities and overall living standards is a large and minimally understood topic. Here is a major research area where the output could be of immediate practical importance. We hope to be able to report major progress on this topic in the future.

ACKNOWLEDGMENTS

It is a pleasure to thank Drs. Carol Vlassoff, Barry Bloom, Elias Sevilla-Casas, and Louis Molineaux for stimulating discussions and suggestions on an earlier draft. Special thanks are due Dr. Tore Godal, Director of the Special Programme for Research and Training on Tropical Diseases at the World Health Organization, who made a splendid oral presentation of this material in my place at this conference.

REFERENCES

1. KITRON, U. 1987. Malaria, agriculture and development: Lessons from past campaigns. Int. J. Health Serv. **17:** 295-326.
2. KITRON, U. &A. SPIELMAN. 1988. Suppression of malaria transmission through source reduction: Anti-anophelene measures applied in Israel, U.S.A. and Italy. Manuscript, Department of Tropical Public Health, Harvard University, Cambridge, MA.
3. SHARMA, V. P. 1987. Community-based malaria control in India. Parasitol. Today **3:** 222-226.
4. JORDAN, P. 1985. Schistosomiasis: The St. Lucia Project. Cambridge University Press. Cambridge, England.
5. WATSON, M. 1953. African Highway: The Battle for Health in Central Africa. John Murray. London.
6. CRUZ MARQUES, A. 1987. Human migration and the spread of malaria in Brazil. Parasitol. Today **3**(6): 166-170.
7. FORD, J. 1971. The Role of the Trypanosomiases in African Ecology. Clarendon Press. Oxford.
8. SCHOFIELD, C.J. 1982. The Problem of Chagas's disease vector control. *In* Perspectives in Trypanosomiasis Research. J. R. Baker Ed.: 71-84. Research Studies Press. Chichester, England.
9. BILSBURROW, R. E., A. S. OBERAI & G. STANDING. 1984. Migration Surveys in Low-Income Countries. Croom Helm. London.
10. HIELSCHER, S. & J. SOMMERFELD. 1985. Concepts of illness and the utilization of health-care services in a rural Malian village. Soc. Sci. Med. **21**(4): 469-481.
11. SRINIVASAN, T. N. 1988. On studying socio-economic change in rural India. Working Paper, Economic Growth Center, Yale University, New Haven, CT.
12. HARRIS, Z. 1987. Language and Information. Columbia University Press. New York.
13. HARRIS, Z., M. GOTTFRIED, T. RYCKMAN, P. MATTICK, A. DALADIER, T. N. HARRIS & S. HARRIS. 1987. The Form of Information in Science: Analysis of an Immunology Sub-language. Reidel. Dordrecht.
14. GIORDANO, R., J. COLE & H. ZUCKERMAN. 1988. Text Retrieval on a Microcomputer. Perspect. Comput. **8**(1): 52-60.

15. SEIDEL, J. V., R. KJOLSETH & E. SEYMOUR. 1988. The Ethnograph: A User's Guide. Qualis Research Associates. Littleton, CO.
16. COHEN, J. E. 1988. Estimating the effects of successful malaria control programmes on mortality. Popul Bull. UN **25:** 6-26.
17. DOLE, V. P., M. E. NYSWANDER, D. DES JARLAIS & H. JOSEPH. 1982. Performance based ratings of methadone maintenance programs. N. Engl. J. Med. **306:** 169-172.
18. SINGER, B. 1986. Self-selection and performance-based ratings: a case study in program Evaluation. *In* Drawing Inferences from Self-Selected Samples. H. Wainer, Ed.: 29-49. Springer-Verlag. New York.
19. SINGHANETRA-RENARD, A. 1987. The combined impact of land pressure and economic needs on the transmission of malaria in Thailand. Paper presented at WHO/TDR Conference on Social and Economic Determinants and Consequences of Malaria and its Control under Changing Conditions. Sitges, Spain, October 26-30, 1987.
20. SCHULTZ, T. P. 1988. Population programs: Measuring their impact on fertility and the personal distribution of their effects. J. Policy Model., **10**(1): 113-149.
21. FINNEY, D. J. 1984. Improvement by planned multistage selection. J. Am. Stat. Assoc. **79:** (387): 501-509.
22. SAWYER, D. R. & D. R. T. O. SAWYER. 1987. Malaria on The Amazon Frontier: Economic and Social Aspects of Transmission and Control. Belo Horizonte: Centro de Desevolvimento e Planejamento Regional, Faculdade de Ciências Econômicas-UFMG.
23. ELLIS, W. S. 1988. Rondônia's settlers invade Brazil's imperiled rain forest. Natl. Geogr. **174**(6): 772-799.
24. HEYNEMAN, D. 1984. Presidential Address: American Society of Parasitologists. J. Parasitol. **70**(1): 2-17.
25. WOODBURY, M. A., J. CLIVE & A. GARSON. 1978. Mathematical typology: A grade of membership technique for obtaining disease definition. Comput. Biomed. Res. **11:** 277-298.
26. MANTON, K. G. & E. STALLARD. 1988. Chronic Disease Modelling: Measurement and the Evaluation of Risks of Chronic Disease Processes. Charles Griffin. London.
27. BERKMAN, L., B. SINGER & K. MANTON. 1989. Black/white differences in health status and mortality among the elderly. Demography. In press.
28. MILLIGAN, P. J. M. & R. BAKER. 1988. A model of tse-tse transmitted animal trypanosomiasis. Parasitology **96:** 211-239.
29. MILLIGAN, P J. M. 1988. Epizootiology of trypanosomiases: Some aspects of mathematical modelling. Presented at the WHO/TDR Workshop on Mathematical Modelling, Trypanosomiases Epidemiology and Control, Antwerp Belgium, 25-29 January, 1988.
30. KAEWSONTHI, S. & A. HARDING. 1984. Cost and performance of malaria surveillance. Soc. Sci. Med. **19:** 1081.
31. KAEWSONTHI, S. & A. HARDING. 1986. Cost and performance of malaria surveillance: The patients' perspectives. Southeast Asian J. Trop. Med. Publ. Hlth. **17**(3): 406-412.
32. BRADLEY, R. 1987. Charisma and Social Structure. Paragon House. New York.
33. AXELROD, R. 1984. The Evolution of Cooperation. Basic Books. New York.
34. COHEN, J. E. 1988. The counterintuitive in conflict and cooperation. Am. Sci. November-December: 577-584.

Investments in Women, Economic Development, and Improvements in Health in Low-Income Countries[a]

T. PAUL SCHULTZ

Department of Economics
Yale University
New Haven, Connecticut 06520

INTRODUCTION

The rate of economic development depends on the mix of investments undertaken by a country and its people. Human capital investments that enhance the productivity of labor and are embodied in the worker are a large and increasing fraction of total investments in most countries.[1] The rates of return on these investments in people are inferred by studies of the productivity of workers who differ in their acquired skills or human capital. These beneficial increases in productivity due to human capital are discounted back to the time when the investments were undertaken to assess whether they are worthwhile, or more precisely to determine the internal rates of return they yield. Comparative studies of worker productivity cannot, in most cases, be based on experimentally induced or randomized variation in human capital investments across a population. For example, persons who acquire more education than others may be different in other respects. There are, consequently, many controversial issues on how to control statistically for extraneous factors that might affect the productivity of workers and also be associated with their human capital investments. With all the limitations that such investigations entail, a large number of studies now exist based on a wide variety of working assumptions that find private and social returns to primary and secondary schooling are relatively high, between 5 and 40% per year, compared with returns on physical capital investments in factories, equipment, inventories and infrastructure. These private rates of returns to basic schooling are also believed to be higher in low-income countries than they are in high-income, industrially advanced countries.[2] The secular increase in investments in education in low-income countries is therefore often interpreted as an economically efficient response of poor people and their governments to the competitively attractive returns they can expect to earn on investments in additional schooling.

It is more difficult to estimate rates of return to public and private health investments and related research and development of new health measures and technologies. The substantial reduction in mortality achieved in the last 30 years strengthens the

[a]This paper summarizes research complete for the Women in Development Division of the Population and Human Resources Department of the World Bank.

impression that these health investments have paid off handsomely, at least in low-income countries. But there are few studies that isolate the role of specific programs or policy interventions in bringing about a major improvement in public health and labor productivity based on data representing the entire population. Even in the most dramatic cases of malaria control in the 1940s and 1950s, the origins of these improvements in health are hard to establish with confidence because broadly based economic advances involving improvements in trade, nutrition, and income occurred at about the same time as the new malaria-control measures were implemented.

There are many reasons why the task of evaluating public health programs in low-income countries is fraught with uncertainty. Many types of human capital investment (such as prenatal health care, child nutrition supplements, and child health care) yield immediate consumption benefits to the family as well as delayed gains in productivity that accrue over the individual's later adult lifetime. As with education, one can conservatively neglect the consumption benefits of health investments, understating their real value, but there still remains the problem of forecasting future gains in productivity and discounting them appropriately. Despite the limitations of our health-evaluation methods, evidence is accumulating that advances in health are responsible for a substantial, if imprecisely measured, part of the unprecedented world economic growth achieved in the period since the Second World War.

A convergence is evident among nations both in years of school investments and in health, proxied by longevity, with the poorer nations closing the *relative* gap that separates them from the richer, industrially advanced nations. This catching up has been widely noted in life expectancy[3] and is equally dramatic if age-specific enrollment rates are summed to provide an analogous single measure of expected years of schooling.[4]

REGIONAL PATTERNS OF INVESTMENT IN SCHOOLING OF WOMEN AND MEN

The human capital investment made in women relative to men is markedly different across countries. Some of these intercountry differences can be rationalized in terms of the economic constraints applicable to these countries. As will be shown, those countries of the world that are poorest tend to be those in which women receive, on average, the smallest share of these human capital investments. The most important human capital investments are, of course, in the two areas already discussed: schooling and health.

In the industrially advanced, high-income countries women receive today nearly the same number of years of schooling as do men, and women often report higher enrollment rates than men through secondary school. Latin America and East Asia are quite similar to the developed countries in this regard. At the other extreme are most of the countries of South and West Asia and North and sub-Saharan Africa, in which women receive about half to three-fourths the years of schooling that men do. This regional pattern is illustrated in column 1 of TABLE 1 using estimates of years of completed schooling from a recent census, and in columns 3 and 4 on the basis of official enrollment rates aggregated across school levels. Although both sources of data on education have their respective shortcomings and probably overstate the real human capital women receive relative to men, the patterns across countries in these

TABLE 1. Years of Schooling Completed and Expected Years of Enrollment Ratios by Sex, for Regions from 1960 and 1980: Selected Available Countries

Region (number of countries observed)	Years of Schooling 1960-1980 Completed at Age 20-24: Female to Male Ratio (1)	Years of Schooling 1960-1980 Completed at Age 20-24: Male Level in Years (2)		Expected Years of Enrollment: Female to Male Ratio 1960 (3)	Expected Years of Enrollment: Female to Male Ratio 1980 (4)	Expected Years of Enrollment: Male Level in Years 1960 (5)	Expected Years of Enrollment: Male Level in Years 1980 (6)
1. High-income industrially advanced countries (including Japan, Israel, and South Africa)	1.00 (24)	8.9 (24)		.94	1.00	10.8	12.6
2. Latin America	.94 (22)	5.5 (22)		.92	.97	5.6	9.8
3. East Asia (excluding Japan)	.83 (8)	6.4 (8)	Asia (excluding Arab)	.65	.75	7.5	9.4
4. South Asia	.45 (5)	3.8 (5)					
5. West Asia (excluding Israel)	.34 (2)	4.7 (2)	Arab States	.49	.73	5.0	9.0
6. North Africa	.39 (2)	3.5 (2)					
7. Sub-Saharan Africa (excluding South Africa)	.44 (7)	3.3 (7)	Africa (excluding Arab)	.56	.73	3.5	7.0
World total	n.a.	n.a.		.75	.82	7.7	9.8

SOURCE: Columns 1 and 2 are derived by averaging the available sample of country estimates reported in APPENDIX TABLE A. Columns 3-6 are derived from UNESCO estimates of enrollment rates by level, with different regional groupings. *1987 Statistical Yearbook,* Table 2.10. See Reference 3 for additional details.

two measures are broadly coincident.[b] Enrollment rates are slowly converging between women and men from 1960 to 1980, as development has proceeded. Are the differences in female and male educational investments that remain explained by the diverse economic conditions in these countries?

An analysis of educational systems from 80 countries for the period between 1960 and 1980 sought to account for differences in public expenditures on education and enrollment rates in terms of real incomes per adult, the relative cost of teachers, and the share and urban composition of the school-aged population. More than 90% of the intercountry variation in public school expenditures per school-aged child and 40 to 70% of the variation in primary and secondary school enrollment rates are explained in this fashion. The proportionate increase in enrollment rates for girls associated with a proportionate increase in income is significantly larger than the analogous income elasticity of enrollment for boys. Price elasticities are also larger in absolute value (negative) for female enrollment rates than for male. With economic growth and long-run expansion of the educational system, which tends to cause the relative price of teachers to decline, educational investments in women appear to increase relative to those in men. But within countries over time this gap between the educational attainment of women and men has narrowed more slowly than would have been expected on the basis of the relationship observed across countries at different levels of development.[4] These findings also suggest that unless special measures are adopted, female enrollments may contract by a larger proportion than male enrollments in periods of economic decline, public sector retrenchment, and macroeconomic adjustment as may now be occurring in many countries of Africa and Latin America.

Holding constant for national income, teacher prices, and demographic structure, one can calculate how many percent above or below average are national enrollment rates, or expenditures on public education at the primary and secondary level for each country. TABLE 2 reports the regional averages of these percentage deviations and reveals a somewhat different pattern from that seen in TABLE 1. Africa is an overachiever, given its low income and high cost of teachers, and these African constraints

[b] Expenditures per year on schooling of boys and girls is frequently not equal, particularly where the schooling system is not coeducational, but also where women are predominantly enrolled in different courses of study. A common arrangement is for women in higher education to be heavily concentrated in teacher training (normal) schools, while men are in academic university-based programs; or else women tend to train as nurses, while men train as doctors, lawyers, and engineers. The public costs and private returns to these courses of study are likely to differ, often substantially. There is also much scattered evidence that females enrolled in school perform more work at home than do males of the same age,[16] and girls are more readily withdrawn from school as temporary requirements for labor in the home increase. Enrollment rates collected at the start of the school year undoubtedly overstate the annual average attendance rates, and the overstatement is probably larger for girls than for boys. Consequently, the census figures on years of schooling completed reported in the first two columns of TABLE 1 are probably a more precise indicator of differences in human capital investment in men and women than the "expected years" measure derived from enrollment rates provided by school systems that are shown in the last four columns of TABLE 1.

Finally, interpersonal or intercountry comparisons based on the *ratio* of years of schooling of women and men may exaggerate gender inequality at low-income levels and understate it at high-income levels. For example, if rates of returns to schooling are constant at, say, 20%, a difference in schooling between women and men may be two years and be then associated with a wage difference of 40% between women and men. As the national level of schooling increases, but the two-year gap remains between men and women, the increase in the *relative* schooling of women and men will not be associated with an increase in the relative wage of women to men, unless, of course, the return on schooling decreases.

TABLE 2. Percentage Deviations in National Educational Investments, Adjusting for the Effects of Income, Teacher Salaries, and Demographic Composition: 1960-1980[a]

	Primary School System				Secondary School System			
	Number of Country/Years	Enrollment Rates		Expenditures per School-Aged	Number of Country/Years	Enrollment Rates		Expenditures per School-Aged
Region	Observed	Females	Males	Child	Observed	Female	Male	Child
Europe, Oceania and North America	36	+6	+6	−6	21	+3	+7	−6
Latin America	43	−10	−15	−5	35	−30	−39	−16
East Asia	21	+22	+12	+9	19	+27	+19	+2
South and West Asia	24	−49	−24	−21	16	−46	−7	−4
Africa	62	+26	+16	+15	49	+43	+34	+17

SOURCE: Schultz[4]; Table 13.

[a] Dependent variables are (1) the logarithm of the number of children enrolled in primary schools divided by the number of children aged 6 to 11, and (2) the logarithm of the secondary enrollment divided by the number of children aged 12 to 17; and the local public expenditures on the school level divided by the number of children in the respective benefitting age class expressed in real 1970 local currency and converted to 1970 U.S. dollars on the basis of IMF exchange rates prevailing on average for 1969 to 1971. See source for more detail.

account for the lower female-to-male enrollments in that continent. Latin America now reports lower than expected enrollment rates, but the adjusted shortfall in this region is greater for males than for females. In the high-income countries, there is a small positive deviation in adjusted enrollment rates, and they tend to be slightly larger for women than for men at the secondary school level. South and West Asia, however, continue to evidence underinvestment in primary and secondary schools, and the adjusted shortfall is significantly larger for females than for males. Consequently, the low levels of income, the high cost of teachers, and the demographic composition of the population do not account for the relatively low level of investment in the schooling of women in South and West Asia or indeed in North Africa.

REGIONAL PATTERNS OF MORTALITY FOR MALES AND FEMALES

Life expectancy also favors women relative to men in the same countries where schooling is more equally distributed by gender, as illustrated in TABLE 3. Biological evidence suggests that women are genetically more viable than men. Given similar consumption opportunities, women experience lower mortality rates at all ages, except perhaps during the childbearing years in countries where women have not been widely enrolled in primary schools. Death due to bearing a child is 20-fold higher in South and West Asia and North and sub-Saharan Africa than in the developed countries, and women in these low-income regions also bear twice as many children as do their high-income counterparts (TABLE 3, col. 7). Nonetheless, infant and childhood mortality is quantitatively a larger factor in the low life expectancy of females in these regions. Estimates of differences in mortality by sex for children are, however, scarce and often unreliable; TABLE 3 illustratively average official figures reported by the 1983 UN *Demographic Yearbook* to suggest regional patterns.[c] Greater confidence can perhaps be placed on the infant and childhood mortality estimates derived from the recent World Fertility Surveys.[5,6] Only two of 29 surveys, those for Jordan and Syria, revealed greater female than male infant mortality, while three—Bangladesh, Pakistan, and Egypt—reported higher female than male child mortality between the ages of 2 and 5. All of these countries fall in the South and West Asian or North African region.

More detailed analyses of mortality trends by sex confirm, as with education, that the prospects for survival are improving more rapidly for women than for men in most regions of the world.[3] The world appears to be converging toward the sex differences in mortality observed in the industrially advanced countries, but the pace of progress differs markedly by regions. Women's education remains the best predictor of the level and sex differences in mortality; female enrollment rates are used by a recent World Bank study to forecast how national mortality schedules are likely to evolve in the next 50 years.[7] Until life expectancy at birth for women exceeds 60 years, the rate of increase in longevity is significantly greater in countries where more than

[c] Because of the scarcity of reliable estimates of mortality rates by age and sex in much of Asia and Africa, TABLE B is appended with only higher quality estimates of life expectancy by sex and age-specific mortality by sex. These are probably more reliable than the regional aggregated estimates of life expectancy and official registration figures for child mortality as reported in TABLE 3. For Latin America and high-income countries the figures in TABLE 3 should be satisfactory.

TABLE 3. Life Expectancy at Birth and Infant Mortality, Ratio by Sex and Maternal Mortality, for Regions in 1960 and 1980

	Life Expectancy at Birth						
	Infant Mortality						
	Female to Male		Male Level		Female to Male	Male Level	Maternal Mortality per 100,000 Live Births
	1960-65 (1)	1980-85 (2)	1960-1980 (3)	(4)	ca. 1980 (5)	ca. 1980 (6)	ca. 1983 (7)
High-income	1.09	1.11	66.6	68.8	.80	17.4	30
Europe	1.05	1.09	67.0	69.7	(22)[a]	(22)	30
Oceania	1.07	1.06	61.7	64.8			
North America	1.10	1.12	66.9	69.4			
Japan	1.08	1.07	66.5	73.8			
Israel	1.04	1.05	68.1	71.0			
South Africa	1.07	1.05	52.1	60.9			
Latin America	1.06	1.07	54.9	62.1	.83	44.09	270
					(11)	(11)	

East Asia (excluding Japan)	1.06	1.05	51.0	64.5	.79 (3)	34.2 (3)	187
South East Asia	1.06	1.05	43.2	53.5			
Other East Asia (e.g. Hong Kong, Korea)	1.07	1.06	54.2	63.4			
China	1.06	1.04	54.4	68.5			
South Asia (middle)	.97	.93	43.3	50.7	.82 (4)	51.0 (4)	618
West Asia	1.05	1.06	48.2	58.2			
Africa	1.07	1.06	40.6	49.3	—	—	
North Africa	1.05	1.05	45.5	54.6	.98 (2)	58.1 (2)	500
Sub-Saharan Africa (excluding South Africa)	1.08	1.07	39.1	47.7	.81 (4)	86.4 (4)	676
World	1.05	1.04	50.9	57.9	—	—	—

SOURCES: First four columns are weighted by populations. Estimates are from United Nations (*Demographic Indicators of Countries,* New York, 1982); columns 5 and 6 are unweighted averages of countries reporting in the *1983 UN Demographic Yearbook* (Table 16); column 7 gives estimates weighted by population of regions from Ross *et al.* (1988, Table 34). For country level estimates that are probably more reliable for Africa and Asia, see APPENDIX TABLE B.

[a] Number of countries averaged in parentheses indicate that they are not necessarily representative of region because of data limitations.

70% of girls are enrolled in primary school (as of 1965-69). In sum, women are especially poor relative to men in their acquired capabilities, such as schooling, in the world's poorest countries, and their relative neglect is also reflected in their shorter lives. Equity calls for increasing the productive capabilities and consumption opportunities of women in these poorest countries. Are there also efficiency gains for a society that might motivate public interventions to equalize investments in women and men?

CONSEQUENCES OF HUMAN CAPITAL INVESTMENT ON ECONOMIC DEVELOPMENT

Efficiency, in an economic sense, implies that investments of the family in each member's food, health, and long-term skill formation is encouraged only if these investments repay the parents or intergenerational family at a rate of return that is at least as high as they can earn on their capital in alternative uses. The current production that the family sacrifices for such an investment or the opportunity cost (for example, in the case of a child attending school, the family's foregone child production) must be repaid with market interest by the child's enhanced future lifetime productivity. A rough rule of thumb suggests that when the allocation of an additional year's time to investment in human capital, such as schooling, raises subsequent lifetime average wage opportunities by a certain percent, then that percent wage gain approximates the private rate of return to schooling.[8,9] Although the wage of the more educated woman may be lower than that of a comparably educated man, the opportunity cost of the time that the woman sacrifices to attend school rather than work is also less than that of a man. It is not the absolute level of wages, therefore, that signals the private efficiency returns to human capital investment, but the *relative* wage differences across groups with a different number of years of time invested in the acquisition of human capital. The question of interest here is whether differences in the private rates of return to schooling of women and men across countries might help to account for why parents and society in some countries invest substantially less in women than in men.

TABLE 4 summarizes this proportionate wage shift associated with a year of completed schooling among workers in several Latin American countries. These separate estimates of the private returns to schooling for men and for women are based on a common conceptual and statistical methodology and take account of variation in labor supply, but make no adjustment for the possibly unrepresentative character of the sample of wage earners. Similar evidence could be reported on the basis of slightly different statistical methods from such places as urban India, China, Taiwan, South Korea, and Thailand. Because underlying samples of wage earners are often small, estimates of the returns to schooling, such as in TABLE 4, are sometimes imprecise. Overall, however, there is no clear evidence from existing studies that private returns to schooling systematically differ by sex, though they differ considerably in overall level across countries and years, depending on macroeconomic conditions in the country and the levels of past investments in schooling.[1]

Relatively few studies have thus far sought to correct for the potentially unrepresentative nature of the samples of wage earners that are generally analyzed to understand the sources of individual productivity gains. Education could be more (or less) productive in wage employment than it is in self-employment or family work.

TABLE 4. Estimates of Private Returns (in Percent per Year) That Men and Women Earn on Investing Their Time in Schooling, in Selected Labor Markets and Years[a]

		Internal Rate of Return in Percent per Year			
		Age 25-44		Age 45-65	
Country and/or Metropolitan Area	Year of Survey	Men	Women	Men	Women
Argentina					
Buenos Aires	1980[b]	9.3	6.6	10.0	11.0
(estimates similar in 1976)					
Bolivia					
La Paz	1980	9.8	11.0	9.6	6.7
(estimates similar in 1976)					
Brazil					
Sao Paulo	1971	5.4	6.3	6.0	6.1
(estimates higher in 1980)					
Colombia					
(estimates lower in 1980)	1973	18.0	18.0	16.0	14.0
Paraguay					
Asunción	1979	11.0	8.0	10.0	11.0
(estimates similar in 1977)					
Peru	1974	14.0	14.0	11.0	19.0

SOURCE: Table in Schultz.[37]

[a] Private returns refer to the estimated coefficient (times 100) on the variable years of completed education in a logarithmic hourly wage rate regression which also includes post-schooling experience, experience squared, and some regional or migration origin variables. Samples vary from 21 to 3,478, but all estimates are statistically significantly different from zero at the .001 confidence level ($t > 2.83$). The selection of the sample of only workers in the labor force for whom wage rate could be calculated is not treated as a specific source of bias in these estimates.

[b] The available age groups in Argentina are 25-49 and over 49.

Farm profits, after payment for the market value of all farm inputs including family labor, tend to be positively associated with the farmer's level of education. This was originally documented in several studies of U.S. farmers and then replicated in a variety of low-income countries.[10] The private rates of return to schooling among farmers estimated in these studies are comparable to the estimated private returns to schooling among wage earners. But these comparisons may also include a sample-selection bias. First, more educated individuals are more likely to leave farming for an urban job than is the less educated rural resident. The remaining sample of farmers that have not left agriculture, as well as the sample of largely urban wage earners are both not precisely representative of the entire cohort of persons who could have benefited from various amounts of schooling. A few studies have attempted to isolate the bias from rural out-migration and they conclude that private returns to rural schooling are downwardly biased unless the returns to schooling collected by leaving agriculture are included in the rural born cohort's lifetime income gains.[1] The second, more intractable problem with studies of farmer education and productivity is that the labor productivity of male and female family farm workers is not separately estimated. Consequently, the increased profits collected by the more-educated farmer are attributed to his (or her) management ability, and the enhanced productivity due to the labor of the spouse or an unpaid family worker, who is also probably better educated, is not distinguished or deducted. Separate calculations of the returns to education for men and women in farming are occasionally available, as for example in Africa, when men and women manage different plots or crops.[11]

A few recent studies have used appropriate statistical methods to correct for the sample-selection bias that might arise because the productive effects of schooling are commonly estimated from an analysis of only wage earners. The tentative findings from these investigations of Thailand, Peru, and Colombia are that the uncorrected private returns to primary schooling inferred from wage earners underestimate the returns received by the representative individual in these low-income countries. But at the secondary school level the private returns to schooling estimated from wage earners may overstate the returns for the representative individual.[d] Refinements in the construction of the wage comparisons between education groups can thus modify the measured private returns to schooling, but these alternative estimation methods have not tended to change systematically the pattern of approximate equality in private returns to schooling to men and women working in the same labor market.

Consequently, there is no statistical basis from many studies of wage earners or farmers to conclude that the efficiency returns to the private individual are lower from educating girls than boys. Moreover, there are several reasons for the social benefits that spill over beyond the individual from educating women to exceed those that are generated from educating men. To the extent that taxation on earnings recoups some of the public outlays on education, the differential labor supply response of women and men should reduce the net social costs of providing education to women and increase it for educating men. This occurs because women tend to work more hours in taxable work as their human capital increases in virtually all populations where labor supply behavior of women has been studied, whereas women and men tend to work fewer hours in taxable activities as the human capital of men increases. The net public cost of extending schooling to women is thus defrayed by the labor supply response of women, and the tax base is eroded and the social costs of schooling increased when men receive more schooling.

Beyond the private productivity return to schooling and the taxes the more productive worker pays, education can have additional consequences on other societal goals that are traditionally subsidized by the public sector. The human capital of parents has distinctive effects on their lifetime fertility, and the health, nutrition, and schooling of their children. Moreover, these linkages tend to be more positive for the mother's education than for the father's education, as discussed below. These social external benefits of women's schooling strengthen the efficiency argument for subsidizing more heavily women's schooling than men's.

[d] To measure the productive returns to investing in the capabilities of either women or men, the special factors underlying the individual's allocation of time to wage employment must be identified, preferably by economic theory. The resulting sample-selection correction procedure then permits one to infer the private rate of return to schooling for the entire population from observing labor productivity for only wage earners. The variables that modify the individual's reservation wage or the value of time in nonwage work will depend on how broadly the relevant resource-pooling family is defined, and how flexibly family labor supply behavior is modeled. Existing studies for low-income countries provide only the beginnings of a basis on which to draw empirical generalization about the magnitude of sample-selection bias in the estimates of school returns, and how they differ for men and women. See, for example, work by Mohan on Colombia, King on Peru, and Schultz on Thailand.[35–37] Though even these three studies employ different rules for model identification, they are moving toward a consensus on appropriate estimation methodology. Replication of this approach is now needed.

Available data thus indicate that private returns earned by investing family resources in schooling are as large for sending girls to school as they are for boys. But the evidence from many countries of Asia and Africa suggests that families are not as willing to sacrifice their resources to provide girls and boys with the same number of years of schooling. To infer why parents value the housework of their daughters more highly than they do the returns from educating their daughters, we need more studies of the general determinants of resource allocations within the family. Why do particular forms of consumption and human capital investments differ for boys and girls? Perhaps family arrangements in some cultures assign the gains from the increased productivity of women only to the family of the woman's husband. It is not clear why the woman's parents are not sufficiently compensated for their daughters' education, but some form of economic "market failure" must be present and warrants corrective measures. If private markets fail to induce individuals to invest socially optimal amounts in the education of certain groups, society is justified on efficiency grounds in subsidizing the schooling of such groups. Women would appear to be such a group in many countries.

The most frequently encountered explanation for the lower level of human capital investment in women than in men is that women participate less in the labor force, on average, and therefore the returns they receive when they work in the labor force should be deflated by the probability that they will assume a job in the market labor force.[8] Although women in high-income countries are rapidly catching up to men in their labor force participation rates,[12] the measured differences between the sexes in many low-income countries remain substantial. But this interpretation of the market returns to schooling implies that the productivity of people working outside of the labor force is not affected by their education. This assumption has recently been challenged by a large number of empirical studies that find education increases the productivity of a worker's time in many nonmarket production processes, particularly those performed by women in the home.[13,14] The practical problem is that there is no measure available to sum up these gains in home productivity.

PRODUCTIVITY IN THE MARKET AND HOME

Because of the difficulty of measuring and valuing nonmarket production, economists have tended to focus on the marketable component of income of families and individuals. In principle, the market value of home-produced and -consumed goods, such as the production and preparation of food, fuel, the fetching of water, and maintenance of housing, for which there are sometimes market-priced equivalents, should be included in personal and national income. But in practice the complexity of imputations leads to their omission, with no attention to untradeable home-production activities such as child-rearing. All of these forms of home production have become neglected because they are relatively unimportant in high-income countries, where economic accounting conventions tend to be first elaborated and refined. But when this omission is replicated in low-income countries, a more serious distortion is introduced that systematically affects one's perception of women's contribution to the economy and transforms the entire quantitative record of modern economic growth. By omitting these nonmarket components of personal income, economists understate sources of income that are larger for poor families, and within families these conventions understate women's economic contribution relative to men's.[15,16] National income appears to grow more rapidly than it should as women allocate progressively more of their time to the market labor force, and no offsetting deduction to national income is made for the time women retract from nonmarket production that would otherwise benefit their families.

Technical change is fostered if it boosts the productivity of workers in the labor force, but may be overlooked if it promises only to raise the productivity of workers engaged in undocumented home production. Public health measures are evaluated with little attention to the critical input of women's time in health care, as though the productive value of women's time is insignificant in comparisons to public sector resources and health inputs privately purchased in the market. It is widely suspected that public investments in agricultural research and development were originally biased toward export crops in many low-income countries because commercial interests are concentrated in these crops and governments view them as a convenient source of tax revenue. Yet these export crops are often managed by males while the family food staples are more often produced by female agricultural workers, particularly in Africa. The gains from technical change in agriculture have thus been shifted toward market workers relative to nonmarket workers or, correspondingly, toward men relative to women.[17–20] This intellectual oversight and resulting distortion in policy will only be corrected when the quantitative importance of nonmarket and in-kind income is estimated and its bearing on public sector priorities explicitly evaluated. In the area of disease control, morbidity reduction, extension of life, and fertility, the importance of women as productive and innovative agents is insufficiently emphasized.[21,16]

CHILD HEALTH AND MORTALITY

The distinctive role of women in managing consumption of and investment in children within the family is a major reason for social intervention to increase specifically her capabilities and control over resources. Improving the productivity of women through human capital investments is a social objective to accelerate economic development, but also to channel that development and new streams of income toward socially desired investments in the food, medical care, and schooling of children. A third set of consequences is associated with raising women's productivity; it involves the reduction of child mortality and the parallel reduction in fertility. Together these two demographic developments constitute the demographic transition that eventually diminishes the rate of population growth and increases the proportion of the population in the more productive labor force ages. Quantitative confirmation of these linkages, however, requires much study and replication at the household level to establish sound generalizations from country-specific empirical regularities. These studies will also help to identify the special features in many societies that modify the magnitudes of these behavioral tendencies.

Studies in the 1970s and 1980s in demography, economics, anthropology, and sociology came to a common conclusion: there was a strong, probably causal, relationship between mother's schooling and decreases in the incidence of mortality among her children. These patterns are widely replicated in dozens of surveys from countries in every region of the world. An added year of mother's education is associated with a 5 to 10% reduction in child mortality. Although the level of mortality tends to be higher in rural than in urban populations of low-income countries, the proportionate reduction in child mortality associated with an additional year of mother's schooling is of a similar magnitude in both urban and rural areas of the same country.[22] On the other hand, the smaller impact of father's schooling on his children's mortality is greatly attenuated in rural populations.[23] Studies in Latin America also found that child mortality differentials associated with maternal education were smaller in Costa Rica and Cuba, and it was hypothesized that the strong public health programs in these two countries had helped even the least-educated mothers to obtain effective health care for their children.[24] This and other economic hypotheses for the differences in the relative magnitude of the mother's schooling effects on child health and mortality have been analyzed with data from Colombia and Philippines.[25–27] It has been observed in several studies that public health outreach programs have their greatest benefit for the children of the least-educated mothers. In economic terms, the management and innovational skills that an educated mother brings to the health care of her family appear to be economic "substitutes" for the preventive health care and extension activities provided by the local health system. Consequently, health outreach activities have their largest payoff among the least-educated portions of the population.

Is education simply associated with having more resources to spend on health inputs or does education provide a mother with the capacity to cope more efficiently with health risks and to better manage her child's environment? In Colombia and Brazil it appears that controlling for household income or husband's education or the marital status of the mother does not eliminate or even greatly reduce the independent partial explanatory role of the mother's education on her children's survival rate.[25,28] Other studies confirmed that it was possible to control for a comprehensive series of life-cycle events and current socioeconomic status variables in a regression equation explaining child mortality rates and still find a strong effect of maternal education.[29]

Demographers were initially confident in the capacity of biomedical and public health technologies to control infectious and parasitic diseases in low-income countries, irrespective of the country's comprehensive socioeconomic development.[30] A major factor in reassessing this conclusion is the quantitative evidence that maternal education is a more important determinant of cross-sectional variation in child mortality than is access to low-cost health services and modern biomedical technologies. Another factor in this reassessment has been the growing evidence that the rate of decline in mortality in low-income countries has slowed down since 1970, while it may have recently accelerated in high-income countries.[3] One conclusion is clear, however: unless the complex roles of mother's education in family health are better understood and properly controlled, evaluation of the cost-effectiveness of a multitude of other health-oriented programs will be extremely imprecise and possibly misleading. One area in which family behavior relevant to child health is strongly affected by the human capital capabilities of women and men is fertility.

FERTILITY: CHANGING REPRODUCTIVE GOALS AND REDUCING UNWANTED BIRTHS

In most societies the level of fertility responds sensitively to women's wage rates. Higher wages for women, which are associated with their human capital, increase their income, but also increase what they must give up for them to bear and rear an additional child. The latter price effect invariably outweighs the former income effect, and the statistical tendency is for fertility to decline as women's market wage opportunities rise. Increases in the labor productivity and wage rates of men, on the other hand, can enhance the attractiveness of a large family and are often associated with higher levels of fertility, at least in low-income agricultural countries.[31]

Because most children work as unpaid family workers, it is difficult to observe in the labor market the productive value of the time of children. But where regional wage rates for children are observed to vary, they are positively related to fertility, as in Egypt, where irrigation opportunities determine what crops are grown and these crops use different amounts of child labor.[32] Nonearned income from land and physical wealth is also generally associated with larger families, because these sources of income are not necessarily related to what it costs to have another child. Nonearned income, therefore, permits parents to have more children, if other things are equal, and empirically we generally observe this pattern holding constant for the separate education or wage opportunities of the mother and the father.[33] But nonearned income also may be dependent on past savings and work behavior of the parents that could increase the opportunity cost of children and mask in nonagricultural societies the expected positive relationship between exogenous sources of nonhuman capital and fertility.

As noted above, major credit for reducing infant and child mortality in low-income countries was initially given to the international transfer of modern public health technologies, such as vaccines, antibiotics, and pesticides, along with institutions to manage their dissemination. By the 1970s, it was becoming evident that fertility declines were closely associated with the declining incidence of infant and child mortality, both when examined in cross-sectional household surveys at the level of the individual woman and when studied across aggregates such as regions or countries.[31] If the association between child mortality and fertility were causal, and child mortality declined in this period only because of the importation of new public health technologies that left economic conditions essentially unchanged, then these data suggested that parents were responding to the increasing rates of child survival by having fewer births. In other words, human fertility exhibited a homeostatic replacement response pattern and could be expected to compensate for child mortality. According to this interpretation of the data, health measures that were successful in reducing child mortality would elicit a compensating reduction in fertility that would dampen any acceleration in population growth caused over the short run by improvements in health conditions in low-income countries.

With more study, however, this explanation of the facts had to be elaborated. Because it is now clear that women's education, among other household endowments, governs a substantial part of the variation in child mortality, it is not accurate to attribute the widespread reduction in child mortality to an exogenously imposed change in public health technology. The association between a mother's education and lower fertility may reflect that more educated women decide to have fewer children because they can effectively shelter their children from many health risks.[27] Even though much of the variation in child mortality appears to be attributable to household socioeconomic resources and the education of parents, fertility appears to respond also to variation in child mortality that is beyond the control of the family household. Thus fertility continues to compensate for the exogenous variation in child mortality, such as might be altered by vaccine availability or disease-eradication programs. But the task of statistically separating the replacement response becomes more difficult because both fertility and child mortality are behaviorally modified by the same class of household variables.

The schooling of women may therefore exert effects on child health and mortality at several levels. Education of mothers is responsible for first reducing child mortality and thereby contributing to a decline in replacement fertility. More-educated mothers also receive higher wages when they work. These improved prospects for employment in the labor market increase the value they assign to their own time at home and thereby raise the total resource costs of having additional children. A reduction in desired fertility follows, with education facilitating competing objectives of providing each of their children with more health care and schooling. At a third level schooling of women improves contraceptive practice and is associated with a reduction in unwanted conception and births. Mother's education and her family's socioeconomic constraints affect fertility and child mortality in these and other synergistic ways. Evaluating the consequences of public health program activities, including family planning, can proceed with greater confidence as these behavioral adjustments of families to their developing opportunities and endowments are explicitly included in the assessment of policy interventions.

CONCLUSION

Women play a central role in determining the health of family members, and the education of women is a powerful, if not yet fully understood, factor affecting child mortality, nutrition, health, and school achievement. The local availability of medical care and public health interventions can be evaluated as independent determinants of health only after the effects of household resources and maternal education are held constant. Analogously, local community expenditures per woman on family planning activities can be assessed as a factor reducing fertility only after the same family socioeconomic resource constraints are taken into account.[34] Unequal investments in the human capital of women and men may have much to do with the differential progress made in various countries in reducing mortality and fertility. Father's education and wage opportunities reduce child mortality modestly and then mostly in urban areas, whereas they are conducive to higher fertility in rural areas. Modern curative health programs, such as clinics and hospitals, appear to confer few health benefits beyond urban populations in many low-income countries. In contrast, mother's education and increased market wage opportunities are associated with reductions in her fertility and in the mortality of her children, whether she resides in an urban or rural area of the low-income world. Those countries that were identified initially in this paper as having invested relatively little in the education and health of women may have paid a high price for this allocation of their resources, both in terms of inefficient slower economic growth in labor productivity and also in terms of slower advances in health.

Unless health policy interventions and pilot programs are implemented according to a randomized design, evaluation of their effectiveness will require a model of the socioeconomic determinants of household behavior. Among health determinants, the education of women and their productive opportunities appear to be important for understanding the family's demand for health care and related behavior such as fertility. The integration of social science models of household behavior and quantitative methods to evaluate public health programs can be of immediate value today in low-income countries. Perhaps in the not too distant future, these methods will also help to set national and international priorities in biomedical research that promise to develop new cost-effective medical technologies that extend the length of human life and raise the productivity of women and men in the Third World.

ACKNOWLEDGMENTS

I appreciate the comments of Barry Bloom and Mauro Guillen on a draft of this paper.

REFERENCES

1. SCHULTZ, T. P. 1988. Educational investment and returns. *In* Handbook of Development Economics, Vol. 1. H. Chenery & T. N. Srinivasan, Eds. North-Holland, Amsterdam.
2. PSACHAROPOULOS, G. & M. WOODHALL. 1985. Education for Development. Oxford University Press, New York.
3. UNITED NATIONS. 1982. Levels and Trends of Mortality Since 1950. Department of International Economic and Social Affairs (ST/ESA/SER.A/74). New York.
4. SCHULTZ, T. P. 1987. School expenditures and enrollments, 1960-1980. *In* National Academy of Sciences Background Papers. D. G. Johnson & R. Lee, Eds. Population Growth and Economic Development, University of Wisconsin Press. Madison, WI.
5. RUTSTEIN, S. O. 1983. Infant and child mortality: Levels, trends, and demographic differentials. WFS Comparative Studies No. 24.
6. HOBCRAFT, J. N., J. M. MCDONALD & S. O. RUTSTEIN. 1984. Socioeconomic factors in infant and child mortality. Popul. Stud. **38**(2): 363-385.
7. ZACHARIAH, K. C. & MY T. VU. 1988. World Population Projection, 1987-88 Edition. Johns Hopkins University Press. Baltimore, MD.
8. BECKER, G. S. 1964. Human Capital, Columbia University Press. New York.
9. MINCER, J. 1974. Schooling Experience and Earnings, Columbia University Press. New York.
10. JAMISON, D. T. & L. I. LAU. 1982. Farmer Education and Farm Efficiency. Johns Hopkins University Press. Baltimore, MD.
11. MOOCK, P. J. 1976. The efficiency of women as farm managers: Kenya. Am. J. Agr. Econ. **58**(5): 831-835.
12. LAYARD, R. & J. MINCER, Eds. 1985. Trends in women's work, education, and family building. J. Labor Econ. **3:** (pt. 2).
13. MICHAEL, R. T. 1982. Measuring nonmonetary benefits of education, *In* Financing Education. W. W. McMahon & T. G. Geske, Eds. University of Illinois Press, Urbana, Ill.
14. HAVEMAN, R. & B. WOLFE. 1984. Education and economic well being: The role of nonmarket effects. J. Hum. Res. **19:** 377-407.
15. KUSNIC, M. W. & J. DAVANZO. 1980. Income Inequality and the Definition of Income: The Case of Malaysia, R-2416-AID. The Rand Corporation. Santa Monica, CA.
16. EVENSON, R. E. 1983. The allocation of women's time: An international comparison. Behav. Sci. Res. **17:** (3/4: Spring-Summer): 196-218.
17. BOSERUP, E. 1965. The Conditions of Agricultural Growth. Aldine. Chicago, IL.
18. BOSERUP, E. 1970. Women's Role in Economic Development. St. Martin's Press. New York.
19. JUDD, M. A., J. K. BOYCE & R. E. EVENSON. 1986. Investing in Agricultural Supply. Econ. Dev. Cult. Change **35**(1): 77-114.
20. EVENSON, R. E. 1987. The International Agricultural Research Centers, CGIAR Study Paper No. 22. The World Bank. Washington, DC.
21. BINSWANGER, H. P., R. E. EVENSON, C. A. FLORENCIO & B. N. F. WHITE, Eds. 1980. Rural Household Studies in Asia. Singapore University Press. Singapore.
22. COCHRANE, S. H., J. LESLIE, D. J. O'HARA. 1980. The effects of education on health. The World Bank Staff Working Paper 405. Washington, DC.
23. MENSCH, B., H. LENTZNER & S. PRESTON. 1986. Socioeconomic Differentials in Child Mortality in Developing Countries. United Nations. New York.

24. BEHM, H. 1980. Socioeconomic determinants of mortality in Latin America. *In* Socioeconomic Determinants and Consequences of Mortality. WHO. Geneva.
25. SCHULTZ, T. P. 1980. Interpretation of the relations among mortality, economics of the household, and the health environment. *In* Socioeconomic Determinants and Consequences of Mortality Differences. WHO. Geneva.
26. SCHULTZ, T. P. 1984. Studying the impact of household economics and community variables on child mortality. *In* Child Survival. W. H. Mosley & L. C. Chen, Eds. Population and Development Review **10** (Suppl.): 215-236.
27. BARRERA, A. 1988. The role of maternal schooling and its interaction with public health programs in child health production. Economic Growth Center Discussion Paper No. 551. Yale University, New Haven, CT. (forthcoming in the *Journal of Development Economics*).
28. THOMAS, D., J. STRAUSS & M. H. HENRIQUES. 1987. Child survival, nutritional status, and household characteristics. Economic Growth Center Discussion Paper No. 542. Yale University, New Haven, Ct.
29. FARAH, A. A. & S. H. PRESTON. 1982. Child mortality differentials in Sudan. Popul. Dev. Rev. **8:** 365-383.
30. STOLNITZ, G. J. 1975. International mortality trends. *In* Population Debate, Vol. I. United Nations. New York.
31. SCHULTZ, T. P. 1981. Economics of Population. Addison-Wesley. Reading, MA.
32. LEVY, V. 1985. Cropping pattern, mechanization, child labor and fertility in a farming economy: Rural Egypt. Econ. Dev. Cult. Change **33**(4): 777-792.
33. MUELLER, E. 1984. Income aspirations and fertility in rural areas of less developed countries. *In* Rural Development and Human Fertility. W. A. Schutjer & C. S. Stokes, Eds. Macmillan. New York.
34. ROSENZWEIG, M. & T. P. SCHULTZ. 1982. Child mortality and fertility in Colombia: Individual and community effects. *In* Health Policy and Education **2:** 305-348. Elsevier. Amsterdam.
35. MOHAN, R. 1986. Work, Wages, and Welfare in a Developing Metropolis. Johns Hopkins University Press. Baltimore, MD.
36. KING, E. M. 1988. Does education pay in the labor force? Population and Human Resource Department. The World Bank. Washington, DC.
37. SCHULTZ, T. P. 1988. Women and development: Objectives, framework and policy. Women in Development Division, Population and Human Resources Department, The World Bank, Washington, DC.

[*See Appendix on pp. 306-310.*]

APPENDIX

TABLE A. Years of Education Completed of Women Relative to Men by Age in the Most Recent Available Census

Region[a] Country	Year	Level of Schooling in Years in Males Aged 20-24	Years of Schooling in Females Relative to Males				
			20-24	25-34	35-44	45-54	55-64
Africa (excluding South Africa)		*3.34*	*.43*				
Malawi	1977	4.40	.49	.44	.33	.32	.35
Mauritius	1962	4.73	.66	.66	.62	.61	.68
Rwanda	1978	2.77	.61	.40	.20	.13	.10
Zambia	1969	4.92	.44	.34	.26	.25	.30
Egypt	1976	3.54	.55	.40	.27	.20	.18
Libya	1973	3.35	.22	.12	.14	.08	.06
South Africa	1970	3.97	1.02	.96	.93	.93	.93
Liberia	1974	4.14	.26	.27	.28	.29	.33
Mali	1976	1.15	.36	.26	.20	.13	.11
Sierra Leone	1963	1.04	.28	.31	.48	.64	.75
Latin America		*5.45*	*.94*				
Cuba	1981	8.79	.99	.93	.85	.88	.81
Dominican Republic	1970	4.19	.95	.86	.81	.81	.81
Haiti	1971	2.06	.68	.53	.52	.56	.99
Jamaica	1960	5.21	1.11	1.08	1.06	1.06	1.05
Puerto Rico	1970	9.37	1.04	.98	.87	.85	.84
Trinidad/Tobago	1980	7.31	1.05	1.00	.94	.88	.84
Costa Rica	1973	6.29	1.02	.95	.97	.96	.98
El Salvador	1961	2.58	.88	.82	.72	.69	.68
Guatemala	1964	1.73	.84	.83	.81	.78	.75
Honduras	1974	3.25	.99	.91	.79	.77	.79
Nicaragua	1950	1.37	1.03	.93	.86	.81	.79
Panama	1980	8.21	1.03	1.00	.98	.98	.95
Argentina	1980	8.64	1.03	1.01	.98	.96	.95
Chile	1960	5.46	.99	.97	.95	.93	.90
Uruguay	1975	7.87	1.08	1.06	1.05	1.02	.99
Bolivia	1976	6.42	.69	.61	.55	.53	.14
Brazil	1980	6.30	1.02	1.00	.96	.94	.94
Colombia[a]	1973	5.18	.92	.92	.92	.92	.92
Ecuador	1974	5.56	.93	.86	.83	.80	.77
Paraguay	1972	5.15	.92	.87	.81	.81	.74
Peru	1972	6.43	.76	.69	.65	.62	.60
Venezuela	1950	2.50	.80	.66	.61	.66	.78
East Asia (excluding Japan)		*6.35*	*.83*				
Hong Kong	1981	8.79	.94	.89	.79	.56	.46
South Korea	1980	10.13	.87	.83	.69	.55	.42
Taiwan	1956	5.00	.58	.48	.33	.21	.16
Indonesia	1980	3.98	.75	.75	.70	.75	.88
Malaysia	1957	4.42	.44	.35	.23	.14	.10
Philippines	1975	7.56	1.05	1.00	.96	.91	.86
Singapore	1980	4.90	1.04	.83	.65	.47	.34
Thailand	1980	6.02	.93	.89	.82	.75	.66

South and West Asia		*4.62*	*.48*				
India	1971	4.29	.40	.32	.28	.23	.17
Iran	1966	3.33	.41	.35	.37	.28	.18
Nepal	1981	2.36	.25	.22	.20	.21	—
Pakistan	1961	2.20	.21	.20	.19	.17	.13
Sri Lanka	1981	6.84	.99	.95	.85	.75	.70
Jordan	1961	4.81	.30	.28	.26	.30	.30
Syria	1970	4.62	.38	.31	.24	.19	.16
Israel	1961	8.52	.90	.84	.84	.82	.75
High-Income Countries		*9.13*	*1.00*				
Japan	1980	13.33	1.01	.98	.95	.95	.94
Australia	1966	9.49	1.01	.98	.96	.96	.97
New Zealand	1981	12.17	.99	1.01	.98	1.00	.87
Canada	1981	11.13	1.01	.97	.94	.96	.97
United States	1980	12.37	1.01	.98	.96	.97	.98
Bulgaria	1975	8.44	1.05	1.03	.95	.89	.84
Czechoslovakia	1980	11.46	.98	.96	.93	.89	.89
GDR	1971	9.97	1.00	.92	.78	.74	.72
Hungary	1970	8.68	1.07	.99	.92	.91	.92
Poland	1970	9.03	1.04	.99	.89	.89	.87
Romania	1966	7.91	.94	.90	.88	.89	.91
Finland	1970	9.88	1.07	1.04	1.05	1.02	1.01
Ireland	1966	6.65	1.11	1.03	1.03	1.03	1.04
Norway	1980	11.01	1.01	.96	.95	.95	.95
Sweden	1970	8.72	1.05	1.01	.95	.93	.91
Greece	1961	6.60	.90	.86	.82	.76	.77
Italy	1971	8.57	.90	.84	.81	.76	.77
Portugal	1970	5.89	1.01	1.01	.99	.96	.92
Spain	1970	6.78	1.00	1.00	1.02	1.01	1.02
Yugoslavia	1971	8.03	.89	.67	.61	.60	.81
Belgium	1970	10.03	.98	.96	.96	.95	.95
France	1975	8.20	1.09	1.05	1.02	.99	.66
Netherlands	1960	7.73	1.02	.97	.96	.96	.97
Switzerland	1960	7.07	.96	.94	.92	.92	.90

SOURCE: Estimated by the author from census and survey tabulations of national populations.
[a] Regional averages are unweighted and, as noted, South Africa is excluded from Africa and Japan is included in high-income category.

TABLE B. Estimates of Life Expectancy at Birth and Mortality for Women and Men from Africa and Asia

		Life Expectation at Birth (yr)			Ratio of Age-Specific Mortality Rates of Males to Females				
Country	Years	Male	Female	Ratio of Female to Male Life Expectation	Less Than 1 Year (infant)	Age 1 to 5	Age 5 to 10	Age 10 to 15	Age 15 to 35[a]
Africa									
Algeria	1948-51	44	49	1.11					
	1954-56	39	45	1.15					
	1969-70	50	54	1.08	1.00	.90	.52	.74	.89
	1970	53	54	1.02					
Egypt	1948-52	40	41	1.03	1.01				
	1958-62	48	49	1.02	.97				
	1963-67	49	50	1.02	.97	.99	1.06	1.04	1.16
Libya	1964-74	51	54	1.06	1.07				
	1968-73	52	55	1.06	1.07				
Morocco	1970	48	49	1.02	1.25				
Sudan	1968-73	43	44	1.02					
Tunisia	1968	52	50	.96	1.00				
	1968-69	54	55	1.02	1.02	.85	1.14	1.14	.82
Burundi	1965	39	42	1.08					
	1970-71	43	46	1.07					
Kenya	1969				.99	.90	.94	1.08	1.22
Madagascar	1966				1.40	1.18	1.19	1.21	1.06
Mauritius	1951-53	50	52	1.04					
	1961-63	59	62	1.05					
	1970-72	61	65	1.07	1.26	.88	.90	1.50	.81
Tanzania (mainland)	1967	39	42	1.08					
Central Africa Republic	1959-60	35	36	1.03					

Chad	1963-64	34	35	1.03					
Congo	1960-61	36	39	1.08					
Gabon	1960-61	40	42	1.05					
Botswana	1971	51	55	1.08					
Lesotho	1966	49	50	1.02					
Benin	1961	34	36	1.06					
Ghana	1968-69	46	48	1.04					
	1975	47	50	1.06					
Liberia	1962	36	39	1.08					
Mali	1960-61	31	33	1.06					
Niger	1960	36	37	1.03					
Sierra Leone	1973	31	35	1.13					
Togo	1961	37	39	1.05					
Asia									
China	1978	67	69	1.03					
Hong Kong	1961	64	71	1.11					
	1971	67	75	1.12					
Malaysia	1956	56	58	1.04					
(peninsular)	1972	63	68	1.08	1.32	1.05			
Philippines	1948	49	53	1.08					
	1969-71	59	64	1.08					
South Korea	1961	54	61	1.13					
	1971-75	59	66	1.12	1.08	.85			
Singapore	1956-58	61	67	1.10					
	1969-71	66	72	1.09	1.21				
Indonesia	1971	45	48	1.07	1.12	1.13			
Malaysia-Sabah	1970	49	45	.92					
Sarawak	1970	52	53	1.02					
Thailand	1947	49	51	1.04	1.19				
	1969-71	59	61	1.04	1.23	.95			
Taiwan	1956	60	65	1.08	1.10	.93	1.22	1.38	
	1975	67	73	1.09	1.36	1.21	1.55	1.56	2.01
Kuwait	1974-76	66	70	1.06	1.15				
Lebanon	1970	62	66	1.06					

TABLE B. *Continued*

Country	Years	Life Expectation at Birth (yr): Male	Life Expectation at Birth (yr): Female	Ratio of Female to Male Life Expectation	Ratio of Age-Specific Mortality Rates of Males to Females: Less Than 1 Year (infant)	Age 1 to 5	Age 5 to 10	Age 10 to 15	Age 15 to 35[a]
Sri Lanka	1945-47	45	43	.96	1.09				
	1962-64	62	63	1.02					
	1970-72	64	67	1.05		.85			
Burma	1954	41	44	1.07					
(urban)	1974	56	60	1.07		.91			
Iran	1973-76	57	57	1.00	.91	.80			
Iraq	1974-75	57	59	1.04		.96			
Afghanistan	1972-73	34	36	1.06					
Bangladesh	1974	46	47	1.02	1.10	1.04			
Democratic Yeman	1973	41	43	1.05					
India	1941-50	33	32	.97	1.09				
	1951-60	42	41	.98	1.11				
	1970-72	49	46	.94	1.01	.76			
Nepal	1952-54	32	29	.91					
	1974-76	45	42	.93	1.04				
Pakistan	1962-65	47	45	.96		.66			
Yeman	1975	38	39	1.03					

SOURCES: United Nations,[3] various tables; Taiwan 1956 figures from Keyfitz and Flieger, and Taiwan 1975 figures from *Demographic Yearbooks* (1984).

[a] Unweighted sum of age-specific mortality rates from age 15 to 35, during which most child-bearing occurs and thus the effect of maternal mortality may be apparent.

Prospects of Paying for Scientific Advances

BRIAN ABEL-SMITH

Department of Social Science and Administration
London School of Economics
London WC2A 2AE, England

Economics has often been described as the dismal science, and what I am going to write will, I am afraid, justify the use of that adjective. But before I talk about the general economic situation of the Third World and the prospects for financing the health sector and new scientific advances within it, I want to thank the organizers of this symposium for allowing a health economist to contribute to the proceedings. It certainly would not have been the custom ten years ago, when those of us who worked in health economics felt ourselves isolated in a small academic ghetto. Today I think that it is recognized that we have something to contribute even if it is not always cheerful.

It is one of the ironies of history that no sooner had the World Health Organization put teeth into its Health for All initiative by producing a detailed strategy in 1981, that the world economic crisis started to overwhelm most of the developing countries. When one rereads that strategy and the other documents produced at the time, one becomes aware that there were three hidden assumptions underlying the Health for All program. The first was that economic growth would continue much as before. The second was that Third World governments, having endorsed Health for All, would be willing and able to mobilize the resources needed to implement it. And the third was that the developed countries, which had also endorsed the program, would find more external aid resources for the health sector. None of these hopes has been fulfilled.

In 1981 it was not unreasonable to be optimistic. After all, developing countries as a whole had achieved an annual rate of growth of 6 percent in the years 1976-78 and nearly this figure over the next two years. Suddenly the growth rate dropped to 1½ percent in 1982—less than the growth of population. Income per head went down not up. But this average for all developing countries conceals enormous variations between and within different regions. Asia continued to grow by 5 percent but this was far from being the case for the least developed countries of that region. In Africa and the Middle East average living standards fell. In Latin America living standards, as measured by Gross Domestic Product per head, fell by 8½ percent over two years. Indeed in these two years it lost all the growth it had achieved since 1976. Sub-Sahara Africa suffered most of all, with a fall in average living standards of around 11 percent over three years. In nine countries living standards fell back to those of 1960. Not surprisingly it has been the oil exporting countries who have suffered most of all over the past seven years.[1]

This change in the fortunes of most of the developing world could hardly have come at a worse time. It followed a decade during which the commercial banks of the developed world had been engaged in what now seems reckless lending. The trouble with debts, as we all know, is that lenders expect to be repaid. And on top of this, interest payments have to be made until this has been done. But what is special about international lending is that the borrower expects the money to come back and the interest to be paid in hard currency. And that is exactly what Third World borrowers were least able to find. The recession in the developed countries had led to a decrease in demand for, and thus the price of, the primary products on which the developing countries so heavily depended to earn hard currency. They found that at these lower prices they had to sell more goods abroad just to maintain the same level of export earnings. And the more they tried to do this, the larger the decrease in prices, so that still more goods would have to be sent abroad to earn the same revenue in hard currency. By 1984 the developing countries would have needed to export 20 percent more to earn the same amount of hard currency as they had earned in 1980.[2] Commodity prices are now lower than they have been for 50 years, and to make matters worse, world interest rates shot up as the United States sucked in money to finance its vast trade deficit. In this situation, finding the foreign currency to service debts, let alone repay them, became a hard struggle. By 1983 Africa was spending more than a quarter of its export earnings on debt service payments and Latin America and the Caribbean were spending nearly 40 percent.

Thus governments of most of the developing countries have been faced with two formidable problems: The first is how to pay for essential exports while keeping their creditors reasonably happy. The second is how to collect the taxes needed for the debt service payments as well as to maintain their public services, including health services, out of declining national resources. Moreover, many of the loans had financed capital projects which now needed tax money to finance their operating costs. More and more countries had to turn to the International Monetary Fund for help, and the price they had to pay for this help was very high, the cost of which is still being felt in the developing countries. First, these countries have often had to devalue their currencies, thus aggravating the burden of debt service payments. Second, they have come under pressure to balance their budgets, and in developing countries, with poorly developed tax systems, this, in practice, meant cutting public expenditure.

Devaluation means that a country has to make itself poorer by lowering still more the prices of its exports in the hope that more will be sold abroad and economic growth resumed. It also means replacing imported food with home-grown food. This is what is called structural adjustment. Latin America managed to balance its imports and exports within only three years, but this was done at a price. The countries had to produce and export goods they had previously made in small quantities. Land previously used to feed the local population became used to grow sugar out of which fuel could be made to save exports. The diversion of products and crops to meet the export market, the high cost of imports, rapid inflation, and often the abandonment of food subsidies increased and deepened poverty. In sub-Saharan Africa few countries could find extra goods that the world market wanted, given the low demand for primary products. Moreover, Africa had become a net food importer. It was bound to take time to replace these imports with home-grown food. The process of structural adjustment was certain to take a long time. At least 17 African countries devalued their currency. Public expenditure had to be cut, subsidies reduced, and capital investments postponed. Poverty increased severely in Africa, as in Latin America. While world attention tends to focus on the success stories of Asia it is often forgotten that at least half of the world's poorer people are in South Asia. As elsewhere, poverty has widened and deepened as countries have devalued and cut public expenditure. The increase in poverty in so many Third World countries has slowed down and in some cases reversed improvements in infant mortality rates.

What has happened as a result of all this to expenditure on health? How far has the health sector been a casualty of public expenditure cuts as countries struggle to promote improvements in the economic infrastructure in the hope of replacing imports, particularly of food, and of promoting exports? There are no hard data to answer this question. One can search all the compendia of international statistics kept by all the international organizations and still find no clear answer.[3] Data are, of course, available for quite a number of developing countries, showing Ministry of Health expenditure as a proportion of the budget or as a proportion of gross national product. But this does not answer the question for four reasons: First, ministries of health generally only finance a part of public expenditure on health. Other ministries may pay for water, sanitation or family planning, and expenditures by lower levels of government is sometimes substantial. Second, in many developing countries private expenditure on health is larger than public expenditure and data on it are hard to find. Third, it is no use knowing that the same proportion of the budget or the gross domestic product is being spent on health services if you do not know whether the budget or gross domestic product has gone up or down. Fourth, the prices paid for health service can and indeed have diverged considerably from prices paid for other goods and services within developing countries. There are extremely few price indices which tell you the trend in prices for the goods and services used by the health sector. In view of the vast amount of information that is systematically collected about the health sector, it amazes me that no regular and reliable source of data is available on whether the sector is becoming larger or smaller, where and in what respects.

In the absence of hard data one has to draw inferences from some of the special economic factors affecting the health sector and generalize from experiences that may not be typical. First, there is no doubt that the economic crisis of the 1980s occurred at a bad time for the health sector. By the end of the 1970s countries were heavily into hospital building. Many large projects were completed at around the time when the money to staff and equip them became short. Not surprisingly governments have lacked the political courage to leave new hospitals unused even if it meant postponing extensions in primary health care. Secondly, the immediate problem confronting countries has been one of foreign exchange. This has caused particular disruption for the health sector. What has tended to be cut has been the money needed to replace and repair equipment. And many countries have had to cut the drug budget severely. It appears to be the case that politically it is thought not possible to lay off trained health manpower, particularly highly trained manpower. So one sees too often the absurdity of doctors and paramedical workers struggling to give some sort of service with equipment no longer in working order and a grossly inadequate supply of drugs. Another heavy casualty is expenditure on the maintenance of buildings. Anything which can be postponed gets postponed whether it is the repair of lifts, vehicles, or electrical fittings. At least this is the impression I have had of the health sector in a number of countries I have visited in all continents over the past few years. And it is the same story I hear from the students we receive from developing countries in all regions of the world and from colleagues from the Third World I meet at international meetings. In those cases where we have managed to look carefully at appropriations for the health sector and develop special price indices, the results suggest the same picture. Of course, there are some notable exceptions. But it is my impression that generally the health sector has suffered heavily from the economic crisis.

How far has the situation been eased by external aid? Has the world endorsement of the Health for All program led to more hard cash in support of it? Some countries have indeed given more, but others have given less. There appears to have been little change in total aid going to the health sector since 1980.[4] Only about 4 percent of bilateral assistance from the OECD countries goes to the health sector. And some donor governments have been redirecting their foreign aid from the poorest countries to those in which they have greater commercial and political interests.[5] There is, of course, the further problem that aid tends to go towards capital expenditure, leaving the recipient country to try and pick up the operating costs. The small relative scale of aid as a whole can be shown from the fact that about twice as much money has been flowing from developing to developed countries in debt service payments than has been flowing into the developing countries in aid and loans.

Is this situation likely to change over the next decade? How far will the developing countries be able to take advantage of new scientific advances? The debt problem hangs like a dark cloud over the prospects of the developing world. Some countries are having to borrow more to keep servicing their debts. One favorable trend is the willingness of some banks to write down the value of some of their debts in their books. And there have been a number of international proposals to relieve the situation. It might well be in the best interests of the developed countries to write off all or most of this debt, which would, of course, require governmental assistance. How can the developed countries hope to sell their goods to developing countries which lack the foreign exchange to buy them? The 17 most indebted countries have had to cut their imports by 40 percent between 1981 and 1987. Thus the debt problem contributes to the high unemployment still to be found in so many of the industrialized countries and to poor levels of world economic growth generally.

The economic situation of a number of developing countries would be notably improved if the industrialized countries were to adopt a free trade policy instead of maintaining, and in some cases strengthening, the protection of their internal markets. The Common Agricultural Policy of the European Economic Community ensures that consumers in the 12 member countries not only have to pay above world prices for food, but cuts the potential exports of the Third World. Farmers also enjoy protection in the United States and rice growers in Japan are heavily subsidized. Farmers seem to mobilize a very strong political lobby throughout the industrialized countries. This restricts the ability of developing countries to earn export revenue from which to get out of debt. Protection by the industrialized countries costs the Third World more than twice the amount provided in official aid.[6]

There is no doubt that most developing countries could find much more money for the health sector if they were prepared to spend much less on their armed forces.[7] But I see no reason to believe that they are likely to do this over the next decade. Indeed this is least likely to happen in countries where the armed forces constitute the government.

What then can the developing countries themselves do to attract more money to the health sector? Considerable interest now exists in the developing countries in finding further sources of finance. The introduction of compulsory health insurance for the regularly employed is being considered in such diverse countries as Nigeria, Malawi, Mauritius, Malaysia and Thailand and is in a pilot stage of development in Indonesia. Often the thinking behind this approach is that if the regularly employed can, with their employers, pay by regular contributions for all the health services they use, the limited tax funds can be used to provide better and more accessible services to those who it is hard to cover by insurance, particularly the rural poor. There is also a renewed interest in a whole variety of community financing schemes such as revolving drug funds, cooperative funding of health services, and informal rural insurance. In addition many countries are introducing charges or higher or further charges for government health services.

In a widely circulated glossy publication, the World Bank has proposed that governments in developing countries should charge virtually the whole running cost of curative services to those who use them and introduce compulsory health insurance for major medical costs in the case of those in regular employment.[8] This extreme proposal of nearly full-cost charging is based on the assumption that only the user benefits from curative services whereas everybody benefits from preventive services. It is intended that the poor should continue to receive free services and the near-poor subsidized services. But the document fails, in my view, to give any really practical guidance of how this could be done, let alone any indication of how much it would cost to try and do it. At least this proposal is beginning to stimulate some badly needed research on the effects of different levels of charges on the use of services by different income groups. What would be the prospects for new scientific advances if most potential users of them in the Third World had to pay for them out of their own pockets?

Many developing countries could make savings by using the resources they presently devote to the health sector more efficiently. There are often weaknesses in management at every level of the system. In view of the shortage of foreign exchange, particular attention needs to be paid to goods, such as drugs, which have a high import content. By no means all developing countries have adopted an essential drugs program; some are still buying drugs at prices far above those available under the UNICEF/WHO contract and the problems of pilferage and overprescribing are endemic in some countries.

But it needs to be recognized that all these ways of improving the resources available to the health sector take time to put into effect. There are no quick solutions. Hastily conceived and rapidly introduced health insurance schemes can go badly wrong and discredit the whole approach for a generation. Community financing schemes require very careful selection of managers and an extended training program if they are to operate efficiently and continue to operate year after year. And poor management cannot be transformed into good management overnight.

This very brief review of the economic scenario and some of the options for developing countries to try and mobilize more resources for the health sector does not lead me to be optimistic. The central question is, of course, the global rate of economic growth. And here the prospect is somewhat better than it was a few years ago. Economic growth in the industrialized countries benefits the developing countries by increasing the demand for and thus the prices of raw materials. But it would be rash to expect the rate of growth to return to that of the 1960s.

Thus I conclude that the finance available to the health sector of developing countries will continue to be tightly limited over the next decade. The only radical change could come from concerted action by the industrialized countries to remove or greatly lighten the debt problem. This means that the developing countries will have to continue to choose their public expenditure priorities with the greatest care. And even if a country made health improvement a central priority of government policy, which few do, it is by no means clear that finding more money to be spent on health services is the surest way of advancing towards that objective. Action to combat poverty, malnutrition, and unsafe water and to promote sanitation, female education, and a better lifestyle may, depending on the situation of the country, offer a more promising way forward.

Within the health sector, governments are often faced with conflicting pressures. The strongest lobby may come from those wanting to offer more sophisticated services to the urban population, including ministers and ministers' wives. And the urban population itself may be demanding better and more convenient services—direct access to the doctor or even to the specialist and the attractively packaged drugs available through the private sector. Less articulated may be the demand of the underserved or the unserved rural population for primary care. It is not unknown for the health plan to back the latter group, while the budget year by year favors the former. But there are many other countries which are putting their money as well as their rhetoric behind the development of primary health care. In this situation new scientific advances may look, at first sight, like a piece of bad news, such as the recognition of the growing problem of AIDS. How many ministers of health in developing countries must have cursed the day such expensive innovations as coronary care units, renal dialysis, and transplants were developed to add to their ethical dilemmas?

The questions of what technologies to use and where and on what scale to use them are among the most formidable problems facing ministers of health of developing countries. The answers to these questions rest upon many major decisions on the equipment of hospitals and health centers, and on the training of specialists, primary care doctors, paramedics, workers, and midwives. Some ministers rightly approach this question with some skepticism, knowing that many routine treatments have been incorporated into world medical practice before systems of careful scientific evaluation, such as random controlled trials, were introduced or without such evaluation ever having been done. Of course, there are opportunities for making such evaluations in a situation where a technology, such as some particularly expensive treatments, cannot be afforded for all who might benefit from it. But these opportunities are rarely taken.

A shrewd minister will ask two questions about any scientific advance. The first is "How many people would it help, where, in what way and at what cost?" The second is whether the innovation will require additional expenditure or be a cheaper way of getting better results than are gotten by the present technology. To prove that a new method works, in scientific terms, is not enough. For example, better diagnosis without hard evidence of better outcome is not a good buy when money is tight. Nor is a form of innovation that can add a few years of life at very high cost when so many are dying early of conditions that could have been prevented at relatively low cost. An innovation that requires expensive and delicate imported equipment may not be a good buy in view of the great stocks of unrepaired equipment that can be found in the basements of hospitals throughout the Third World. On the other hand a kind of innovation that is effective, can be made from local materials, prescribed by paramedical workers, and that replaces a more expensive older treatment is an ideal candidate for adoption. In this respect oral rehydration therapy (ORT) met all these criteria and has, of course, been widely adopted and I was delighted to find that the sophisticated medical service beneath WHO's Geneva Headquarters prescribed ORT for me when I returned recently to Geneva with chronic diarrhea. Are there no further opportunities for finding cheaper ways of prevention and cure that are reliable, simply taught, and use local materials and do not depend on a reliable electricity supply?

Over the next decade the developing countries will be searching for more cost-effective solutions to their health problems, including solutions that communities can learn to apply themselves. There is, of course, much simple, cost-effective knowledge and has not yet been applied all over the Third World. The priority is to take this within reach of everyone. This is what the Health for All program is about. But the challenge also is to extend the range of low-cost solutions to health problems wherever it is possible to do so.

REFERENCES

1. WORLD BANK. 1984. Towards Sustained Development in Sub-Saharan Africa: 10. World Bank. Washington, D.C.

2. Centre for Policy Research. 1985. Bulletin. April: 2.
3. Abel-Smith, B. Health and the world economic crisis! Health Policy and Planning **1**(3): 208-212.
4. OECD. Development Co-Operation Review. Annual report (1984-7 editions). Paris.
5. McNamara, R. S. 1985. The Challenge for Sub-Saharan Africa: 27. World Bank, Washington, D.C.
6. *The Times* (London), September 27, 1988: 1.
7. Sivard, R. L. 1983. World Military & Social Expenditure: 32. Washington, D.C.
8. World Bank. 1987. Financing Health Services in Developing Countries. World Bank. Washington, D.C.

The Roles of the World Health Organization in Tropical Disease Research

TORE GODAL

Special Programme for Research and Training in Tropical Diseases
World Health Organization
Geneva, Switzerland

The World Health Organization represents a unique focus of health for countries, particularly in the developing world, and its mission has been to emphasize the importance of primary health care throughout the world. Perhaps less appreciated is the fact that this effort has been supported in the past 10 years by a series of special programs designed to develop new tools and strategies, or "interventions," ultimately to improve the primary health care effort. This requires new tools, new tools require new knowledge, and new knowledge requires research. To the question of how relevant research is likely to be to the practical goals of an international organization like WHO, let me remind you that it is precisely research that made it possible to discard the enormously expensive "iron lungs" used for poliomyelitis victims, and to develop effective and inexpensive vaccines to prevent the disease.

The aims of the Special Programme for Research and Training in Tropical Diseases (TDR), as is implicit from its title, is two-fold. In an area poorly served by research priorities in the developed nations, one aim is to establish through research and development new weapons against tropical and parasitic diseases primarily in the developing world. The second objective is the training and strengthening of biomedical research capability in tropical countries. Under the leadership of WHO's Director General, Dr. Halfdan Mahler, and now Dr. H. Nakajima, and my predecessor, Dr. Adetokunbo Lucas, we have tried to build up a strong scientific program, not so much to be measured in financial resources, but in human resources. Scientists from all over the world, fieldworkers, sympathetic officials in ministries of health, development experts, and a dedicated WHO Secretariat have all given generously of their knowledge and time to this program and have dedicated major portions of their activities to problems of tropical diseases. The program started with a scientific approach to six major diseases—malaria, schistosomiasis, trypanosomiasis, leishmaniasis, filariasis and leprosy—and was intent on bringing the most advanced knowledge of immunology, pharmacology and epidemiology to the tropical diseases. The program is now moving to encompass areas ranging from molecular biology and biotechnology to field research and applications to control. The challenge remains.

PERCEPTIONS OF PARASITES

The implicit premise of the TDR program was that by bringing the new biology to bear on the problem it would be possible to identify new targets for drugs and protective antigens from parasites, and to develop new drugs and vaccines to the tropical diseases. We accepted, of necessity, the reductionist view of science of analyzing the parts and focusing on the weak links, and the fact that 60 new products have followed from this approach in a sense justifies this approach, at least on a practical level. On the other hand, after 10 years, we have been humbled to appreciate the subtlety and sophistication of the parasites, which have evolved over millions of years to survive in their hosts and in the biosphere. We are now beginning to understand the complexities of the parasites and vectors—and of people. We are now even forced to revise our scientific dogmas and strategies.

As an illustration, let me argue that research in parasitic diseases has in the last two years forced the world of biology to change its fundamental paradigm, namely, that all the genetic information for making proteins is encoded in DNA. Recent discoveries in trypanosomes have revealed that an organism can make proteins from mRNA, the sequence of which does *not* correspond to original nucleotide sequences in the genes. The discovery of editing, the inserting of uridines and other nucleotides in RNA, not specified by the DNA, is revolutionizing our understanding of the transmission of genetic information and the generation of biological diversity.

PARASITES AND US

We have learned other things no less surprising. The problem of designing new drugs to prevent proliferation or pathogenesis by parasites has become strikingly similar to that required for new drugs against many other human conditions, including cancer and heart disease. Although designing drugs for tropical diseases can seem an esoteric enterprise, not only are the overall problems similar, but also many of the specific problems and details are common. For example, in the case of African trypanosomes, the parasites express receptors for growth factors (EGF) which have phosphokinase activity, just as do many mammalian growth factors and oncogenes. A trypanosome also needs considerable quantities of cholesterol for its growth. This it obtains from its human host through specific receptors in its flagellar pocket for low-density lipoprotein (LDL), a target for drug design in preventing atherosclerosis. The malaria parasite provides another illustration, for it needs iron to survive. While there is plenty of iron in the human blood, neither the parasite nor the mature human red cell it infects has the capability of extracting or making it available directly in usable form. The parasite apparently solves the problem by making for its host red cell a receptor molecule for the iron-transporting protein, transferrin, from which it can now acquire iron. My point here is that the pharmaceutical industry screens thousands of compounds every year in search of drugs against cancer or cardiovascular disease. Hundreds of compounds that act by blocking growth factor receptors on cancer cells or ionic channels on cardiovascular tissue cells are sought for high specificity against the disease target cells and low toxicity for healthy cells. Since there are similar receptors used by parasites for growth factors, for lipids, for ions, it may well be that among compounds screened and found to have effects on such receptors and functions, but that have insufficient specificity, some might have a higher specificity and effectiveness against the comparable receptors or enzymes in parasites. One example in recent years would be verapamil, a calcium channel blocker used to treat cardiovascular diseases and which is known also to block multi-drug resistance in cancer cells. Two years ago verapamil was also reported to inhibit chloroquine-resistance in malaria parasites. Further work has now identified analogues of verapamil that act selectively on malaria parasites, and not on host cells. Just as compounds that are not effective in man may well be effective in parasites, similarly, it may be easier in some cases to modify drugs effective in parasites to render them specific for mammalian cells. It could be, indeed, that the study of by-products of the massive research effort on cancer, heart disease, and other chronic diseases of man may well point to a rich source of new antiparasitic drugs.

The powerful tools of modern immunology and molecular biology offer the means to identify and clone genes encoding important antigens and enzymes as targets for vaccines and drugs. But how will the appropriate target be identified? One approach to answering that question is the study of the mechanisms of pathogenesis, the molecules required for the parasite to enter and damage cells of their hosts. It is clear from recent studies of *Leishmania,* for example, that more than one molecule can act as a ligand for attachment of the parasite to the host cell. Blocking one such ligand, as by antibodies, is not sufficient to block infection. Further, one of those ligands binds to a receptor on cells of the immune system for complement, one of the host's immunologically important weapons. Hence the parasite has evolved a way to mimic and exploit a molecule important in the immune system. From this simple analysis, two things become evident. To deal with these complex parasites, vaccines of the future will have to reflect the complexity of the pathogenic process of the parasites. I envision multi-antigen vaccines derived from matrix analysis of different parasite molecules involved in pathogenesis or required for protection. Also, if parasites evolve structural motifs similar or identical to those found in the host's immune mechanisms, then we must eliminate these motifs in the vaccine so autoimmune reactions will not be produced in the host. In essence, then, we are learning new rules for the game, namely, that vaccines designed to block penetration of parasites into a host cell will probably be more complex than simple virus vaccines and will require multiple antigens in their makeup and deletion of epitopes similar or identical to those of the host. We must create antigens that provoke better protective responses than natural antigens.

CONFRONTING COMPLEXITY

Faced with the complexity of the parasites, the vectors, and the hosts, the TDR strategy must explore multiple points of attack against the diseases with which it is concerned. Too often in the past, we have been so seduced by the development of a new technology to control disease that we have seen the research halted by the assumption that there only remains a question of "implementation."

Leprosy is a case in point. Dapsone was the first drug with a direct action on the leprosy bacillus, and from the mid-1940s the control of leprosy consisted of the application of this drug to patients around the world. Twenty years later, as would hardly be a surprise to a first-year graduate student in genetics, leprosy bacilli became resistant to dapsone monotherapy. There is virtually no country in the world reporting leprosy that does not now have cases of primary and secondary drug-resistance to dapsone. In the late 1970s, under TDR's Scientific Working Group on the Chemotherapy of Leprosy (THELEP), with great help from the WHO Leprosy Unit, studies on a multidrug strategy were initiated to overcome and prevent drug-resistance. Multidrug therapy (MDT) has now revolutionized the treatment of leprosy. Hundreds of thousands of patients are being taken off treatment registers and are now considered cured after relatively short courses of treatment. Follow-up studies to date have indicated almost no incidence of relapse or emergence of organisms resistant to MDT. In many parts of the world, this is not adequate to the need. For example, only about 9 percent of the patients in Africa currently receive multidrug therapy. Thus, basic research is necessary to address the emerging challenges of these diseases, but operational and field research is needed to make it possible to implement the results of this research.

As another example, in 1949 Jules Freund immunized monkeys against malaria. In 1952, pesticides were shown to be effective in control, and the research on the immunology of malaria virtually stopped for 20 years in the United States. Pesticide-resistant vectors and drug-resistant parasites are now the reality and the current complexity.

Finally, there is the success story of onchocerciasis. TDR takes pride in its association with the development of ivermectin (Mectizan; Merck and Company, Inc.) and the Mectizan Donation Program. In less than 2 years, we have planned and put into execution in collaboration with the Onchocerciasis Control Programme final (Phase IV) trials of this drug in more than 70,000 onchocerciasis patients in rural Africa and Guatemala and have confirmed its safety and efficacy. Its potency and duration of efficacy are remarkable and it may well be that a single tablet a year may be sufficient. But can we assume that onchocerciasis treatment is now only a question of implementation? We need to know the minimum coverage required to reduce transmission in the areas of low as well as high rates of transmission, and we need to know how it can be most cost-effectively deployed for the prevention of blindness.

As parasites have been and are continually evolving, control strategies must keep up and anticipate changes, including those of global arming and massive patterns of human migration. A different level of research is needed to uncover and solve problems concerning national commitment and priorities, health infrastructure training and needs, treatment-seeking behavior of patients, compliance, case-finding, and drug distribution and availability. Potent combinations of drugs, by further shortening therapy, could dramatically ease these logistic and compliance problems. These concerns are now priority research issues for TDR.

RESEARCH CAPABILITY STRENGTHENING

To address these problems, TDR has taken new initiatives in the area of research capability strengthening. At the beginning of this program, many countries of the world had virtually no scientific research institutions, infrastructures or material resources to address local problems of tropical diseases. The research-strengthening group in the TDR program has aimed to provide resources and guidance to help initiate and to upgrade existing research institutions in the disease-endemic countries. This has accounted for 25 percent of our budget. The goal is to help countries to meet their needs for self-sufficiency in areas of their highest medical and health priorities. In order to leave as much room for initiative and imagination to applicants as possible, we have outlined a set of guiding principles that can be summarized as follows: (1) Indigenous approaches to problem-solving must be stimulated. Because poorer countries have limited resources and major needs, it is essential that they use their available strengths to do what can best be done within the disease-endemic country and what would be more difficult for scientists in Paris or London or Bethesda to do. (2) Even without all of the material resources of the more developed laboratories, a major part of research training requires "learning by doing." For the application of new drugs and vaccines, it is essential to have knowledge of the disease problems in the local countries and the laboratories and research and epidemiologic capabilities to be able to meaningfully intervene and evaluate the process of intervention. A basic challenge is therefore to link training to the advancing frontier of knowledge, without losing sight of the needs and opportunities to apply that knowledge to problems in disease-endemic countries.

The TDR program has taken new initiatives to accomplish this. We are now deliberately using workshops and field trials as training mechanisms to upgrade the role of science in disease-endemic countries. Secondly, we have embarked upon a TDR-Rockefeller Joint Venture, an activity we developed in response to repeated calls for linkages between institutions in the North and the South. The aim is to provide support for linked scientific programs, providing for rapid exchange of knowledge and training and the application of different institutional capabilities to problems of tropical diseases. The response has been enormous, far beyond anyone's expectations. We received letters of intent from 208 persons, from which 23 were selected to compete with full applications. All of these proposals were superb and it was very difficult to select only 12, the limit of our available resources for funding. It has been gratifying that these programs span the range from basic research to field research and we hope that with a very rapid evolution of scientific knowledge, these linkages will narrow the knowledge gap between scientists in developing and developed countries. The fact that there were so many outstanding applications for this program indicates that there is a burning need of means to allow scientists in the developing world to maintain contacts with the frontiers of science. After many years of strengthening institutions, we are emphasizing investment in human beings, in training scientists, locally as much as possible. It is unrealistic to expect that everyone who is trained will remain in research. The TDR program for a long time realized that the period when students return from training experiences to their countries and laboratories is a critical one and therefore we have enhanced the re-entry grant and introduced a new grant, the career development grant, to give ample support for five years for the most promising students to return home and engage in research. Finally, the Research Strengthening Group has introduced program-based grants, which is a way of helping institutions to develop multidisciplinary programs to provide training for areas needed, but not presently available, such as in immunology, epidemiology, and social science, so that these institutions can take on a broader range of activities. With the program-based grants we are also stimulating linkage formation between institutions in the South, in what we believe to be a second phase of strengthening towards research output. With this mechanism, we hope to stimulate joint efforts to solve common problems, and in local and regional ways to increase the critical mass of science and inquiry and to stimulate collaboration between different institutions and different disciplines in the disease-endemic countries. This involves not only the biomedical sciences, but social sciences and disease control as well. Program grants will no longer only be judged by their institutional needs, but by their scientific progress. The hope is to make it possible for young scientists receiving training abroad to continue their research in the disease-endemic countries and to reward them for their scientific progress, as well as providing institutions with a broader range of expertise.

FIELD RESEARCH NETWORKS

As mentioned above, over the past two years the TDR program, in collaboration with the Onchocerciasis Control Programme, has launched five major field trials of ivermectin. In addition to learning of the safety and effectiveness of this drug, we learned some more broad lessons as well. In field research, in contrast to laboratory research, one has to take initiatives at a much earlier stage, notably in formulating questions and developing careful study protocols. At the same time we were disappointed that these projects required such heavy input from expatriate scientists. If, in fact, the TDR program succeeds in developing new drugs and vaccines, we are going to have an urgent need for the capability of carrying out field trials against multiple tropical diseases in the disease-endemic countries. Yet nowhere is it easy to generate field research or to attract qualified scientists to it. Regrettably, this absolutely vital area of research does not bring with it the visibility and recognition often found in laboratory research, and this must be changed.

As was described by Peter Smith in this symposium, our aim is to develop field research networks. These networks will be multidisciplinary, based on field research projects that are directly related to the control of tropical diseases and that will encourage the formation of linkages between investigators associated with research institutions and members of disease control programs under the ministries of health of the countries concerned. The training will be adapted to the nature of each project, and the networks will ultimately be assessed by their impact on disease control strategies. In this context, field research includes both epidemiology and social sciences, and linkages where appropriate to laboratories. Our TDR scientific steering committees will be responsible for the projects, and the Research Strengthening Group will be responsible for training of these networks. Early on in TDR's development, its planners established a social and economic research component. This component will be expanded and will work very closely with the newly established field research programs and increasingly focus on research related to intervention and evaluation of disease control, making use of the most recent advances in social science and statistical methods.

THE CHALLENGE FOR THE 1990s

Product development—in the broadest sense from basic laboratory to disease control in the field—has always been a feature of TDR's work. The emphasis to date, which has largely been on academically based research, understandingly derives from the sharp demarcation that has existed between academic institutions and industry in willingness to conduct biomedical research on diseases of developing countries. In the past ten years the situation has changed considerably, and there are now much closer relations between the two. Nevertheless, the pharmaceutical industry is showing little interest in building upon drug and vaccine development deriving from TDR's and other agencies' investments in basic research for the tropics. If anything, industry investment in tropical diseases is shrinking, and companies are frequently handing over their own leads to the TDR program for further exploitation. We are grateful, however, that while companies may be loath to commit themselves to entire development processes for drugs of interest, they appear increasingly willing to carry out, under contract to TDR or often at no cost to the program, certain well-defined parts of the process for which they have particular expertise. One example is the development of the artemisinin derivative, arteether, an antimalarial drug which is expected soon to reach clinical testing under TDR auspices.

Clearly a major long-term objective of the TDR program must be to facilitate product development in the disease-endemic countries themselves. Thus far, this has been pursued largely by trying to strengthen their academic research capabilities. Because of the enormous potential of biotechnology for addressing problems of vaccines and diseases and because of the potential of biotechnology to contribute to the economies of the developing countries themselves, TDR has launched an Initiative for Biotechnology Implementation. The aim is to provide support to selected centers in disease-endemic countries to scale up their facilities for the production of biological reagents that the TDR program has helped to develop, such as DNA probes, monoclonal antibodies and recombinant antigens, and which are now ready for small- or large-scale field testing. We are pleased that the need has been imposed on us by the progress within the laboratories, and that this initiative provides an example of how two of TDR's objectives—the development of new tools for disease control and research capability strengthening—can be harnessed together for the benefit of the disease-endemic countries.

As this century comes to a close, the North and South are being more and more closely linked together in a biosphere with limited capability of absorbing human activities and increasingly common human problems. Individually and collectively, we will increasingly have to make rational decisions and correctly assign priorities. Let us hope that we will make them in the direction of improving the quality of life of all people on this planet. Among the many problems that confront mankind, from the destruction of the environment, to epidemic diseases, from war to hunger, combatting tropical diseases in the developing world represents an important and hopeful aspect of our common future.

Biotechnology and the Third World: Development Strategies in Cuba

MANUEL LIMONTA

Centro de Ingenieria Genética y Biotecnología
Havana, Cuba

INTRODUCTION

The possibilities for the growth of science and biotechnology in any country directly depend on the level of general development in that country. Political will and economic organization determine possibilities for development. Biotechnology in the developed world is essentially supported by private investment. Guided by the profit motive, this creates a situation of disadvantage and dependency for the Third World. Cuba, a Third World country in development, stands as a singular exception to that general rule. Scientific concepts have guided Cuba's growth, and problem resolution is based on the application of those scientific concepts to create a scientific base. Cuba has thus achieved a startlingly high level of scientific and biotechnological development, unmatched by that of any other developing Third World country.

The most adequate response of the countries of the Third World, faced with the exponential development of biotechnology in the developed world and its private nature, is without doubt to develop concrete activities with well-defined, practical objectives which can directly influence the epidemiology of each country and offer less costly solutions for diagnoses, treatment, drugs and medicines, without having to make purchases from large transnational companies. Those who do not genuinely struggle to change this correlation produce a negative feedback mechanism for scientific development and therefore for the economy. To avoid dependence, a serious approach that allows for the development of science in the Third World is needed.

BIOTECHNOLOGY IN THE DEVELOPING WORLD

The problem that some pose is how to begin, but certainly in our evaluation of the facts, one has to begin with an effort of sufficient magnitude to allow the possibility of the coordination of forces, with the necessary resources and the political will to create a base for definitive change and keep things moving on course.

Each country has its own characteristics and a single schema which defines the percent, quantity or size of the needed commitment to build the base is impossible. There are many roads to development: one could define a policy to concentrate efforts or to decentralize them; a mixed strategy might combine the concentration of efforts on long-term objectives as well as the reinforcement of the infrastructure to achieve short-term objectives in other areas. Objectives could be aimed at the development of products that could be exported to other countries. Whatever the mix, the factors need to be determined by the nature of the objectives.

The definition of objectives is probably one of the most important things to consider in changing the course of Latin American biotechnology. It is essential to choose an objective that not only relates to the problems of the country in question (whether they be in the area of health, agriculture or industry), but that also complements existing characteristics and permits the creation of a positive feedback loop. For example, fulfilling some objectives may resolve an important problem at the national level. As the work proceeds, an infrastructure evolves, and people develop technical skills and learn to think differently, which in turn allows them to undertake new models of work, tackle new and/or different objectives, and so on. These interactions produce a positive feedback loop.

Recognizing that different countries need to solve problems in their own style, we recognize three essential aspects to consider in deciding how to focus development. These three elements are personnel, equipment and installations, whether they begin with advanced technologies, and whether they are biotechnological, microelectronic, or other. In the developed countries these three elements are well defined. What happens in the underdeveloped countries with these three elements? With the exception of Cuba, these countries lack the following advantages:

1. Personnel:

(*a*) An educational system that permits maximum intellectual development, beginning in primary school;

(*b*) A critical mass of researchers who enjoy the richness of regular scientific interchange, which can also generate a scientific culture and style, encouraging constant feedback;

(*c*) Efficient methods of communication among researchers in different scientific institutions, aided by an efficient telephone system and extensive and effective computer equipment with appropriate application possibilities;

(*d*) The possibility of travel to places with adequate development;

(*e*) Facility in other languages. The reality is that in large part the scientific literature is written in English, and this can be a limiting factor for some researchers of the Third World; and

(*f*) Libraries with varied, timely and relevant materials.

2. Reagents:

(*a*) Difficulties obtaining supplies of endonuclease enzymes and radioisotopes necessary to work in today's biotechnology; and

(*b*) Difficulties importing needed plastic material not produced in these countries.

3. Equipment:

(*a*) Equipment such as mass spectrometers, gamma counters, ultra-centrifuges, DNA automatic sequencers, and electron microscopes can be difficult to obtain;

(*b*) Equipment maintenance, which requires a highly qualified work force, which does not exist in most countries of the Third World; and

(*c*) Replacement parts, which are often difficult to get when they are needed, resulting in long waiting periods.

Other aspects of the problem of development of biotechnology in the Third World are: (1) research centers are often in bad condition and frequently have problems with electricity and adequate water supplies; (2) the rules of the game related to patents and industrial protection are often unclear; (3) the relationship between the productive and scientific sectors is often difficult; and (4) real credit and market incentives to support the sector's firms are frequently absent. An additional aspect needs also to be mentioned, the "brain drain."

The well-known brain drain from the less to the more developed world has always played an important role and is currently exacerbated by the economic crisis battering the Third World; it is also aggravated by the lack of a coherent policy for scientific development. Scientific researchers see in the developed world a possibility for economic solvency which is impossible in their own countries, and, aware of the lack of vision in many of their official institutions, they lose confidence in the possibility of achieving the truly applicable scientific results that could compensate them for their efforts at work and as men and women of science. Taken together, this creates a vicious cycle which generates scientific underdevelopment, which in turn leads to greater economic and social underdevelopment, and greater dependence on the developed countries.

The biotechnological industry, as such, really does not exist, and indeed mainly consists of product-packaging firms.

Local industries in the Third World are accustomed to inheriting discoveries and innovations from the developed countries. Often this pattern produces a lack of self-confidence which delays results and little by little generates a habit of waiting for outcomes from the developed world. This not only works against the development of indigenous science, but also does not help to bridge the gap between the two worlds.

The approach to problem-solving in the developed world does not generally take into consideration the needs of the Third World. This is largely due to the profit motive, which guides the large, private companies of the developed world. These big companies only develop products important to the Third World (i.e. vaccines) when those products are, at the same time, important for the developed world.

The case of Cuba is an exception. The country has produced and has begun to commercialize medicines and diagnostic systems based on recombinant proteins. These include interferons (alpha and gamma), diagnostic kits for HIV antibodies, and epidermal growth factor. There are no other examples in the Third World of countries that have completed the cycle from cloning-expression to large-scale production, application, and commercialization of recombinant proteins. Possibilities for development exist, but when we look at the modern bioindustrial infrastructure needed to produce recombinant proteins in the Third World, we note that there is a considerable distance between them and similar facilities in the developed countries. This confirms the idea that minimal conditions are necessary to produce a turnabout in this situation. The minimal requirements include sufficient personnel, equipment, and installations. These conditions will permit work to begin and the achievement of essential concrete ends. Incompetent efforts, insufficient personnel, and lack of clear objectives will only aggravate the existing breach. Without a sufficient base, a negative feedback loop is created, because added to the objective situation of lack of material resources insufficient to redress scientific underdevelopment, the subjective problem of discouragement is added, which arises when real results cannot be produced.

THE CUBAN EXAMPLE

In 1981 the government of Cuba took steps to develop biotechnology as one of the principal industries of the country. A nation-wide program of biological research was launched, and that year a group of leading scientists from various centers began to work on the production of human leukocyte alpha interferon. Its production was stabilized and its use in medicine for treatment of viral diseases was introduced. The production of interferon had a specific objective: to use the drug in clinical tests for the treatment of cancer and viral diseases. Production began in April 1981, and by May production methods were established that guaranteed adequate supplies for use in clinical studies. In June 1981 interferon produced in Cuba was used to treat patients affected by an outbreak of dengue fever, type II. Months later it was applied in the treatment of patients affected by an epidemic of acute hemorrhagic conjunctivitis.

In June 1981 the president of the country, Dr. Fidel Castro, organized and presided at a meeting of the directors of Cuban scientific institutions doing biological work, and organized the Frente Biológico or the Biological Group.

This Group coordinates work among various centers in order to solve the problems of the country, by appropriately utilizing the potential and possibilities of each, across ministerial lines. For example, the Group includes centers that belong to the Academy of Sciences, the Council of State, the Ministry of Higher Education, the Ministry of Public Health, the Ministry of Sugar, and others. The directors of these institutes and centers meet monthly to analyze and exchange ideas concerning problems in the country and to assign tasks based on an annual work plan that they themselves generate.

Subsequently, a decision was made to create an institution for the production of alpha interferon on a larger scale and to promote the development of molecular biology. As a result the Centro de Investigaciones Biológicas (the Center for Biological Research or CIB) was officially inaugurated in January 1982, with the principal objective of developing modern biotechnology by using interferon as a model. That is, the main strategy was to start in the field of the new biotechnology by using a specific production goal to achieve the objective.

The CIB undertook the production of human alpha and gamma interferons by so-called conventional methods. Concomitantly, they began the development of genetic engineering in Cuba, and were successful in the cloning, expression, and production of alpha and gamma interferons by recombinant methods. Between 1982 and 1986 activity at the CIB was intense. The center undertook the production of monoclonal antibodies, the chemical synthesis of gene fragments, and the development of virology and tissue cultures and new diagnostic methods. The researchers gained experience in enlarging the scale of fermentation and purification of biomolecules.

The CIB expanded its staff and hired outstanding university graduates who engaged in intense training in different areas and adopted the work style of the institution, where excellence in performance by each member is expected.

From the beginning, the CIB developed an exchange with institutes of different countries, and almost all the researchers of the Center participate in courses and training and attend international meetings. In addition, the Center has promoted several scientific international events, of which the following deserve mention. The First Cuban Seminar on Interferon was held in 1983 and was attended by more than 600 national and foreign delegates. The Second Cuban Seminar on Interferon and the First Cuban Seminar on Biotechnology were held in Havana in 1986, at which more than 900 delegates from 44 countries participated. And in 1989, the Third Cuban Seminar on Interferon, the Second Cuban Seminar on Biotechnology, and the First Iberoamerican Meeting on Biotechnology attracted more than 1,200 delegates from 51 countries.

Centro de Ingeniería Genética y Biotecnología

The decision was made in 1983 to build a new, larger center capable of applying the most advanced techniques of modern biology in laboratory research to practice. The Centro de Ingeniería Genética y Biotecnología (Center for Genetic Engineering and Biotechnology or CIGB) was inaugurated on July 1, 1986. The Center is located in the outskirts of Havana, close to other important scientific institutions, hospitals, and a school of medicine, which, when taken together, embody a powerful array of institutions dedicated to scientific progress.

The CIGB is a complex of buildings designed to unite all stages of work ranging from cloning and expression studies at the laboratory level, production in the pilot plant, design of the industrial production standards (including product evaluation in corresponding biological systems), and large-scale production of monoclonal antibodies to micropropagation of plant cells and plant culture, all under controlled conditions. As such, it constitutes an original and exceptional complex within its class, comparable to the most modern genetic engineering and biotechnological centers in highly developed countries.

Structure and Objectives of the CIGB

The CIGB is structured into divisions, which each address a particular aspect of biotechnology. The divisions and their principal objectives are as follows:

A division for *proteins and hormones* deals with protein production by recombinant methods or use in human and veterinary medicine. The division develops chemical synthesis of oligonucleotides and genes.

A division for *vaccines and diagnostics* handles the production of vaccines for diseases present in Cuba and in other tropical and subtropical countries by so-called unconventional methods, such as cloning surface proteins of the viruses, parasites of bacterium, or bacteria which cause the disease. It works on the development and practical introduction of new specific, diagnostic methods for the detection of pathogenic DNA.

A division for *hybridomas and animal modeling* is concerned with the development and applications of murine, human, and bifunctional monoclonal antibodies; second-generation antibodies obtained by genetic engineering techniques; the development of transgenic animals and animal models for vaccine testing; and toxicology and evaluation of recombinant and nonrecombinant products.

A division for *energy and biomass* works on biomass utilization, its transformation by chemical-enzymatic methods, and the development of industrial enzymes for use directly or in biotechnological processes.

A division for *plants and fertilizers* deals with the application of genetic engineering of plant cells for species improvement. This division has five greenhouses and 2.5 hectares of land for work on experimental parcels.

A division for *mammalian cell genetics* is concerned with the use of cells from higher organisms for gene cloning and protein production by changing the corresponding expression systems; it is also concerned with the search of transgenic animal systems for gene regulation studies and animal improvement.

A division for *restriction and modification enzymes* manages the production of these enzymes.

The *analytic unit* engages in protein analysis and purification by HPLC; protein characterization through mass spectrometry, protein crystallography, electronic microscopy, and immunomicroscopy; and evaluation of specific biologic activity of peptides and proteins.

The *pilot plant* has sections dedicated to the production of proteins for pharmaceutical uses and the purification of biomolecules.

The division of *quality control* verifies purity, structural integrity, molecular composition, functioning, clinical and pharmacologic properties as well as immunologic response and undesirable side effects for all Center products. Protein verification is carried out according to the most advanced gene and amino acid sequencing techniques and through the use of a mass spectrometer of peptide fragments. All new pharmaceutical substances are subjected to pharmacotoxicologic evaluation using established norms. *In vitro* and *in vivo* preclinical trials as well as clinical tests of the final products are performed.

The *computer division* was designed to set up a computerized system for the control and supervision of the fermentation process. It has a multichannel automatic system for data memorization in fluid chromatography. The analytic process and comparison of sequences of amino and nucleic acids have been assured by the use of computers. The management infrastructure and the leadership of the Center can count on appropriate information as well as programs which rationalize management activities.

The Center relates closely to all of the other principal scientific institutions of the country which work in biology. The CIGB is in close contact with university centers in Havana with whom it develops different projects. In addition, the CIGB acts as a training center for Cuban researchers at both university and postgraduate levels.

As part of the Cuban development program for biotechnology, new scientific centers have been created. These include the following:

1. The Centro de Immunoensayo (Immunoassay Center or CIE) was inaugurated in 1987 and produces SUMA (Sistema Ultramicroanalítico or the ultramicroanalytic system), which is a sophisticated and unique piece of equipment which reads results through an ELISA system developed in Cuba that uses a very low amount of reagent in comparison with the standard systems in the rest of the world. SUMA is being used in Cuba for prenatal testing of almost all pregnant women to diagnose congenital malformations such as neural tube defects and hypothyroidism.

2. The Instituto Nacional de Medicina Tropical Pedro Kouri (the Pedro Kouri National Institute for Tropical Medicine or IPK) is an epidemiologic and biotechnological national institute providing clinical service, teaching and research in the field of tropical diseases. A new complex to house the Institute is currently under construction.

3. The Centro Nacional para la Producción de Animales de Laboratorio (National Center for Laboratory Animal Production or CENPALAB) has as a main objective to provide animals for scientific research; they are currently constructing a new center.

4. The Centro Nacional de Biopreparados (National Center for Biopreparation or BIOCEN) is another center that is housed in temporary quarters until their new buildings are completed. They will be in charge of vaccine production and other biopreparations of national interest.

In addition to the CIGB's coordination with the Biological Group, there are permanent connections with other Cuban institutions for purposes of scientific exchange and coordination. These include the following:

1. The Centro Nacional de Investigaciones Científicas (the National Center for Scientific Researches or CENIC), founded in 1965, has done scientific research for the benefit of the country and has provided technical-analytic and technical services to many institutions in the country. This center leads the country in postgraduate

education for several branches of science, and they have trained more than 8,000 professionals.

2. The Centro Nacional de Sanidad Agropecuaria (National Center for Animal and Plant Health or CENSA) works for animal health and genetic and animal reproduction. Since 1981 this center has protected plants and has paid special attention to exotic diseases for different crops in the country.

3. The Instituto Cubano de Investigaciones de Caña de Azucar (Cuban Institute for Sugar Cane Research or ICIDCA) has made important contributions to the research in and applications of sugar cane byproducts.

4. The Instituto Cubano de Ciencia Animal (Cuban Institute for Animal Sciences or ICA) has made important contributions to the country in animal nutrition. Recently they produced zacharine, a promising substance for animal nutrition because of its high protein content.

The CIGB also coordinates with centers and research institutes that belong to the following scientific institutions of ministries: the Academy of Sciences of Cuba, the Ministries of Agriculture, Basic Industry, Nutrition, Fishing, Sugar, Education and Higher Education. The work with the Ministry of Public Health is of particular note because of CIGB's connections with their research institutes in oncology and radiology, hematology, gastroenterology, nephrology, and rheumatology, and with the pediatric cardiac center and various hospitals, such as the general medical and surgical hospital, "Hermanos Ameijeiras" and "Calixto Garcia" Hospital.

The main achievements of the CIGB are listed in TABLE 1, and they also include the following:

1. Characterization and quality control by means of mass spectroscopy of the proteins listed in TABLE 1.

2. Identification of protein sequences through the use of protein sequence equipment.

3. Production of transgenic mice.

4. Production of human monoclonal antibodies.

5. Production of more than 40 types of monoclonal antibodies for diagnosis, characterization, and purification and research.

6. Production of more than 35 types of restriction and modification enzymes.

7. Diagnosis by hybridization techniques of various viruses (hepatitis B, papilloma).

8. Crystallization of various recombinant proteins.

9. Expression of genes in plants to resist attacks of lepidopters.

10. Production through large-scale fermentation procedures (300, 500, 1,000 liters) of different recombinant proteins with adequate downstream procedures, fulfilling all the requirements of G.M.P. and G.L.P. established for these productions.

Personnel

The CIGB's most valuable asset is its staff. Of the 400-plus scientists and other highly skilled workers at the Center, 80 percent are directly involved in research, while the rest are administrative and support personnel. More than 230 are university graduates, many with postgraduate degrees from Czechoslovakia, the Federal Republic of Germany, Finland, the German Democratic Republic, Japan, Great Britain, Hungary, the Soviet Union, Sweden, Switzerland and the United States. One-third of the staff are assigned to full-time research.

TABLE 1. Main Achievements of the CIGB: Cloning and Expression of Genes in *E. coli* and Yeast

Product	Host
Human alpha interferon	*E. coli*
	Yeast
Human gamma interferon	*E. coli*
Interleukin-2	*E. coli*
Epidermal growth factor	Yeast
gap41	*E. coli*
HIV-1	
gap24	*E. coli*
HIV-1	
gap36	*E. coli*
HIV-2	
Proquimosine of calf	*E. coli*
	Yeast
Human insulin	*E. coli*
Toxine of *C. haemoliticum*	*E. coli*
Pvu II	*E. coli*
PNK	*E. coli*
T7 Polymerase	*E. coli*
Thiorredoxin	*E. coli*
Streptoquinase	*E. coli*
Human gonadotrophic hormone	*E. coli*
HBsAg	Yeast
	Mammalian cells
t-PA	Mammalian cells
Human beta interferon	Mammalian cells

The CIGB has the most advanced equipment available in the biological industry including mass spectrometers, scanning and transmission electron microscopes, ultraviolet infrared spectrometers, electrophoresis facilities, and DNA synthesizers and fermenters with downstream facilities.

Installations

The CIGB covers an area of 62,200 square meters. The main six-story air-conditioned building, of modern, functional design, houses all the divisions except the pilot plant. All have low-temperature laboratories, cold chambers at +4°C and −20°C, and P-4 laboratories for the manipulation of high-risk biological agents, which satisfy all international requirements for installations of this type. It also has a 400-seat theater with a simultaneous translation system for four languages, five 50-seat seminar rooms, a library, language laboratory, computer center with access terminals, supporting facilities for workshops, as well as a laundry, kitchen, cafeteria, and offices.

The pilot plant (area, 6,300 square meters) has areas for animals in a controlled environment, stables, five greenhouses, a radioisotope laboratory with its own warehouse, power plant, general warehouse, and a solvent-purification laboratory.

SUMMARY

In March 1981, six researchers started production of natural interferon in a modest building adapted as a laboratory. By May the first yields of this protein were achieved. Applications of this interferon were already taking place in 1981 in the first clinical trial with the drug in the country. In June, the top level of the government decided to organize the Biological Group.

In January, 1982, a new institution (CIB) began work with about 30 scientists and developed activities in gene manipulation, molecular virology, work with monoclonal antibodies, immunochemistry and tissue cultures. By 1983 interferon genes were cloned and expressed, and the group continued working, increasing the number of personnel. A decision was made in 1984 to build a new center, the CIGB. In July 1986, the center was officially inaugurated. Between 1986-89 important results were achieved by members of the biological group, among which was a vaccine against meningococcal meningitis. Three years later, in July 1989, the CIGB produced 15 new recombinant proteins, drugs, enzymes and antigens for diagnostic purposes.

With the application of the most advanced technology, research has been conducted in areas such as gene regulation, bacterial and yeast genetics, protein structure and mammalian development.

In addition, 43 types of monoclonal antibodies were produced as were 38 types of restriction enzymes (three of them recombinant), as well as several linkers, markers, and phages. Interferons, monoclonal antibodies, restriction enzymes, and epidermal growth factor, among others, are all being marketed.

The CIGB became the leading institution in the country for work in modern biotechnology, generating new work styles in the country and developing a special selection procedure to include young scientists on the staff, simultaneously providing intense training in the center and abroad. This provided the stimulus of participating in the achievement of important results for the country, producing a positive feedback loop to maintain high standards.

Interferon has been applied in more than 10,000 cases in the country. The diagnostic kit for AIDS based on recombinant proteins has been used in millions of tests and epidermal grow factor is already registered as a drug after fulfilling all the requirements of the preclinical and clinical testing with hundreds of patients in different clinical trials. A close connection with different institutions working in the field of biotechnology and with different universities has provided a greater strength for the work in modern biotechnology in Cuba.

BIBLIOGRAPHY

1. BIFANI, P. Desafios de la Biotecnológia para la politica cientifica y tecnológica. Presented at Segundo Seminario Ibero-Americano "Jorge Sabato" de Politífica Científica y Tecnológica, June 2-7, 1986, Madrid, Spain.
2. BIFANI, P. 1988. Biotecnologia, Quimica Fina y Farmoquimica en América Latina. Informe preliminar preparado para el Banco Interamericano de Desarrollo.
3. DEMAIN, A. L. 1981. Industrial microbiology. Science **214:** 987.
4. DEMBO, D., C. DIAS & W. MOREHOUSE. 1987. Biotechnology and the Third World: "Caveat emptor." Development **4:** 11.
5. GÁLVEZ TAUPIER, L. O. 1988. Ciencia, Tecnológia y Desarrollo. Ed. Científico-Técnica. Havana, Cuba.

6. LIMONTA, M DE J. 1986. Desarrollo de la Biotecnologia en Cuba. Interferon como modelo. Memorias II Seminario Cubano sobre Interferon y I Seminario Cubano sobre Biotecnologia. 1ra. parte. 31.
7. QUINTERO RAMIREZ, R. Evaluación de oportunidades en Biotecnologia para América Latina. Taller de Biotecnologia, Organizado por el Centro Internacional de Ingenieria Genética y Biotecnologia/ONUDI y el Centro de Ingenieria Genética y Biotecnologia de Cuba. February 8-12, 1987, Havana, Cuba.
8. QUINTERO, R. La Biotecnologia Latinoamericana: Oportunidades y Desafios. *In* La Biotecnologia en el Grupo Andino, Año 2000. G. Montaño and R. Franco, (Eds). Corporacion Andina de Fomento. Caracas, Venezuela.
9. RAW, I. 1970. An Effort to Improve Science Education in Brazil.
10. SASSON, A. 1984. Las Biotecnologias: Desafios y Promesas. UNESCO. Paris.
11. ZELEDÓN, R. Significado de la nueva Biotecnológica para America Latina y el Caribe. IICA/OPS/OEA/OIE. Grupo de estudio interamericanao de la nueva Biotecnologia en agricultura y salud. El uso y seguridad de las técnicas de Ingenieria Genética, January 26-29, 1988, San José, Costa Rica.
12. ZILINKAS, R. A. 1988. Biotechnology and the Third World: The missing link between research and applications. Genetic Engineering and Biotechnology Monitor **24:** 105.
13. Memorias del I Seminario Cubano sobre Interferon, 1983, Havana, Cuba.
14. Informe final de la reunión del grupo de trabajo sobre impactos de la Revolución Tecnológica en el desarrollo de América Latina. CEPAL, December 10-11, 1987, Santiago, Chile.
15. Industrialización y desarrollo tecnológico. División Conjunta CEPAL/ONUDI de Industria y Tecnología. Informe No. 4, July, 1987, Santiago, Chile.
16. Las transformaciones tecnológicas mundiales y sus consecuencias para America Latina y el Caribe. Vigésimo segundo periodo de sesiones de la Comisión Ecónomica para América Latina y el Caribe. ONU, April 27-29, 1988, Rio de Janeiro, Brazil.
17. Memorias del III Seminario Cubano sobre Interferon y II Seminario Cubano sobre Biotecnologia. Havana, Cuba. In press.

Index of Contributors